Fertility and Occupation

POPULATION PATTERNS IN INDUSTRIALIZATION

This is a volume in

STUDIES IN SOCIAL DISCONTINUITY

A complete list of titles in this series appears at the end of this volume.

Fertility and Occupation

POPULATION PATTERNS IN INDUSTRIALIZATION

Michael Haines

Department of Economics
Cornell University
Ithaca, New York

Academic Press
New York San Francisco London

A Subsidiary of Harcourt Brace Jovanovich, Publishers

ACADEMIC PRESS, INC.
111 Fifth Avenue, New York, New York 10003

United Kingdom Edition published by
ACADEMIC PRESS, INC. (LONDON) LTD.
24/28 Oval Road, London NW1 7DX

Library of Congress Cataloging in Publication Data

Haines, Michael R
Fertility and occupation.

(Studies in social discontinuity)
Bibliography: p.
1. Fertility, Human. 2. Population--Economic aspects. 3. Occupations. I. Title. II. Series.
HB901.H34 301.32'1 79-6936
ISBN 0-12-315550-9

PRINTED IN THE UNITED STATES OF AMERICA

79 80 81 82 9 8 7 6 5 4 3 2 1

To my wife, Patricia, and to my children, J. J. and Molly, who endured my frequent absences from home and my even more frequent academic absentmindedness, I dedicate this book.

Contents

Preface

As is mentioned at the beginning of Chapter 1, this book grew out of an initial curiosity about demographic differentials between coal-mining and heavy-industrial populations, and rural, agrarian populations in nineteenth-century Prussian Upper Silesia (now part of Poland). My doctoral dissertation, written with Professor Richard A. Easterlin at the University of Pennsylvania, was about economic and demographic change in Prussian Upper Silesia over the period 1840–1914. It revealed that mining and heavy-industrial populations and regions had fertility higher than that of surrounding agricultural populations and areas, which ran counter to the expectation from standard demographic transition theory. The conventional transition theory stated that the movement to urban areas and to nonagricultural employment was part of the process whereby fertility declined to the relatively low levels characterizing modern, developed, industrial societies. This apparent anomaly led to further research which indicated that others, notably E. A. Wrigley, had noticed the same phenomenon. Furthermore, the differentials extended beyond fertility to mortality, nuptiality, migration, age–sex structure of the population, and patterns of labor-force participation. The investigation led to work on published census and vital statistics material for other areas of Germany and for France, Belgium, Britain, and the United States, in both the nineteenth and twentieth centuries.

This preliminary research resulted in my hypothesis that particular economic structures lead to particular demographic behavior patterns and differentials—hence, the interest in occupation as a way of discussing different economic structures. Most of the results of these initial inquiries are presented in Chapter 1. Chapter 2 represents the distillation of my views on the subject of the interaction between economic structures and demographic behavior or events in the form of an informal (i.e., nonrigorous) verbal model.

Available published evidence clearly indicated that two further courses of research were necessary: the study of small, more economically homogeneous geographic units and, wherever possible, the use of samples from original census enumerators' schedules. Both were pursued. The results from the former are presented in Chapter 3 (for Prussia, 1875–1910; for England and Wales, 1851–1871) and from the latter in Chapters 4 (on the eastern Pennsylvania anthracite region, 1850–1900) and 5 (on Durham and Easington, England, and Merthyr Tydfil, South Wales, 1851–1871). The material in Chapter 6 (on the U.S. Commissioner of Labor Survey of 1889–1890) would be most clearly similar to work with census samples, although the survey results themselves were actually published.

The inquiry has been restricted to an emphasis on mining and heavy-industrial populations and regions, because they exhibited some of the most extreme differential demographic behavior. Other occupational and industrial groups have, of necessity, been chosen for comparison, but the choice of regions was dictated by a heavy concentration in coal mining and metallurgy. The investigation remains essentially historical for three reasons. First, there was a practical consideration of time and resources. Second, it was felt that the early development stages of the presently developed, industrial economies, which form the basis for this study, were most likely to provide the contrasts and differentials useful for this study. Finally, I find historical research intrinsically interesting. None of this means that the work should not be carried to the present, utilizing, for example, public-use census samples and the wealth of survey materials which have become available for both developed and developing nations in the past several decades. On the contrary, evidence indicates that differential demographic behavior by occupational group, which is really a proxy for socioeconomic status group and for economic and social structures, continues to exist. It will undoubtedly play a role in the demographic evolution of developing countries. For these reasons and for others, I feel that this book is addressed not just to historians, economic historians, or historical demographers, but also to demographers, economists, sociologists, and to any others who share the view of the complex interrelatedness of all social science disciplines. Viewed with the proper perspective, the past can furnish lessons for the present and the future.

Acknowledgments

There are many acknowledgments that must be made in connection with the publication of this book. First, a substantial portion of the research was funded by a grant from the National Institutes of Child Health and Human Development (Grant No. RO1-HD07599), whose support is gratefully acknowledged. Three small grants from the Western Societies Program and its parent organization, the Center for International Studies, at Cornell University sustained my work in its early stages. Finally, a small grant from the Cornell University Small Grants Program (administered by the Office of Academic Funding, now the Office of Sponsored Programs) was helpful in preparing some of Chapter 3. Cornell University was generous in supplying computer funds through the Department of Economics, which also made available secretarial help, support services, and a working paper series.

Some of the material in the volume has appeared in various forms at previous times. An original statement of many of the ideas and some of the materials for Chapters 1–3 was given as a paper at the meetings of the Population Association of America in New York City in April, 1974. This was distributed as "Fertility and occupation: Coal mining populations in the nineteenth and early twentieth centuries in Europe and America," *Cornell University Western Societies Occasional Paper* No. 3 (July, 1975). Permission to reprint all or part of the following publications by the author is gratefully acknowledged: "Fertility, marriage, and occupation in the Pennsylvania anthracite region, 1850–1880," *The Journal of Family History*, Vol. 2, No. 1

(Spring, 1977), pp. 28–55. "Fertility, nuptiality, and occupation: A study of coal mining populations and regions in England and Wales in the mid-nineteenth century." Reprinted from *The Journal of Interdisciplinary History*, VIII (1977), pp. 245–280, by permission of *The Journal of Interdisciplinary History* and the M.I.T. Press, Cambridge, Massachusetts. (Copyright © 1977, by the Massachusetts Institute of Technology and the editors of *The Journal of Interdisciplinary History*.) "Mortality in nineteenth century America: Estimates from New York and Pennsylvania census data, 1865 and 1900," *Demography*, Vol. 14, No. 3 (August, 1977), pp. 311–331. "Age specific and differential fertility in Durham and Easington registration districts, England, 1851 and 1861," *Social Science History*, Vol. 2, No. 1 (Fall, 1977), pp. 23–52. "Fertility decline in industrial America: An analysis of the Pennsylvania anthracite region, 1850–1900, using own-children methods," *Population Studies*, Vol. 32, No. 2 (July, 1978). Some material in Chapter 6 was originally published as "Industrial work and the family life cycle, 1889–1890," *Research in Economic History*, Vol. 4 (copyright JAI Press, Inc., Greenwich, Connecticut). The Johns Hopkins University Press has granted permission to reprint an extended passage from Clifton K. Yearly, Jr., *Enterprise and Anthracite: Economics and Democracy in Schuyllkill County, 1870–1875* (copyright The Johns Hopkins University Press, 1962).

Many individuals also deserve thanks. Foremost among these is Richard A. Easterlin of the University of Pennsylvania, who originally spurred my interest in economic demography and historical demography and guided me through my studies in economic history. He suggested my original thesis, carefully supervised the work, and later encouraged me to seek grant support for my further research interests. For his help as a teacher, mentor, and role model, I am most deeply grateful. Another individual who has contributed a great deal is Roger C. Avery of the Sociology Department at Cornell University. He was a willing listener and helpful critic who shared his time, his computer programs, and his interest in historical demography with me. Erik Thorbecke, when he was chairman of the Department of Economics at Cornell University, actively urged me to undertake this book. Peter Lindert helped me to obtain a machine-readable version of part of the Commissioner of Labor Survey and provided many suggestions concerning its use. Sidney Tarrow, when he was director of Cornell's Western Societies Program, provided the opportunity to publish a lengthy occasional paper and allowed me the use of an excellent editor, Barbara Lynch. J. M. Stycos, director of the International Population Program at Cornell, has made the useful resources of his program easily available. Michael Anderson of the University of Edinburgh and Roger Schofield of the Cambridge Group for the History of Population and Social Structure were of great assistance in obtaining copies of the enumerators' manuscripts of the British censuses. Maris Vinovskis, Paul Uselding, Peter McClelland, Mary Katzenstein, Rob Masson, Davydd Greenwood, and several anonymous referees provided useful criticisms of some of the work. Theodore Hershberg, director of the Philadelphia Social History Project, gave considerable moral and intellectual support during the time I was actually writing.

Among the unsung heroes of any empirical undertaking such as this are the support personnel. Therefore, extra thanks go out to my tireless research assistants over the past several years (William Hogan, Thomas Wheeler, Eileen Driscoll, David Rubashkin, and Michael Strong) and to the many coders, work–study students, and student employees who were the mainstays of my data collection. Also, the departmental secretaries (Lois Brown, Jan Collins, Shirley Graham, Lynn Rabenstein, Josephine Velez), who worked many hours over the difficult text and turgid tables, deserve special plaudits. Having thanked a large number of people, I must reserve the responsibility of errors for myself.

Fertility and Occupation

POPULATION PATTERNS IN INDUSTRIALIZATION

I

Introduction

The origins of this book stretch back to my doctoral thesis, originally completed in 1971, on the mining areas of Prussian Upper Silesia and the surrounding agricultural regions in the late nineteenth and early twentieth centuries (Haines, 1978). For that area in that period, the differences between the industrial region, based on coal mining and metallurgy, and the adjacent agrarian regions were striking. Mortality was considerably higher in the industrial region, although age structure played some role in this, and migration was strikingly different. Most interesting of all, however, was the higher fertility of the industrial *Kreise* (Haines, 1976, 335–345). Much of the prevailing literature has contended that urbanization and industrialization led to declining fertility and that lower fertility could be expected in urban, industrial areas. (See, for example, Hawthorn, 1970, pp. 106–107; U.N., 1953, pp. 85–87, 94–95; 1973, pp. 91–92, 95–97.) This was patently not the case for Prussian Upper Silesia and, as it turned out, not for the coalfield areas of western Germany, northern France, and Belgium over the same period (Wrigley, 1961, Part II).

The finding that this was a more general phenomenon led to an investigation of individual occupational groups. Among other conclusions, the United Nations stated:

> *Analyses of mortality by occupation reveal higher mortality in the manual and lower paid occupations. . . . Generally, it has been found that the population engaged in agriculture has particularly large families; miners have also been shown to be a*

> *highly fertile group in those censuses where information for them was tabulated separately. At the other extreme, professional workers and clerical workers have particularly low fertility. The various groups of manual workers outside of agriculture, forestry, and mining differ widely in their level of fertility* [U.N., 1953, pp. 62, 87–88. See also U.N., 1973, 99–101, 137–140].

After some perusal of the available historical evidence, it became apparent that individual occupations were associated with quite distinct patterns of residence, income opportunities, family employment, risks of mortality and morbidity, marriage, labor-force structures, and family composition. Those "intrinsic" characteristics were frequently overlaid by circumstantial patterns, such as different ethnic or religious mixtures, but the basic behavior expected from the intrinsic characteristics was usually dominant. It was felt that a more detailed investigation, building on the pathbreaking work of Wrigley (1961), was warranted and would hopefully lead to a clearer understanding of general demographic behavior not only in the past but also in the present.

In this book it will be shown that occupational fertility differentials have existed historically and have remained throughout the modern era. It is argued that these differentials can be partly, and even largely, explained by economic factors, although the general social and status norms surrounding each occupation obviously play a role. In addition, the mortality, morbidity, and geographic mobility associated with different occupational groups and their environments also interact with this differential fertility. Evidence from Germany, England and Wales, and the Pennsylvania anthracite region in the nineteenth century will be used to support the case for an economic interpretation of these fertility differentials. Case studies of individual regions using micro-level data will be presented for the major Pennsylvania anthracite counties for 1850 through 1900, for Durham and Easington registration districts in the Durham coal field in northern England for 1851–1871, and for the mining and metallurgical center of Merthyr Tydfil in South Wales, also for 1851–1871. These will be supplemented by data on individual families in nine industries (bar iron, pig iron, steel, coal, coke, iron ore, cottons, woolens, and glass) in the United States and five Western European countries (Britain, France, Germany, Belgium, and Switzerland) from an 1889–1890 U.S. Commissioner of Labor Survey. The principal emphasis will be on mining and metallurgical populations and regions, but other occupational groups will, necessarily, be used for comparison.

There are several reasons for this emphasis on mining and heavy industry. First, coal mining and ferrous metallurgy were in the nineteenth century, and remain today, among the most basic activities of the industrial revolution.[1] According to David Landes, as the nineteenth century progressed,

[1] On the importance of energy, particularly coal, to the industrial revolution, see Cipolla (1965, Chap. 2) and Cottrell (1955). For extensive discussion of the technologies of mining and

"it was heavy industry—coal and iron—that was the leading sector [Landes, 1969, p. 174]." Second, for this reason and because of production conditions, mining and metallurgical populations were often numerous and geographically highly concentrated. When demographic information on separate occupations is lacking, as it frequently is, then small areas containing high concentrations of a particular occupational groups can be used in its stead. Third, as has already been stated, mining and heavy-industrial populations have had differentially high fertility. This makes them interesting as an extreme case.

The major emphasis here will be on fertility and, to a lesser extent, marriage. But mortality and migration cannot be separated from these. Demographic events of all kinds can well be regarded as parts of an interconnected whole. That is the approach adopted here.

The study of occupation can be a useful one, beyond the traditional areas of labor-force studies and of social stratification and mobility analysis. The area of fertility and marriage is one such application. It may be true, as Bogue points out, that once the effects of education, income, age, and residence are removed, occupation itself appears to have little effect on fertility (Bogue, 1969, p. 705). But historical data on education and income are often not available, whereas those on occupation are frequently obtainable. Furthermore, the peculiar attributes of each occupational group along such dimensions as income, education, and residence are important in and of themselves to understanding the effects of modernization and industrialization on the population, economy, and society. Finally, some of the ambiguities in occupational titles themselves might be clarified by more comprehensive studies of particular groups.[2]

EVIDENCE OF DEMOGRAPHIC DIFFERENTIALS BY OCCUPATION

The particular demographic behavior of miners and heavy-industrial workers and their families has been noted for a number of countries over time. Peter Stearns, for example, has remarked for Europe that

---

ferrous metallurgy and their vital role in industrial development, see Landes (1969, passim); Deane and Cole (1969, pp. 214–229); Wrigley (1961, Part I, and especially pp. 3–11) argues for the central importance of heavy industry to all aspects of life in Western Europe. See also Gillet (1969); Cameron (1958); Clapham (1936, pp. 232–245, 278–289); Pounds and Parker (1957). For the U.S., see Temin (1964); Davis *et al.* (1972, Chap. 12); and Williamson (1951, pp. 172–189, 454–494).

[2] For a discussion of the applications of occupational data for historical and sociological purposes, see Armstrong (1972). The conclusion of this article is that occupation is usable both as an industrial grouping for the study of the economic features of society and as a social ranking. For some of the problems in using occupation, see Hershberg *et al.* (1974); Katz (1972); and Griffin (1972).

> *Everywhere miners and the unskilled had the largest families, metallurgical workers were next, and so on to the skilled artisans. Child raising patterns followed similar industrial lines. . . . Miners' families were far more structured, albeit highly traditional, while skilled artisans were moving toward essentially bourgeois family patterns including quite a late marriage age* [Stearns, 1970–1971, p. 120].

Historically, coal miners, as well as metallurgical workers and some other industrial–occupational groups, have appeared more to resemble their counterparts in other countries than their fellow citizens. This was particularly true of demographic, family, and social characteristics.

General occupational fertility differentials have been observed in both historical and contemporary populations. The United Nations noted certain consistencies in the data for France, England and Wales, the United States, Sweden, Norway, Denmark, Germany, Canada, Italy, and Hungary (United Nations, 1953, pp. 87–88). As a rule, populations in agriculture, forestry, fisheries, and mining have relatively large families, whereas at the other extreme, professional and clerical workers have relatively low fertility. In between there is a general ranking from manual, blue-collar to nonmanual, white-collar occupations.

Unfortunately, occupation is frequently used as a principal indicator of social class, and much detail is lost when a few broad categories of social class are created from large groups of occupations. This is particularly true for Great Britain, where, following the pioneering work of Charles Booth in the late nineteenth century, considerable attention has been paid to fertility differentials by social class.[3] The censuses of England and Wales of 1911, 1946, 1951, and 1961 did, however, furnish information on fertility for detailed occupations, as well as for social classes (England and Wales, 1923; Glass and Grebinik, 1954; Great Britain, 1949, 1959, 1966).

One of the difficulties in approaching occupation from the viewpoint of social class is the ambiguous nature of the concept of social class itself. While it can be useful in dealing with factors related to tastes, attitudes, and "norms," it obscures the possible role of economic and even straightforward demographic factors. Here the analysis deals with more detailed occupational groups, for which data related to fertility, age, sex, marital status, and other characteristics are available. These data cover a number of countries at a number of points in time.

Table I-1 presents some materials from the Census of Marriage and Fertility of 1911 of England and Wales, a remarkable historical social document. As may be seen from the first panel, there was a general progression from the low fertility of high professional and business occupations (Class I) to the high fertility of unskilled manual workers (Class V). Of special note were the relatively small families among textile workers (Class VI) and the

[3] Among the various works exploring this, see Innes (1938, 1941); Hopkin and Hajnal (1947); and Stevenson (1920). In general, see Armstrong (1972, pp. 198–203, 226–237).

large families among coal miners (Class VII) and agricultural laborers (Class VIII). These differentials held true both for women above and below age 45 and also both for total children born and children surviving.

Since different socioeconomic groups in the population experienced differing patterns of age at marriage, the rates in Table I-1 were also standardized to the age and duration pattern of the female population as a whole.[4] The fertility differentials nonetheless persisted, although they were narrowed after compensating for the earlier average age at marriage and longer average marital duration among the working classes. The same was also true for average surviving children.

More detailed breakdowns of completed fertility by date of marriage indicate that those differentials not only persisted over time, but they widened from at least the 1850s. Table I-2 presents some evidence on this. Married females of completed fertility (i.e., over age 45 of 1911) were tabulated by date of marriage and social class and then the rates were standardized for age of marriage within each group. For higher socioeconomic groups (I and II) completed fertility was declining relative to the national average whereas that of unskilled, manual workers (V) was rising relative to the average, which itself was declining for successive marriage cohorts. Completed fertility among miners' and agricultural laborers' families (Groups VII and VIII) rose sharply relative to the national average. The rates of decline of children ever born for marriage cohorts after 1851 were greatest among the highest social classes and least among the lower groups. Completed fertility declined from the marriage cohort of 1852–1861 to that of 1882–1886 at an average annual rate of 1.21 and 1.08% per annum, respectively, for social classes I and II but only by .51% per annum for social class V and by .32% and .47% per annum, respectively, for coal miners' and agricultural laborers' wives. The national decline was .69%. The bottom panel of Table I-2 shows that a similar divergence was taking place for effective fertility (i.e., surviving children). Thus, during the fertility decline in late nineteenth-century Britain, class differentials widened as the lower socioeconomic groups, and especially coal miners, lagged behind the national average.[5]

Returning to Table I-1, the selected detailed occupations also suggest a ranking similar to social class; but certain occupations, especially coal mining and metallurgy, were notable. For wives over 45 in 1911, children ever born per 100 couples where husband's occupation was in coal mining was 630 (and 652 for workers at the coal face). This was 129% (and 134%) of the national average and ranked miners' wives first among all occupational

[4] For an explanation of the standardization techniques, see the note to Table I-1. For women above age 45, standardization was only for the age of marriage and no standardization was done for surviving children.

[5] This feature of the fertility decline was noted by Innes (1938, pp. 41–52).

groups, closely followed by wives of blast furnace workers, iron puddlers and rollers, ship platers and riveters, iron miners (not shown), and glass workers. In contrast, wives of higher-level civil service officers and clerks were only 72% of the national average, wives of indoor domestic servants only 58%, wives of merchants only 74%, and wives of cotton textile workers only 94%. Adjusting for infant mortality (i.e., ever-born children surviving), fertility for miners' wives dropped to 446 for women aged 45 and over (and 462 for wives of workers at the coal face). For this measure of "effective fertility," coal miners dropped slightly behind that of agricultural laborers (but not farmers), blast furnace workers, puddlers and rollers, ship platers and riveters, shipyard workers, some construction laborers, and some unskilled gen-

TABLE I-1 Fertility and Child Mortality in Relation to Husband's Social Class and Occupation: England & Wales, 1911. (Children Ever Born & Children Surviving Per 100 Couples)

	Wife under 45 At Census				
Category	Children born per 100 couples		Children surviving per 100 couples		Standardized child mortality per 1000 born
	Actual	Standardized	Actual	Standardized	
Total population	282	282	233	233	174
Total occupied	282	282	233	233	174
Total unoccupied	236	215	194	179	167
Social class I	190	213	168	187	123
II	241	250	206	212	150
(occupied only)					
III	279	278	232	231	167
IV	287	285	237	236	173
V	337	317	268	253	202
VI	238	247	191	197	203
VII	358	348	282	274	212
VIII	327	320	284	278	129
Selected occupations					
Coal miners (total)	360	349	283	274	213
Coal miners at the coal face	368	356	289	280	214
Iron and steel workers	354	336	274	262	222
Puddlers; rollers	357	340	275	262	229
Blast furnace workers	376	354	294	278	214
Builders' laborers	384	333	302	265	205
General laborers	370	330	293	263	203
Ship platers/ riveters	372	340	293	270	206
Glass manufacture	362	328	284	259	210
Agricultural laborers	330	323	285	279	135
Civic service officers and clerks	190	210	171	187	110
Indoor domestic servants	151	189	134	164	131
Farmers	276	283	248	254	104
Merchants	198	201	178	180	101
Cotton textile workers	232	242	182	190	218
Tailors	286	273	244	233	147
General shopkeepers	292	271	235	220	187

eral laborers. When these rates were standardized by the age structure of marriage for the female population of England and Wales aged 45 and over, then the first rank of coal-mining populations was regained and the rates became 123% (and 125%) of the national average. It is notable that many of the industrial occupations with high fertility had similar locational and economic characteristics to coal mining. For women under 45 at the 1911 census (and hence with incomplete fertility), whose fertility had been standardized to the age at marriage and the duration of marriage characteristic of all women under 45 in England and Wales in 1911, the ranking remained roughly the same. Coal miners were second only to blast furnace workers and agricultural laborers. For children surviving and standardized for age of marriage and marital duration (a calculation not performed in the

TABLE I-1 (Continued)

Wife over 45 at census			All ages of wife			
Children born per 100 couples		Children surviving per 100 couples	Children born per 100 couples		Children surviving per 100 couples	Social Class
Actual	Standardized		Actual	Standardized		
487	487	368	353	353	280	
489	487	372	350	353	278	
465	489	334	445	310	322	
365	389	294	249	274	210	I
435	451	341	311	319	255	II
504	489	382	350	351	279	III
498	492	379	356	357	283	IV
533	528	388	399	390	306	V
457	444	331	308	315	235	VI
626	585	445	423	430	321	VII
572	556	457	433	402	359	VIII
630	588	446	423	432	321	VII
652	604	462	427	442	325	VII
603	559	426	422	414	316	IV&V
622	571	434	436	420	322	V
625	578	451	442	432	336	V
536	540	384	435	405	320	V
542	548	396	441	406	335	V
614	555	442	432	415	330	III
600	537	429	426	401	323	IV
574	561	455	451	405	369	VIII
351	369	292	236	265	205	I
282	357	225	192	247	162	III
467	503	387	378	359	322	II
362	367	309	265	258	232	I
459	446	326	296	313	223	VI
496	484	379	355	346	288	III
467	469	339	361	340	276	II

TABLE I-1 Fertility and Child Mortality in Relation to Husband's Social Class and Occupation: England & Wales, 1911. (Children Ever Born & Children Surviving Per 100 Couples)

Ratios to total population averages (total population = 100)

Category	Wife under 45 At Census				
	Children born per 100 couples		Children surviving per 100 couples		Standardized child mortality per 1000 born
	Actual	Standardized	Actual	Standardized	
Total population	100	100	100	100	100
Total occupied	100	100	100	100	100
Total unoccupied	94	76	83	77	96
Social class I	67	76	72	80	71
II	85	89	88	91	86
(occupied only)					
III	99	99	100	99	96
IV	102	101	102	101	99
V	120	112	115	109	116
VI	84	88	82	85	117
VII	127	123	121	118	122
VIII	116	113	122	119	74
Selected occupations					
Coal miners (total)	128	124	121	118	122
Coal miners at the coal face	130	126	124	120	123
Iron and steel workers	126	119	118	112	128
Puddlers; rollers	127	121	118	112	132
Blast furnace workers	133	126	126	119	123
Builders' laborers	136	118	130	114	118
General laborers	131	117	126	113	117
Ship platers/ riveters	132	121	126	116	118
Glass manufacture	128	116	122	111	121
Agricultural laborers	117	115	122	120	78
Civic service officers and clerks	67	74	73	80	63
Indoor domestic servants	54	67	58	70	75
Farmers	98	100	106	109	60
Merchants	70	71	76	77	58
Cotton textile workers	82	86	78	82	125
Tailors	101	97	105	100	84
General shopkeepers	104	96	101	94	107

census for women over 45), miners' wives were only behind wives of agricultural laborers, blast furnace workers, and iron miners (not shown). Wives of workers at the coal face were, however, still first despite the relatively high child mortality among the mining population. Child mortality,[6] standardized for duration of marriage and age at marriage of woman, was among the highest for coal-mining families at 122% of the national average, but this was compensated by high total fertility. The same was true for most of the other occupations with extremely high total fertility. The overall effects of differentials in child mortality was to cause some slight con-

[6] See note to Table I-1.

TABLE I-1 (Continued)

Wife over 45 at census			All ages of wife			
Children born per 100 couples		Children surviving per 100 couples	Children born per 100 couples		Children surviving per 100 couples	Social Class
Actual	Standardized		Actual	Standardized		
100	100	100	100	100	100	--
100	100	101	99	100	99	--
95	100	91	126	88	115	--
75	80	80	71	78	75	I
89	93	93	88	90	91	II
103	100	104	99	99	100	III
102	101	103	101	101	101	IV
109	108	105	113	110	109	V
94	91	90	87	89	84	VI
129	120	121	120	122	115	VII
117	114	124	123	114	128	VII
129	121	121	120	122	115	VII
134	124	126	121	125	116	VII
124	115	116	120	117	113	IV&V
128	117	118	124	119	115	V
128	119	123	125	122	120	V
110	111	104	123	115	118	V
111	112	108	125	115	120	V
126	114	120	122	118	118	III
123	110	117	121	114	115	IV
119	115	124	128	115	132	VIII
72	76	79	67	75	73	I
58	73	61	54	70	58	III
96	103	105	107	102	115	II
74	75	84	75	73	83	I
94	92	89	84	89	80	VI
102	99	103	101	98	103	III
96	96	92	102	96	99	II

vergence toward the national average for "effective" fertility, but the effect was minimal and was often altered by standardization procedures.[7]

[7] It is important to note that the census of 1911 presents only surviving married women with surviving spouses. If their marital fertility were systematically different from those who did not survive, a bias is introduced. Of course, couples who do not make it through childbearing without one or both partners dying *will* have lower fertility, in general, because of the interruption of the marriage. The question is what their completed fertility would have been. Also, couples having completed childbearing but not surviving to 1911 might have been different from those who did survive. Innes and T. H. C. Stevenson, the man who conducted the 1911 Census of Marriage and Fertility, both argued that no important bias was introduced by inclusion only of surviving married women with surviving spouses (Innes, 1938, pp. 22–24; England and Wales, 1923, XIII, vciv). Counterarguments are advanced by R. R. Kucynski (1935, pp. 95–96).

TABLE I-1 (Continued)

Source: England and Wales, Registrar General, *Census of England and Wales: 1911*, Vol. XIII, "Fertility of Marriage," Part II (London: H.M.S.O., 1923), Table XLVIII.

NOTE: The standardization procedure for wives under age 45 involved taking the actual rates (of children ever-born per woman) in each category of wife's age of marriage cross-classified by duration of marriage for a particular occupation of husband and then multiplying each rate by the number of ever-married women in each age/duration category for the total population of England and Wales. The marriage age categories used were 15-19, 20-24, 25-29, 30-34, and 35-44. The duration categories were 0-2, 2-5, 5-10, 10-15, 15-20, 20-25, and 25-30. The "expected" children ever-born were then summed and divided by the total number of married women for all marriage ages and durations at the census who were below age 45. This procedure was repeated for surviving children to women aged under 45. Standardized child mortality per 1000 born was then calculated as:

$$\frac{\left(\text{Standardized Children Ever Born per 100 couples}\right) - \left(\text{Standardized Children Surviving per 100 couples}\right)}{\left(\text{Standardized Children Ever Born per 100 couples}\right)}$$

For wives over age 45 at the census, children ever born per 100 couples was standardized only for age of marriage since duration was much less important for older women. (Standardizations for duration and age of marriage were done for the eight social classes and little difference appeared between those standardizations only for age). Children surviving per 100 couples was not standardized since child mortality for older women was greatly influenced by factors external to the family and therefore had much less significance for fertility. Thus, standardized child mortality per 1000 born could not be computed for women over 45.

The biases involved in choosing the total national population of married females of different marriage ages and durations as the standard population are evident and were noted by the compilers of the census (pp. lxxx - lxxxii).

Social classes may be roughly categorized as follows:

I: High skill level and high income professional and business occupations (e.g., scientists, artists, lawyers, physicians, managers, high level civil servants).

II: Lower skill and income professional and business occupations (e.g., small shopkeepers, agricultural employers and less skilled professional, scientific and artistic workers).

III: Skilled manual laborers

IV: Semi-skilled manual laborers

V: Unskilled manual laborers

VI: Textile workers

VII: Miners

VIII: Agricultural laborers

Descriptive evidence for nineteenth-century England conveys the same impression. For example, Arthur Redford remarked in his pioneering work on labor migration in England in the first half of the nineteenth century:

> *In general the evidence for any strong influx of labour into coal mining is not plentiful. A large part of the supply of new labour required by the expansion of the industry probably came from the natural increase of a* notoriously prolific section of the population. *To contemporary observers the coal mining population afforded "an example of the principle of population in full vigour, in the absence of external influence, and (hitherto) of internal checks. Pitmen must be bred to their work from childhood . . . their*

TABLE I-2 Completed and Effective Fertility per 100 Wives by Social Class and Marriage Cohort. Wives over Age 45 at Census, 1911. Rates Standardized for Marriage Age. Total Rates Standardized for Class Composition.

Date of marriage	I[a]	II	III	IV	V	VI	VII	VIII	Total	Total occupied population
				Children Born Per 100 Couples						
1851 and earlier	605[c]	728	681	740[c]	698[c]	—[b]	—[b]	746	697	700
1852-1861	625	700	707	700	718	654	759	738	690	701
1862-1871	593	650	679	673	698	633	760	702	662	673
1872-1881	497	567	615	616	652	567	717	667	605	611
1882-1886[d]	422	493	556	562	609	513	684	632	551	554
				Percentage of national average						
1851 and earlier	86	104	98	106	100	—[b]	—[b]	107	100	100
1852-1861	91	101	102	101	104	95	110	107	100	102
1862-1871	90	98	103	102	105	96	115	106	100	102
1872-1881	82	94	102	102	108	94	119	110	100	101
1882-1886[d]	76	89	101	102	111	93	124	115	100	100
				Annual percentage decrease						
1852/1861 to 1862/1871	.52	.74	.40	.39	.28	.33	+.01	.50	.41	.41
1862/1871 to 1872/1881	1.77	1.37	.99	.92	.68	1.10	.58	.51	.90	.97
1872/1881 to 1882/1886	2.18	1.86	1.34	1.22	.91	1.33	.63	.72	1.25	1.30
				Children surviving per 100 couples						
1851 and earlier	378[c]	452	420	464[c]	405	—[b]	—[b]	490	432	436
1852-1861	433	492	471	472	466	436	465	527	464	478
1862-1871	440	479	481	482	480	423	505	535	473	482
1872-1881	393	438	460	464	470	406	502	534	454	458
1882-1886[d]	345	393	430	434	451	379	497	521	425	428
				Percentage of National Average						
1851 and earlier	88	105	97	107	94	—[b]	—[b]	113	100	101
1852-1861	93	106	102	102	100	94	100	114	100	103
1862-1871	93	101	102	102	101	89	107	113	100	102
1872-1881	86	96	101	102	104	89	111	118	100	101
1882-1886	81	92	101	102	106	89	117	123	100	101

Source: J.W. Innes, *Class Fertility Trends in England and Wales, 1876-1934*, (Princeton, N.J.: Princeton University Press, 1938), pp. 43-42. England and Wales, Registrar General, *Census of England and Wales, 1911*, Vol.XIII, "Fertility of Marriage," Part II (London: H.M.S.O., 1923), Table XLIV.

[a] Includes only wives of occupied husbands.

[b] Fewer than 10 cases available.

[c] Based on fewer than 100 cases.

[d] Includes a few women not quite age 45 in 1911 (i.e., wives married at ages 15-19 in 1881/1886).

numbers cannot be recruited from any other class . . . the increase of the pit population solely from internal sources has in consequence been such that . . . one hundred and twenty-five families attached to a single colliery were capable of annually supplying twenty to twenty-five youths fit for hewers (P.L.C. Report, *1834, Appendix* A, *Part I, No. 5, p. 130)*" [Redford, 1964, pp. 56–57, emphasis added].

It is notable that similar features are observable in the mid-twentieth century. In the Census of England and Wales of 1951, for example, the mean number of children ever born per woman aged 45–49 (i.e., with completed fertility) was 2.60 children for women whose husbands were in mining and quarrying (see Table I-3). Those in metal manufacture, construction, and agriculture were also well above the national average of 2.01.

TABLE I-3 Mean Family Size (Children Ever Born) and Proportions Infertile by Industry Group of Husband: England and Wales, 1951[a]

Industry group	Mean family size: Unstandardized	Mean family size: Standardized for marriage: Age	Mean family size: Standardized for marriage: Age and socio-econ. group	Proportion infertile: Unstandardized	Proportion infertile: Standardized for marriage: Age	Proportion infertile: Standardized for marriage: Age and socio-econ. group
1. Agriculture, horticulture and forestry	2.25	2.31	2.25	.19	.18	.19
2. Mining and quarrying	2.60	2.37	2.13	.14	.17	.18
3. Metal manufacture	2.33	2.23	2.15	.17	.18	.19
4. Engineering and vehicles	1.97	1.99	1.99	.21	.21	.20
5. Textiles	1.74	1.77	1.75	.25	.24	.24
6. Clothing	1.69	1.73	1.81	.24	.23	.22
7. Food, drink, and tobacco	2.01	1.99	1.99	.19	.20	.20
8. Other manufacturing industries and utilities	2.00	1.99	1.95	.20	.20	.21
9. Buildings and construction	2.34	2.29	2.25	.17	.18	.19
10. Transport and fishing	2.13	2.07	2.01	.18	.19	.20
11. Distributive trades	1.72	1.77	1.97	.23	.22	.22
12. Professional services	1.65	1.81	1.91	.24	.21	.21
13. Other services	1.83	1.87	1.93	.23	.22	.22
Ratios to total population (%)						
1. Agriculture, horticulture and forestry	112	115	112	94	88	94
2. Mining and quarrying	130	118	106	68	82	87
3. Metal manufacture	116	111	107	81	89	92
4. Engineering and vehicles	98	99	99	101	101	100
5. Textiles	87	88	87	120	118	116
6. Clothing	84	86	90	116	112	108
7. Food, drink, and tobacco	100	99	99	95	97	97
8. Other manufacturing industries and utilities	100	99	97	98	100	101
9. Buildings and construction	117	114	112	85	89	92
10. Transport and fishing	106	103	100	89	95	98
11. Distributive trades	85	88	98	113	110	105
12. Professional services	82	90	95	120	103	101
13. Other services	91	93	96	111	107	105

Source: Great Britain, General Register Office, *Census: 1951, England and Wales*, "Fertility Report," (London: HMSO, 1959), pp. 207-210.

[a](Women aged 45-49 at census. All marriage ages combined. Once married women with husband present).

Only 14% of miners' wives remained childless, and only 17% of those in metal manufactures, as opposed to a national average of 20.8%. These above-average rankings for parity remained even when standardized for age at marriage and socioeconomic composition.[8] The rank for miners' wives

[8] Standardization for socioeconomic groups involved standardization of rates for the individual socioeconomic groups within an industrial classification to the national socioeconomic group composition. The 13 socioeconomic groups were: farmers; agricultural workers; higher administrative, professional and managerial; shopkeepers (including proprietors and managers of wholesale businesses); clerical workers; shop assistants; personal service; foremen; skilled workers; semiskilled workers; unskilled workers; armed forces (Great Britain, 1959, viii, 178, 208).

was first among all industrial–occupational classifications for unstandardized mean number of children ever born and was still first even when standardized only for age at marriage. The rank dropped to fourth (among 13 industrial–occupational classifications) when fertility was standardized both for age at marriage and socioeconomic composition. The higher groups were, however, agriculture, construction, and metal manufactures. Clearly, heavy industry and mining possessed distinct patterns. Also, the completed fertility of wives of semiskilled and especially skilled workers in mining and quarrying (i.e., mostly workers at the coal face) was high relative to that of other socioeconomic groups *within* the mining industry. Since semiskilled and skilled workers made up the bulk of the mining industry, standardizing to the national socioeconomic composition, with its lower share of skilled and semiskilled workers, would tend to lower the relative standardized fertility in mining and quarrying.[9]

The same pattern of differentially high fertility among these occupational–industrial groups seems to have persisted in 1961 in England and Wales (Great Britain, 1966, Table 16). For women who were married before reaching age 45, mean parity at the time of the census was 2.15 children for mining and quarrying, and only 14% of all couples were infertile. This was the highest level of fertility and the lowest percentage infertile. When standardized for marital age and duration, mining and quarrying dropped to second rank behind agriculture with regard to fertility and proportion of all marriages fertile. Among the other fertile groups were families with husbands' employment in metal manufactures and construction, as before.

Some French data also point to similar fertility differentials in the nineteenth and twentieth centuries. The 1911 Census of Dwellings and Families noted that, among all classes of employment (managers, professional employees, workers, and self-employed) and all occupations, miners and quarry workers had the highest numbers of children surviving per family headed by a married male (254 and 255 children per 100 families, respectively). This was 162% of the national average for each of the occupational groups. Other occupations with large families were agricultural laborers (232), glass workers (232), metallurgical workers (230), day laborers (231), road workers (236), brewers (228), farmers (243), self-employed masons (243), and terracers (236). Heavy industrial employments, mining and quarrying, construction, and laborers seemed to dominate. Among men 50 to 60 years of age who had been married more than 15 years, the average number

[9] This fact was noted in the census: "The high fertility of the mining group as a whole was evidently due to the exceptionally large families of those actually employed as miners (i.e., skilled and semiskilled), while the unskilled workers attached to the industry . . . had slightly smaller families than the average of [unskilled workers] [Great Britain, 1959, p. vix]." The share of skilled and semiskilled workers in this sample of married couples was 84.18% for mining and quarrying as compared with 46.12% for all occupational/industrial categories.

of surviving children per 100 families for coal miners was 361. This was the highest of any occupational–employment group and was 138% of the national average of 261. Again, the largest families were also found among agricultural laborers (304) and carters (310), quarrymen (310), brewers (310), iron and steel workers (309), terracers (315), and glass workers (342). Heavy industry and extractive professions were well represented (France, 1918, pp. 57–113).

The high relative fertility of the coal-mining departments of the Nord and the Pas-de-Calais has been noted by Wrigley (1961, pp. 132–171; 1969, pp. 180–193) and by Ariès (1948, pp. 202–267) for the late nineteenth and early twentieth centuries. Ariès found that, although the population had a higher proportion of young adults than most areas of France (due to heavy net in-migration), it also had a higher mortality. High fertility was thus partially a compensation for high mortality, but there was also a true differential in "effective" fertility, especially in the late nineteenth century (Ariès, 1948, pp. 226–233). Although part of his evidence rests on the uncertain basis of the views of Emile Zola in his novel *Germinal* (1885), Ariès' conclusions are plausible. Recent work by Louise Tilly (1977, p. 22) with manuscript census returns found higher age-specific marital fertility among miners' wives in the mining town of Anzin for 1872 than for the remainder of the population.[10] An investigation of fertility in the arrondissement of Lille (in the department of the Nord) by Spagnoli (1977) found that fertility was quite high relative to the fertility of the nation. Also the communes which were more industrial often had higher fertility.[11] These differentials have continued to exist in France. For example, the Census of Families of 1946 gave the number of children surviving per 100 families with head aged 45 to 54 and occupied as a miner or terracer as 272, the highest of any occupational group and well above the national average.[12]

For Germany, similar observations have been made. E. A. Wrigley, in his study of the coal-mining and industrial regions of northern France, southern Belgium, and the Rhineland in Germany in the nineteenth century, found higher fertility in the industrial areas than in the surrounding agricultural areas (Wrigley, 1961, pp. 134–136, 145–151; 1969, pp. 181–183). Furthermore, industrial areas with considerable coal mining and ferrous metallurgy had higher fertility than other types of industrial areas. High fertility in the coal-mining and metallurgical center of Upper Silesia relative to the surrounding agrarian areas may also be observed for the late nineteenth and

[10] It must also be noted that she found higher overall fertility in the textile-dominated town of Roubaix than in the mining town of Anzin (Tilly, 1977, p. 20).

[11] Comparing the list of industrial cantons given in Wrigley (1961, p. 66) for 1901 with the constituent communes given in Maps 1 and 3 in Spagnoli (1977), it is notable that the industrial communes almost always exceeded the median index of marital fertility (I_g) where data are available. For definition of I_g, see Coale (1967).

[12] See Girard (1955). The following table (page 15) is taken from the 1946 census:

twentieth centuries (Haines, 1978, Chap. 2; 1976, pp. 339–341). Contemporary writers pointed to the high fertility of miners relative to other occupational groups (Fircks, 1889; Berger, 1912; Manschke, 1916). The work by Berger in 1912 was the only one to cover detailed occupational groupings: He found for 1907 the highest number of legitimate births per 100 married men in mining and metallurgy (27.8), followed by metal fabrication (22.1), construction (19.5), and agriculture–forestry–fisheries (18.8). The national average was 19.7. Not all heavy industries had a high rank with this crude measure (e.g., machine building and chemicals), but age distribution was also not taken into account here (Berger, 1912, p. 229).

John Knodel, in his study of the fertility decline in Germany, has noted the high fertility of miners when legitimate births are related to married males. Notable in Germany was, however, the persistent high differential fertility in agriculture (Knodel, 1974, pp. 112–127). Table I-4 indicates that for crude male marital fertility (legitimate births per 1000 married men) miners' fertility was higher than that of other major occupational groups in Prussia for 1877–1886, 1894–1896, 1906–1908, and 1924. The general category of mining, manufacturing, and construction was also relatively high. On the other hand, when general male marital fertility (legitimate births per 1000 married men under age 50) is considered, then miners' fertility is high but not the highest. The especially low level in 1877–1886 may be, in part, accounted for by depressed conditions in the German mining industry in the late 1870s and the early 1880s. The differences in ranking between crude and refined marital fertility implies that the age distribution of married men within occupations played a role in differential fertility levels. This appears particularly true for farmers who had larger proportions of married men at older ages than in other groups (Knodel, 1974, p. 116).

A lack of vital statistics, or even adequate census tabulations, makes it difficult to identify the phenomenon of differential occupational fertility until the mid-twentieth century, although there is some contemporary

(a) Occupational group	(b) Children surviving per 100 married men, aged 45–54
1. Miners and terracers	272
2. Farmers	253
3. Common laborers, foremen	189
4. Small employers, artisans	181
5. Higher employees, liberal professions, employers of more than five workers	170
6. Tradesmen, shopkeepers	165
7. Office staff	162
8. Sales, clerks	139
National average	213

[Cited in Kindleberger, 1964, p. 77.]

TABLE I-4 Male Marital Fertility Rates by Branch of Industry, Prussia, 1877-1924

Industry	Period			
	1877-1886	1894-1896	1906-1908	1924
I. Crude male marital fertility rates[a]				
1. Agriculture	204	203	190	134
2. Mining, manufacturing, construction	224	215	197	99
a. Mining only	239	276	278	156
3. Trade and transport	225	201	165	77
4. Professional, government, military	179	171	139	74
II. General male marital fertility rates[b]				
1. Agriculture	317	332	308	236
2. Mining, manufacturing, construction	290	278	246	137
a. Mining only	277	321	315	194
3. Trade and transport	303	270	213	104
4. Professional, government, military	262	237	188	103

Source: John Knodel, *The Fertility Decline in Germany, 1871-1939,* (Princeton, N.J.: Princeton University Press, 1974), p. 115.

[a]Legitimate births (including stillbirths) per 1000 married men.

[b]Legitimate births (including stillbirths) per 1000 married men under age 50. The age distribution by occupation and marital status was only available for Prussia in 1882. Thus, the number of married men below 50 for each occupational group 1895, 1907, and 1925 were estimated from the German age distribution by sex, occupation, and marital status for these dates.

qualitative and statistical evidence of the high fertility of the wives of miner and industrial workers for the nineteenth and early twentieth centuries. Fo example, it has been noted that in the western Maryland coalfields, "Men as a rule, marry young. . . . Women and girls attend exclusively to house hold duties. . . . Large families are the rule in the mining districts, si children to a household being a low average [Harvey, 1969, p. 29]."[13] A notable sociological study of the Pennsylvania anthracite region by Pete Roberts indicated a very high current fertility, although no standard o comparison for the United States was given[14] (Roberts, 1904, pp. 68–76). Fo

[13] Harvey was quoting from the Maryland Bureau of Industrial Statistics, *Report 1884–85* pp. 77–78, and *Report 1890–91*, p. 214.

[14] Roberts apparently either took a survey or, more likely, gained access to the enumerator' schedules for the 1900 census. The data were from Olyphant Borough in Schuylkill County, mining community. The sample included 492 women, of whom 109 had been married over 2 years.

women in the coal-mining areas who had been married over 20 years in 1900, there was an average of 8.3 children ever born per woman and an average of 5.4 children surviving. To gain perspective, this may be compared to an average of 4.454 children ever born per native-born white woman aged 45–54 in 1910. A more relevant cohort, women aged 55–64 in 1910, had 4.805 children ever born per woman for native-born whites and 5.836 for foreign-born whites. For the northeastern states (including Pennsylvania) urban fertility was 3.161 children, and rural nonfarm fertility was 3.378. For ever-married foreign-born women aged 55–64 in 1910, urban fertility in the northern and western states was 5.228 and for rural nonfarm it was 5.496. In Massachusetts, native-born married mothers (i.e., women who had at least one child) aged 50–59 in 1885 had had 3.835 children ever born while foreign-born mothers had 6.328 children ever born. For all women (in 1885) the numbers were 3.269 and 5.470 children ever born, respectively (U.S. Bureau of the Census, 1943b, Tables 16, 18; Massachusetts, 1888, Part 2, pp. 1174–1181). Thus, comparing the anthracite region in 1900 with the United States in 1910 and Massachusetts in 1885, there is at least some evidence of higher fertility in the mining–industrial area. The most appropriate comparison is with foreign-born women since most of the miners and their wives were foreign born.[15]

Available quantitative evidence, in the form of children ever born and children surviving per married woman, cross-classified by occupation of husband, also points to higher fertility among coal miners and industrial workers. Table I-5, based on a sample of enumerators' schedules for seven counties of the anthracite mining region,[16] shows that, in 1900, miners' wives of completed fertility (aged 45–54) or nearly completed fertility (aged 35–44) had cumulative births and numbers of surviving children in excess of the other groups. The category of manufacturing–crafts–construction was in second rank for women aged 35–44 and close behind laborers for women aged 45–54. For women aged 45–54 in 1900, the completed fertility of miners' wives was 124% of the overall average, while the group manufacturing–crafts–construction was 104% of the overall figure. This is in contrast to only 88% and 74% for wives of farmers and professionals, respectively. The differentials were less for surviving children, however, pointing to higher child mortality among mining populations.

Interestingly, these differentials have persisted up to the present for the United States as well as Britain. As Tables I-6 and I-7 show, as of 1960,

[15] According to samples of the U.S. Census enumerators' schedules for the main Pennsylvania anthracite counties (Lackawanna/Luzerne, Schuylkill, and Northumberland), in 1850, 86.6% of miners or mine workers were foreign born, and 86.2% of foreign-born family heads with spouses present were married to foreign-born spouses. For 1880 the percentages were 74.5% and 91.5%, and for 1900 they were 63.10% and 77.83%.

[16] Lackawanna, Luzerne, Northumberland, Schuylkill, Susquehanna, Wayne, and Wyoming counties.

TABLE I-5 Children Ever Born and Children Surviving to Married Women Aged 35-44 and 45-54 by Occupation of Family Head. Lackawanna, Luzerne, Northumberland, Schuylkill, Susquehanna, Wayne, and Wyoming Counties, Pennsylvania, 1900 (Families with Both Husband and Wife Present).

	Women aged 35-44			Women aged 45-54		
	Average children ever born	Average children surviving	*N*	Average children ever born	Average children surviving	*N*
1. Farmers and farm workers	3.943	3.443	70	5.086	3.810	58
2. Laborers	4.409	3.172	93	6.205	4.273	44
3. Miners and mine workers	5.869	4.330	176	7.186	4.457	70
4. Manufacturing-crafts-construction	4.853	3.780	109	6.017	4.153	59
5. Mercantile-food-lodging-servants-transport	4.481	3.443	106	4.849	3.396	53
6. Professional and other	4.098	3.195	41	4.304	3.130	23
TOTAL	4.859	3.708	595	5.805	3.967	307
Index (Overall Average = 100)						
1. Farmers and farm workers	81	93		88	96	
2. Laborers	91	86		107	108	
3. Miners and mine workers	121	117		124	112	
4. Manufacturing-crafts-construction	100	102		104	105	
5. Mercantile-food-lodging-servants-transport	92	93		84	86	
6. Professional and other	84	86		74	79	

Source: Sample of manuscript enumerators' schedules.

among white wives aged 35–44 at the time of the census, coal miners' wives had fertility 143% of the national average of 2.596 children ever born per woman and 136% of the national average of 2.906 children ever born per mother. The differential was even higher for white wives aged 45–54 (166% and 150% of the national average of children ever born per woman and mother, respectively). The differential was smaller but high for nonwhite women aged 45–54. Nonwhite coal miners' wives were, however, only a small part of this population.[17] The fertility of coal miners' wives ranked third among all the detailed occupational categories given in the census and was behind only farm laborers and lumbermen–raftsmen–woodchoppers. It is notable that this latter occupational group is an extractive industry similar in many respects to coal mining. In addition, coal miners' wives had the

[17] Of the total wives 35–44 whose husbands were in coal mining, only 5.8% were nonwhite. The percentage was 6.0 for wives 45–54 (U.S. Bureau of the Census, 1964, Tables 33 and 34).

lowest proportion of childless marriages (9.1% for white wives aged 45–54). For whites, wives (aged 45–54) of farmers and professionals had fertility only 86% and 82% of the national average, respectively, whereas manufacturing operatives and nonfarm laborers had fertility 109% and 129% of the national average. There did not seem to be especially high completed fertility among workers in heavy industry in the United States by 1960. For example, operatives in primary metals only had fertility at 114% of the national average, and laborers in manufacturing were at 125% of the national level. High fertility continued to be found among transportation and construction workers, farm laborers, and other workers in extractive industries. By 1960, however, the character of manufacturing employment had changed a great deal since the late nineteenth century. The rankings in 1970 were much the same although the differentials had narrowed considerably (U.S. Bureau of the Census, 1973a, Table 48).

Although it appears that the traditionally high fertility rate of coal miners is gradually converging toward the national average, this may not be so. First of all, mean number of children ever born to white wives of coal miners aged 35–44 fell from 3.723 in 1960 to 3.525 in 1970, whereas the national average actually rose from 2.596 in 1960 to 3.062 in 1970. (All other occupations in Table I-7 showed increases between 1960 and 1970 for children ever born to women 35–44.) The same is also true when mothers and not just total married women are considered. The cohort of women aged 35–44 in 1960 were born during 1916–1925 and passed through their peak childbearing years (i.e., 20–29), on the average, during the period 1936–1944, before the baby-boom had really begun. In contrast, wives of miners in 1970 aged 35–44 had passed through their peak childbearing years on average during the period 1945–1954, when the postwar baby-boom was well underway. If one accepts Easterlin's explanation of the baby-boom (Easterlin, 1968, Chaps. 4 and 5), that it was largely a function of favorable labor-market conditions for young adults, then there is a possible explanation for coal miners' fertility falling while the national average rose. Coal mining was a "depressed" industry following World War II (Hendry, 1961), with declining employment after 1948 and a history of poor labor relations. While most young adults were entering a market characterized by rising demand for labor among the youngest labor-force entry cohorts, potential coal miners were not. It is possible that as a result young adults deferred marriage and/or childbearing in an attempt to compensate. However, it is also possible that psychological, economic, or institutional impediments to occupational and geographic mobility lowered miners' fertility. Thus, conditions peculiar to the mining industry may have caused the dramatic lowering of miners' differential fertility, rather than some general convergence of class fertility differentials as miners finally caught up with the rest of the population in levels of education, economic well-being, health, etc. This latter might have been a partial cause, but probably not the only one.

TABLE I-6 Mean Number of Children Ever Born per Woman and per Mother and Percent Childless by Husband's Occupation. United States, 1960. (Married White and Non-white Women with Husband Present and Aged 35-44 and 45-54)

Occupation of husband	*Wives 35-44*						*Wives 45-54*					
	Children ever born per				Percentage childless		Children ever born per				Percentage childless	
	Woman		Mother				Woman		Mother			
	White	Non-White	White	Non-White	White	Non-White	White	Non-White	White	Non-White	White	Non-White
Total U.S.	2.596	3.216	2.906	4.025	10.7	20.1	2.321	2.890	2.811	3.972	17.4	27.2
1. Professional, technical, etc.	2.417	2.198	2.723	2.733	11.2	19.6	1.892	1.953	2.364	2.903	19.9	32.7
2. a) Farmers and farm managers	2.431	5.572	2.712	6.129	10.4	9.1	1.999	5.073	2.445	5.957	18.3	14.8
b) Other managerial and proprietors	2.431	2.567	2.712	3.188	10.4	19.5	1.999	2.249	2.445	3.108	18.3	27.6
3. Clerical, etc.	2.302	2.340	2.648	3.070	13.1	23.8	1.913	1.909	2.446	2.870	21.8	33.5
4. Sales Workers	2.354	2.613	2.656	3.194	11.4	18.2	1.871	2.145	2.356	3.074	20.6	30.2
5. Craftsmen, foremen, etc.	2.607	3.001	2.897	3.752	10.0	20.0	2.368	2.740	2.835	3.718	16.5	27.1
6. Operatives	2.730	3.156	3.040	3.961	10.2	20.3	2.540	2.662	3.017	3.675	15.8	27.6
a) Coal miners	3.723	4.736	3.967	5.259	6.1	9.9	3.843	2.881	4.228	3.632	9.1	20.7
b) Sawyers	3.412	4.591	3.760	5.217	9.3	12.0	3.540	3.827	3.985	4.743	11.2	19.3
c) Others related to mining	3.092	4.054	3.353	4.862	7.8	16.6	3.021	3.125	3.417	4.264	11.6	26.7

7. Manufacturing operatives	2.678	3.100	2.993	3.837	10.5	19.2	2.523	2.678	3.009	3.689	16.1	27.4
a) Saw and planing mills	3.517	4.226	3.443	4.843	8.3	12.7	2.855	3.109	3.401	4.021	16.0	22.7
b) Primary metals	2.744	3.131	3.010	3.745	8.8	16.4	2.658	2.317	3.100	3.444	14.2	32.7
8. Private HH workers	2.290	2.188	2.820	3.236	18.8	32.4	2.080	1.907	2.775	3.079	25.0	38.0
9. Other service workers	2.484	2.719	2.843	3.575	12.6	23.9	2.304	2.240	2.849	3.389	19.1	33.9
10. Farm laborers and foreman	3.988	5.078	4.351	5.866	8.3	13.4	4.024	4.634	4.534	5.481	11.2	15.5
11. Other laborers	2.008	3.458	3.364	4.305	10.6	19.7	2.992	3.064	3.542	4.203	15.5	27.1
a) Fishermen	3.139	3.593	3.458	4.400	9.2	18.3	2.686	3.835	3.373	4.813	20.4	20.3
b) Lumbermen, Raftsmen, Woodchoppers	3.998	5.092	4.258	5.711	6.1	10.8	3.932	4.793	4.439	5.721	11.4	16.2
c) Manufacturing	2.907	3.552	3.245	4.363	10.4	18.6	2.895	3.112	3.416	4.212	15.3	26.1
d) Non-manufacturing	3.079	3.365	3.431	4.249	10.3	20.8	3.131	2.988	3.668	4.169	14.6	28.3
i) RR's	3.321	3.705	3.672	4.450	9.5	16.8	3.396	2.931	3.926	4.127	13.5	29.0
ii) Construction	3.103	3.530	3.453	4.382	10.2	19.4	3.192	3.085	3.712	4.208	14.0	26.7

Source: U.S. Bureau of the Census, *U.S. Census of Population: 1960. Subject Reports. Women by Number of Children Ever-Born.* PC(2)-3A. (Washington, D.C.: GPO, 1964), Tables 33 & 34.

TABLE I-7 Index of Mean Number of Children Ever Born per Woman and per Mother and Percent Childless, United States, 1960. (Married White and Non-White Women with Husband Present Aged 35-44 and 45-55. Selected Occupations.)

Occupation of Husband	Wives 35-44						Wives 45-54					
	Children ever born per				Percentage childless		Children ever born per				Percentage childless	
	Woman		Mother				Woman		Mother			
	White	Non-White	White	Non-White	White	Non-White	White	Non-White	White	Non-White	White	Non-White
Total U.S.	100	100	100	100	100	100	100	100	100	100	100	100
1. Professional, technical, etc.	93	68	94	68	105	98	82	68	84	73	114	120
2. a) Farmers and farm managers	94	173	93	152	97	45	86	176	87	150	105	54
b) Other managerial and proprietors	94	80	93	79	97	97	86	78	87	78	105	101
3. Clerical, etc.	89	73	91	76	122	118	82	66	87	72	125	123
4. Sales workers	91	81	91	79	107	90	81	74	84	77	118	111
5. Craftsmen, foremen, etc.	100	93	100	93	93	100	102	94	101	94	95	100
6. Operatives	105	98	105	98	95	101	109	92	107	92	91	101
a) Coal miners	143	147	136	131	57	49	166	100	150	91	52	76
b) Sawyers	131	143	129	130	87	60	152	132	142	119	64	71
c) Others related to mining	119	126	115	121	73	82	130	108	122	107	67	98
7. Manufacturing operatives	103	96	103	95	98	96	109	93	107	93	92	101
a) Saw and planing mills	122	131	118	120	78	63	123	108	121	101	92	83
b) Primary metals	106	97	104	93	82	82	114	80	110	87	82	120
8. Private HH workers	88	68	97	80	176	161	90	66	99	78	144	140
9. Other service workers	96	84	98	89	118	119	99	78	101	85	110	125
10. Farm laborers and foreman	154	158	150	146	78	67	173	160	161	138	64	57
11. Other laborers	116	108	116	107	99	98	129	106	126	106	89	100
a) Fisherman	121	112	119	109	86	91	116	133	120	121	117	75
b) Lumberman, raftsmen, woodchoppers	154	158	146	142	57	54	169	166	158	144	66	60
c) Manufacturing	112	110	112	108	97	92	125	108	122	106	88	96
d) Non-manufacturing	119	105	118	106	96	103	135	103	130	105	84	104
i) RR's	128	115	126	111	88	84	146	101	140	104	78	107
ii) Construction	120	110	119	109	95	96	138	107	132	106	80	98

Source: U.S. Bureau of the Census, *U.S. Census of Population: 1960. Subject Reports. Women by Number of Children Ever-Born.* PC(2)-3A, (Washington, D.C.: GPO, 1964), Tables 33 and 34.

TABLE I-8 Mean Age at First Marriage by Occupation of Husband. England and Wales, 1884-1885.

Occupation of husband	Mean age at first marriage	
	Males	Females
Miners	24.06	22.46
Textile hands	24.38	23.43
Shoemakers, tailors	24.92	24.31
Artisans	25.35	23.70
Laborers	25.56	23.66
Commercial clerks	26.25	24.43
Shopkeepers, shopmen	26.67	24.22
Farmers and sons	29.23	26.91
Professional and independent class	31.22	26.40

Source: England and Wales, Registrar General, *Forty-Ninth Annual Report: 1886* (London: Eyre & Spottiswoode, 1887), p. viii.

So far we have only been discussing marital fertility. Marriage practices also appear to have been related to occupation, although the evidence is less clear. For England and Wales, mean age at first marriage for both males and females seems to have been among the lowest in miners' families and in mining regions. In a special study in 1884 and 1885 by the Registrar General, miners and their wives had the lowest mean age at first marriage (24.06 and 22.46, respectively) among all nine occupational groups studied. The results are given in Table I-8. The rankings for age of marriage by occupational groups were similar to the ranking by marital fertility. Unfortunately, other than miners, no workers in heavy industry were included; but marriage ages among blue-collar workers were less than those among clerks, shopkeepers, farmers, and professionals.

For a sample of 61 mining and metallurgical districts in England and Wales for 1861,[18] Coale's index of proportion married (I_m)[19] was significantly higher than for a random sample of 125 registration districts. The same was true for 1871. (See Chapter III, this volume.) The highest proportion of persons married at ages 15–24 in 1861 was found in Durham, a county heavily populated with coal miners. A paper by Crafts (1978) found that County Durham had among all the counties of England the lowest estimated mean age of marriage (23.0 years) and median age of marriage (22.2 years) for females in 1861. It also had the second highest proportion ever

[18] These districts were defined as those with more than 10% of the male population aged 20 and over in coal mining/iron mining, and/or ferrous metallurgy.

[19] For a definition, see Coale (1967).

married at age 45–59 (91.8%). Of the five counties with the lowest marriage ages, four (Durham, Staffordshire, Lancashire, and the West Riding of Yorkshire) were strongly represented in mining and heavy industry. Lancashire was also a major textile center. Anderson found that for registration districts in 1861 "a clear relationship existed between living in areas dominated by textiles, coal-mining, engineering and metal manufacturing . . . and one's statistical chances of marriage and of an early marriage age [Anderson, 1976, p. 64]." Anderson used as his indicators of marriage the proportion unmarried at 25–34 (males and females), the proportion unmarried at 45–54 (females only), the singulate age of first marriage (males and females), and I_m (females).

In 1834, the Poor Law Commissioners stated that "miners assumed the most important office of manhood at the earliest age at which nature and passion prompted."[20] The census of 1911 noted that only 7% of middle-class husbands and one-third of their wives were married before age 25, whereas for coal miners, those proportions were 57% and 75% for their wives (England and Wales, 1923, p. xvi). This differential marriage pattern has persisted up to the mid-twentieth century, especially among mining populations. The census of 1951 reported that "[e]arly marriage is known as a matter of common experience to increase in frequency down the social scale [Great Britain, 1959, p. xlvii]." As Table I-9 shows, among women aged 45–49 at the time of the 1951 census, the highest proportions married by age 25 were among wives of men in mining and quarrying (64%), metal manufacture (58%), and construction (56%). The lowest proportion was among wives of professionals (39%). Wives of semiskilled and unskilled manual workers were most likely to marry early among the various socioeconomic groups.

As for other Western European countries, Wrigley found in his investigation of census data on Germany, France, and Belgium that female proportions married were demonstrably higher for the mining and heavy-industrial areas than for adjacent agricultural areas or for large cities. This was not, however, generally the case for males[21] (Wrigley, 1961, pp. 140–157). There is some evidence of earlier male marriage among certain occupational groups, however. Table I-10 presents labor-force data cross-classified by age and marital status for males in three leading industrial administrative areas (*Regierungsbezirke*) of Prussia in 1882. Oppeln (Upper Silesia) was a predominantly Polish-speaking area in southeastern Prussia, whereas both Arnsberg and Düsseldorf were located in the Ruhr industrial region of western Prussia. As Column 7 indicates, all were reasonably industrial, although Oppeln was still heavily agricultural in 1882. Column 4 gives the percentage of ever-married males aged 20–29 in particular indus-

[20] *British Parliamentary Papers*, Vol. XXXVII, p. 125. Quoted in Hewitt (1958, pp. 40–41).
[21] This issue will be taken up in Chapter II.

TABLE I-9 Proportions of Women Married by Age, England and Wales, 1951
(Women Married Only Once, Aged 45-49 at Census, Husband Present)
(per 1000)

Occupational group of husband	Under 20	20-24	Under 24
1. Agriculture, etc.	80	409	489
2. Mining and quarrying	155	484	639
3. Metal manufacturing	109	467	576
4. Engineering and vehicles	81	439	520
5. Textiles	74	450	524
6. Clothing	72	448	520
7. Food, drink, tobacco	81	457	538
8. Other manufacturing and utilities	83	449	532
9. Construction	98	460	558
10. Transport and fishing	97	477	474
11. Distributive trades	67	428	495
12. Professional Services	44	343	387
13. Other Services	80	418	498
Socio-economic group of husband			
1. Farmers	64	394	458
2. Agricultural workers	90	422	512
3. Higher administration and professional and managerial	27	338	365
4. Other administration and professional and managerial	47	395	442
5. Shopkeepers (including managers of wholesale business)	61	426	487
6. Clerical	54	387	441
7. Shop assistants	55	407	462
8. Personal service	97	440	537
9. Foremen	83	479	562
10. Skilled workers	89	462	551
11. Semiskilled workers	123	468	591
12. Unskilled workers	129	456	585
13. Armed forces	93	353	446

Source: Great Britain, General Register Office, *Census: 1951, England & Wales,* "Fertility Tables," (London: HMSO, 1959), p. xlvii.

tries. As is apparent, mining and metallurgy showed considerably higher proportions of males ever married than did other industrial groups. Metal working–machine building also exhibited high proportions in the Ruhr. These were in marked contrast to agriculture (mostly farmer–owners in these areas) which had uniformly the lowest proportions. Other industries ranked in between. It is also notable that mining–metallurgy and metal working–machine building were also younger men's industries, as seen in

TABLE I-10 Male Labor Force by Age, Selected Regierungsbezirke of Prussia, 1882

(1) Region/industry	(2) Males in labor force aged 20-29	(3) Ever-married males in labor force aged 20-29	(4) (3) as percentage of (2)	(5) Total males in labor force	(6) Percentage of (5) aged 20-29	(7) Percentage of total male labor force in occupation
R.B. Oppeln						
Agricultural, forestry, fishery	36,319	10,838	29.84	180,376	20.13	44.12
Mining and metallurgy	19,010	7,457	39.23	60,553	31.39	14.81
Metal working/machine building	3,557	1,071	30.11	13,044	27.26	3.19
Textiles and clothing	6,126	2,035	33.22	25,832	23.71	6.32
Construction	6,132	2,002	32.65	23,618	25.96	5.78
Trade, transport, banking	4,238	1,328	31.33	19,521	21.70	4.78
Food and beverages	3,596	984	27.36	13,438	26.76	3.29
R.B. Arnsberg						
Agricultural, forestry, fishery	11,840	2,037	17.20	62,477	18.95	18.43
Mining and metallurgy	30,120	11,148	37.01	94,600	31.84	27.91
Metal working/machine building	11,907	3,534	29.68	40,794	29.19	12.03
Textiles and clothing	5,066	1,363	26.91	21,046	24.07	6.21
Construction	6,432	1,666	25.90	22,282	28.87	6.57
Trade, transport, banking	5,731	1,504	26.24	24,480	23.41	7.27
Food and beverages	3,705	751	20.27	11,550	32.08	3.41
R.B. Düsseldorf						
Agricultural, forestry, fishery	17,917	2,812	15.69	90,903	19.71	18.18
Mining and metallurgy	13,290	4,737	35.64	45,930	28.93	9.19
Metal working/machine building	14,754	4,409	29.88	50,235	29.37	10.05
Textiles and clothing	27,870	8,116	29.12	105,860	26.33	21.18
Construction	8,253	2,370	28.72	28,678	28.78	5.74
Trade, transport, banking	10,538	2,818	26.74	46,453	22.68	9.29
Food and beverages	6,516	1,461	22.42	21,240	30.68	4.25

Source: Prussia. Statistisches Landesamt, *Preussische Statistik*, Bd. 76, Teil II, (1885).

Column 6. The different social context of predominantly Polish-speaking Upper Silesia versus the predominantly German-speaking Ruhr is illustrated by the consistently greater proportions of younger males married for each industrial grouping in Oppeln. Analogous results may be seen in the occupational censuses of 1895[22] and 1907 for Germany as a whole. The results for the 1907 census are given in Table I-11.

There is very little published evidence on marriage by occupation for the United States, either from the census or from vital statistics. What information is available, in the form of proportions of males married by age and occupation or industry derived from census data, indicates that there were also occupational nuptiality differentials by age for the United States. For example, as may be seen in Table I-12, the census of 1940 reveals that mining operatives had the highest proportions married in the age group 14–24 (35.3%) among all nonagricultural manual workers. Only farmers and farm managers (53.2%) and, somewhat surprisingly, other managers and proprietors (38.0%) showed higher proportions married by this age. The high proportion in agriculture was, however, undoubtedly affected by nonwhites in the South. Iron and steel operatives also showed reasonably high proportions married at an early age.

Two other demographic phenomena, migration and mortality, also deserve comment. They too are related to industrial and occupational composition and change. The rapid growth of mining and industrial regions, both urban and semiurban, was accomplished partly by net in-migration. The high fertility of mining and heavy-industrial regions meant, however, that natural increase could supply a larger portion of total increase. This feature of mining areas has been noted by Redford for England and Wales (Redford, 1964, pp. 56–57) and by Wrigley for France and Germany (Wrigley, 1961, pp. 163–164). It was rather the very large cities (e.g., London, Paris, Berlin, Hamburg, New York), administrative and cultural as well as commercial and industrial centers, that experienced the heaviest net in-migration. And yet mining areas did attract huge numbers of migrants. For example, net

[22] The 1895 census was analyzed by Wrigley (1961, p. 155) who reported:

Industry	Males 20–29 ever married (%)
Coal mining and associated industries	46.5
Iron manufacture	42.5
Metal working (smithying, etc.)	31.4
Spinning and ancillary textile industries	41.4
Weaving	38.3
Brewing	31.4
Shoemaking	33.6
Building (masons)	35.2
Farming and forestry	27.8

TABLE I-11 Labor Force by Age, Sex, and Marital Status, Germany, 1907

Occupation/industry	(2) Males in labor force aged 20-29	(2a) Males in labor force aged 20-24	(3) Ever married males in labor force aged 20-29	(3a) Ever married males in labor force aged 20-24
Total Labor Force	4,941,011	2,536,226	1,508,103	242,772
1. Agriculture, forestry, fisheries	965,149	468,877	253,728	38,585
2. Mining and metallurgy	282,720	132,620	121,262	23,062
a. Coal mining	179,105	85,161	78,767	15,189
b. Metal refining	70,948	32,236	27,962	4,506
3. Industries of stone and earth	177,004	82,898	68,664	12,592
4. Metal working	321,215	162,035	118,603	21,744
5. Chemical industries	52,030	21,210	21,957	3,531
6. Textile industries	116,698	54,498	40,119	9,065
7. Machinery industries	273,641	131,249	104,481	18,558
8. Paper and leather industries	89,048	41,599	33,928	5,948
9. Wood products industries	191,203	88,897	72,049	11,660
10. Food and beverage	244,625	113,739	74,487	10,146
11. Clothing	184,705	80,553	64,992	8,859
12. Construction	562,077	262,306	211,662	38,540
13. Other industry	65,468	31,173	21,929	3,759
14. Commerce and insurance	303,038	141,164	84,810	11,388
15. Transport and communications	254,748	94,349	110,109	13,279
16. Food and lodging services	71,532	30,017	21,679	2,390
17. Domestic and day labor	35,307	14,963	14,231	2,302
18. Professional, government, military	757,909	589,281	60,677	7,406

migration to the mining and industrial region of Upper Silesia averaged well over 2% per annum from the 1830s up to the 1870s (Haines, 1976, p. 337).[23] The Pennsylvania anthracite region had over 26.8% of its population born outside Pennsylvania and 21.3% born outside the United States in 1850. For 1900 the percentages were 27.3 and 23.2, respectively.[24] The relative importance of migration varied with particular areas and the stage of development. In the early stages of rapid growth, substantial net in-migration was usually necessary to ensure adequate labor supply. Later, natural increase became more important while growth rates of production and labor force usually began to decline.[25] An important aspect of migration, which will be dealt with later, was the selectivity bias by age and sex. Mining and heavy-industrial areas tended to attract large numbers of single, young adult males, because of the structure of employment. This tended to raise sex ratios in these age groups and influence nuptiality and overall fertility (Wrigley, 1961, Table 42).

[23] Another example is that of the Ruhr. See Brepohl (1948).

[24] Calculated from samples of manuscript enumerators' schedules. For details, see Chapter IV, this volume.

[25] An example of this is Upper Silesia (Haines, 1976).

TABLE I-11 (Continued)

(4)	(4a)	(5)	(6)	(7)
(3) as a percentage of (2)	(3a) as a percentage of (2a)	Total males in labor force	Percentage of (5) aged 20-29	Percentage of total males in labor force in occupation
30.52	9.57	18,583,864	26.59	——
26.29	8.23	5,284,271	18.26	28.43
42.89	17.39	943,494	29.96	5.08
43.97	17.83	592,980	30.20	3.19
39.41	16.11	237,605	29.85	1.27
38.79	15.18	642,250	27.56	3.46
36.91	13.42	1,113,060	28.87	5.99
40.76	16.64	199,596	26.06	1.07
34.37	16.63	529,008	22.06	2.84
38.18	14.13	863,789	31.68	4.64
38.10	14.30	338,103	26.33	1.82
37.68	13.12	739,726	25.85	3.98
30.44	8.92	878,962	27.83	4.73
35.19	11.00	808,885	22.83	4.35
37.66	14.69	1,887,055	29.79	10.15
33.51	12.05	208,810	31.35	1.12
27.99	8.07	1,251,437	24.22	6.73
43.22	14.07	983,474	25.90	5.29
30.31	7.96	311,342	22.97	1.68
40.30	15.38	263,108	13.41	1.41
8.00	1.26	1,867,763	40.58	10.05

Source: Germany, Statistisches Reichsamt, *Statistik des deutschen Reichs*, Bd. 203, Teil I, (1910), Table 3.

Mortality is also potentially related to industry and occupation. It might be expected that industrialization would lead to higher adult male mortality and morbidity and that the new urban and industrial environments would have unfavorable effects on mortality of the whole population. Again, the evidence is mixed. In an extensive survey of age and cause specific death rates by occupation for the period 1860–1882 for England and Wales, the Registrar General found below-average death rates for coal miners and workers in iron and steel manufacture. For metal workers generally, death rates were 93.8% of the national average for all males (employed and unemployed) aged 25–65 and 97.0% of that for employed males of the same ages. Coal miners of the same age group had mortality only 89.1% of the national average for all males and 92.1% for employed males. Copper, lead, and tin mining were apparently much more dangerous, because of the increased volume of hard rock dust inhaled. Coal miners did indeed suffer from above-average mortality from respiratory infections and accidents, but this was not excessive. Table I-13 gives some selected results for England and Wales. The same was apparently also true for Belgium and Upper Silesia (England and Wales, 1885, Tables J and L and pp. xxv–xxvi, xxviii–xxx).

TABLE I-12 Labor Force by Age, Sex, and Marital Status, United States, 1940[a]

Occupation/industry	(2) Males in labor force aged 14-24[c]	(3) Married[b] males in labor force aged 14-24	(4) (3) as a percentage of (2)	(5) Total males in labor force	(6) Percentage of (5) aged 14-24	(7) Percentage of total male labor force in occupation
Total labor force	5,648,384	1,257,220	22.26	34,027,905	16.60	--
1. Professional and semi-professional workers	148,474	32,408	21.83	1,875,387	7.92	5.51
2. Farmers and farm managers	325,484	173,031	53.16	4,991,715	6.52	14.67
3. Other managers and proprietors	121,696	46,242	38.00	3,325,767	3.66	9.77
4. Clerical and sales	868,336	147,411	16.98	4,360,648	19.91	12.81
5. Craftsmen and foremen	423,332	139,052	32.85	4,949,132	8.55	14.54
6. Operatives	1,239,673	348,232	28.09	6,205,898	19.98	18.23
a. Mining	103,445	36,531	35.31	649,226	15.93	1.91
b. Industrial operatives	473,104	132,910	28.09	2,303,054	20.54	6.77
i. Food products	43,634	12,395	28.41	200,298	21.78	.59
ii. Wood products	34,238	10,515	30.71	150,344	22.77	.44
iii. Iron and steel	46,962	13,680	29.12	263,837	17.80	.78
c. Non-manufacturing operatives	64,019	15,417	24.08	366,175	17.48	1.08
7. Domestic service	24,439	4,317	17.66	142,231	17.18	.42
8. Other services	405,985	55,637	13.70	2,196,695	18.48	6.46
9. Farm laborers and foremen	1,384,952	144,371	10.42	2,770,005	50.00	8.14
10. Other laborers	634,903	159,564	25.13	2,965,693	21.41	8.71
a. Fishermen	9,741	2,074	21.29	54,876	17.75	.16
b. Lumbermen, raftsmen, woodchoppers	31,394	7,559	24.08	127,497	24.62	.37
c. Industrial laborers	552,431	140,092	25.36	2,497,885	22.12	7.34
i. Construction	87,450	22,396	25.61	435,808	20.07	1.28
ii. Manufacturing	294,723	79,885	27.10	1,237,239	23.82	3.63
I. Food	34,008	8,996	26.45	133,945	25.39	.39
II. Wood	71,785	22,167	30.88	252,922	28.38	.74
III. Iron and steel	48,894	12,540	25.64	260,725	18.75	.77
iii. Non-manufacturing	170,258	37,811	22.21	824,838	20.64	2.42
I. Railroads	24,787	8,144	32.85	211,660	11.71	.62

Source: U.S. Bureau of the Census, *U.S. Census of Population: 1940*, Vol. III, "The Labor Force," Part I, "U.S. Summary," (Wash., D.C.: GPO, 1943), Table 67.

[a] Employed males (excluding experienced males seeking work and emergency workers).

[b] Married with wife present.

[c] Excludes widowed, divorced or separated.

TABLE I-13 Death Rates by Occupation for Males, Aged 25-65. England and Wales, 1860-1871 and 1880-1882

Occupation	Mean annual death rates per 1000 living				Comparative mortality figure 1880/1882
	1860/1861-1871 Years of age		1880/1882 Years of age		
	25-45	45-65	25-45	45-65	25-65
All males	11.27	23.98	10.16	25.27	1000
Occupied males	--	--	9.71	24.63	967
Unoccupied males	--	--	32.43	36.20	2182
Males in selected healthy districts[a]	--	--	8.47	19.74	804
1. Clergy, priest, minister	5.96	17.31	4.64	15.93	556
2. Barrister, solicitor	9.87	22.97	7.54	23.13	842
3. Physician, surgeon, general practitioner	13.81	24.55	11.57	28.03	1122
4. Schoolmaster, teacher	9.82	23.56	6.41	19.84	719
5. Artist, engraver, sculptor, architect	11.73	22.91	8.39	25.07	921
6. Musician, music master	18.94	34.76	13.78	32.39	1314
7. Farmer, grazier	7.66	17.32	6.09	16.53	631
8. Laborer in agricultural counties[b]	--	7.13	5.52	17.68	701
9. Gardener, nurseryman	6.74	17.54	5.52	16.19	599
10. Fisherman	11.26	15.84	8.32	19.74	797
11. Cab, omnibus service	15.94	35.38	15.39	36.83	1482
12. Bargeman, lighterman, waterman	14.99	30.78	14.25	31.13	1305
13. Carter, carrier, haulier	--	--	12.52	33.00	1275
14. Groom, domestic coachman	--	--	8.53	23.28	887
15. Commercial traveler	12.28	29.00	9.04	25.03	948
16. Brewer	19.26	36.86	13.90	34.25	1361
17. Innkeeper, publican, spirit, wine, beer dealer	18.01	34.14	18.02	33.68	1521
18. Inn, hotel servant	21.91	42.19	22.63	55.30	2205
19. Maltster	7.04	22.26	7.28	23.11	830
20. Law clerk	18.75	37.05	10.77	30.79	1151
21. Commercial clerk and insurance service	14.28	28.88	10.48	24.49	996
22. Bookseller, stationer	10.84	21.36	8.53	20.57	825
23. Chemist, druggist	13.92	23.56	10.58	25.16	1015
24. Tobacconist	13.19	21.76	11.14	23.46	1000
25. Grocer	9.49	17.15	8.00	10.16	771
26. Draper and manchester warehouseman	14.34	26.33	9.70	20.96	883
27. Ironmonger	10.38	22.95	8.42	23.87	895
28. Coal merchant	8.83	22.59	6.90	20.62	758
29. General shopkeeper	--	--	9.12	21.23	865
30. Cheesemonger, milk, butter-man	--	--	9.48	26.90	1009
31. Greengrocer, fruiterer	11.41	24.51	10.04	26.57	1025
32. Fishmonger, poulterer	15.62	29.21	10.53	23.45	974
33. Shopkeepers as represented by the above eleven (22-32)	--	--	9.04	21.90	877
34. Butcher	13.19	28.37	12.16	29.08	1170
35. Baker, confectioner	10.72	26.39	8.70	26.12	958
36. Corn miller	--	26.65	8.40	26.62	957
37. Hatter	12.81	31.76	10.78	26.95	1064
38. Hairdresser	15.11	30.10	13.64	33.25	1327
39. Tailor	12.92	24.79	10.73	26.47	1051
40. Shoemaker	10.39	22.30	9.31	23.36	921
41. Tanner, fellmonger	10.43	26.57	7.97	25.37	911
42. Currier	11.32	25.09	8.56	24.07	906
43. Saddler, harness maker	12.29	25.21	9.19	26.49	987
44. Tallow chandler, soap-boiler	11.75	27.24	7.74	26.10[c]	920
45. Tallow, soap, glue, manure manufacture	--	--	7.31	27.57	933
46. Printer	13.02	29.38	11.12	26.60	1071
47. Bookbinder	12.76	31.56	11.73	29.72[c]	1167
48. Watch and clock maker	10.78	24.90	9.26	22.64	963
49. Watch, clock, phil. instrument maker and jeweller	--	--	9.22	23.99	932
50. Paper manufacture	10.33	20.19	6.48	19.62	717
51. Glass manufacture	13.19	29.32	11.21	31.71	1190
52. Earthenware manufacture	12.59	41.75	13.70	51.39	1742
53. Cotton, linen, manufacture (Lancashire)	10.65[d]	27.90[d]	9.99	29.44	1088

TABLE I-13 (Continued) Death Rates by Occupation for Males, Aged 25-65. England and Wales, 1860-1871 and 1880-1882

Occupation	Mean annual death rates per 1000 living: 1860/1861-1871 Years of age 25-45	1860/1861-1871 45-65	1880/1882 Years of age 25-45	1880/1882 45-65	Comparative mortality figure 1880/1882 25-65
All males	11.27	23.98	10.16	25.27	1000
Occupied males	--	--	9.71	24.63	967
Unoccupied males	--	--	32.43	36.20	2182
Males in selected healthy districts	--	--	8.47	19.74	804
54. Silk manufacture	9.89	20.08	7.81	22.79	845
55. Wool, worsted, manufacture (West Riding)	9.35[d]	23.26[d]	9.71	27.50	1032
56. Carpet, rug-manufacture	9.92	25.57	9.48	24.10	945
57. Lace manufacture	--	--	6.78	20.71	755
58. Hosiery manufacture (Leicestershire, Notts)	--	--	6.69	19.22	717
59. Dyer, bleacher, printer, etc. of textile fabrics	11.19	25.99	9.46	27.08	1012
60. Rope, twine, cord-maker	9.19	29.35	7.95	22.25	839
61. Builder, mason, bricklayer	11.43	27.16	9.25	25.59	969
62. Slater, tiler	10.66	30.76	8.97	24.93[c]	942
63. Plasterer, whitewasher	9.50	27.90	7.79	25.07	896
64. Plumber, painter, glazier	12.48	34.66	11.07	32.49	1202
65. Upholsterer, cabinet maker, french polisher	11.09	24.09	9.55	24.77	963
66. Carpenter, joiner	9.44	21.36	7.77	21.74	820
67. Sawyer	8.67	21.27	7.46	23.74	852
68. Wood turner, box maker, cooper	11.80	26.13	10.56	28.55	1091
69. Coach builder	10.43	29.57	9.13	24.72	944
70. Wheelwright	8.40	21.17	6.83	19.21	723
71. Shipbuilder, shipwright	10.68	26.26	6.95	21.29	775
72. Locksmith, bellhanger, gasfitter	11.04	27.90	9.15	25.66	967
73. Gunsmith	10.62	25.32	10.62	25.78	1031
74. Cutler, scissors maker	--	--	12.30	34.94	1309
75. File maker	16.27	42.30	15.29	45.14[c]	1667
76. Cutler, scissors, file, needle, saw, toolmaker	11.88[e]	32.74[e]	11.71	34.42	1273
77. Engine, machine-maker, fitter, millwright	--	--	7.97	23.27	803
78. Boiler maker	--	--	9.27	26.65	994
79. Last two together (Nos.77-78)	10.61	23.81	8.23	23.89	888
80. Blacksmith	10.07	23.88	9.29	25.67	973
81. Other iron and steel workers	--	--	8.36	22.84	869
82. Tin workers	10.36	23.67	8.00	24.17	885
83. Copper, lead, zinc, brass, etc. workers	10.74	26.17	9.15	26.79	992
84. Metal workers (Nos. 72-83)	--	--	8.30	25.03	938
85. Miner, Durham, Northumberland	11.30[f]	22.01[f]	7.79	24.04	873
86. Miner, Lancashire	--	--	7.91	26.30	929
87. Miner, West Riding	--	--	6.59	21.80	772
88. Miner, Derbyshire, Nottinghamshire	--	--	6.54	20.23	734
89. Miner, Staffordshire	11.33[f]	30.45[f]	7.81	26.50	929
90. Miner, South Wales, Mommouthshire	14.72[f]	20.66[f]	9.05	30.87	1081
91. Coal miners as represented by the above six (Nos. 85-90)	--	--	7.64	25.11	891
92. Miner (North Riding and other iron stone districts)	--	--	8.05	21.85	834
93. Miner, Cornwall	11.94[f]	41.73[f]	14.77	53.69	1839
94. Stone, slate quarrier	10.88	28.67	9.95	31.04	1122
95. Railway, road, clay, sand, etc. laborer	--	--	11.01	24.80	1025
96. Coalheaver	--	--	10.22	23.77	968
97. Chimney sweep	17.53	42.87	13.73	41.54[c]	1519
98. Messenger, porter, watchman (not government)	--	--	17.07	37.37	1565
99. Costermonger, hawker, street seller	20.09	37.82	20.26	45.33	1879
100. General laborer (London)	18.35	40.04	20.62	50.85	2020

For the United States, on the other hand, data for the registration states analyzed by Uselding point to generally (though not consistently) above-average age-standardized death rates for males 15 and over engaged in mining and also in manufacturing and mechanical industries for the census years 1890 and 1900 and for 1908–1910 (Uselding, 1976, p. 347). These results are presented in Table I-14. Up to the present day, higher mortality continues to be found among semiskilled and unskilled manual workers and lower mortality among professional and clerical workers. But mortality among coal-mining and some industrial populations and among laborers seems to be more closely correlated with socioeconomic status, since mortality among wives is often as high as among husbands. On the other hand, some specific occupations, such as glass workers, hard rock miners, machine tenders, and chemical workers, have mortality for husbands significantly above those of their wives (Benjamin, 1965, pp. 32–34; Dublin, Lotka, and Spiegelman, 1949, Chap. 11; Kitagawa and Hauser, 1973, Chap. 3; Moriyama and Guralnik, 1956). One problem with occupational mortality per se is that persons who die in one occupation or, more likely, while unemployed, may have contracted the condition in another occupation or industry. The problem is comparable for morbidity. In sum, it may be that miners and heavy-industrial populations experience higher than average mortality and morbidity, but the evidence is ambiguous.

A related issue is whether mortality in mining and industrial *regions* might be higher than average. In an extensive investigation of just this issue, Wrigley concluded that mining districts in France and Germany seldom had mortality that differed much from that in nearby rural areas. The higher mortality was generally found in large cities (Wrigley, 1961, Chap. VI).

TABLE I-13 (Notes)

Source: England and Wales, Registrar General, *Supplement to the Forty-Fifth Annual Report (1882)*, "Mortality 1871-1880," (London: Eyre and Spottiswoode, 1885), Table J.

[a] The selected healthy districts were all those registration districts in which mean annual death rates (males and females together) was under 17.00 per 1000 for 1871/1880.

[b] Includes agricultural laborers in Hertfordshire, Oxfordshire, Befordshire, Cambridgeshire, Suffolk, Wiltshire, Dorsetshire, Devonshire, Herefordshire, and Lincolnshire.

[c] Rate based on less than 5000 person years.

[d] These rates relate to England and Wales.

[e] 1871 only.

[f] Based on a return to an inquiry into the condition of miners in Great Britain made in connection with the census of 1861. Covers 1860/1862 only.

TABLE I-14 Male Standardized Death Rates and Comparative Mortality Figures by Occupational Class, Registration States, 1890, 1900, and 1908/1910

Occupational class	Standardized death rates per 1000			Comparative mortality figures		
	1890	1900	1908/1910	1890	1900	1908/1910
Professional	14.15	14.60	12.56	1.01	.97	.99
Clerical and official	11.10	14.35	10.93	.79	.95	.86
Mercantile and trade	12.78	13.27	8.34	.91	.88	.66
Entertainment, personal service, police, military	15.74	13.75	11.31	1.13	.91	.89
Laboring and servant	24.54	25.12	18.45	1.76	1.67	1.45
Manufacturing and mechanical	14.62	14.23	14.22	1.05	.95	1.12
Agriculture	7.72	11.75	11.22	.55	.78	.88
Forestry and fishing	7.80	9.67	7.82	.56	.64	.61
Mining	9.94	15.78	13.06	.71	1.05	1.03
Transportation and communication	16.13	14.92	13.59	1.15	.99	1.07
Overall death rate	13.98	15.06	12.73	1.00	1.00	1.00

Source: Paul Uselding, "In Dispraise of the Muckrakers: United States Occupational Mortality, 1890-1910," *Research in Economic History*, Vol. I (1976), p. 347.

Mortality in industrial slums was very high,[26] but "in more strictly industrial areas, although very large populations in aggregate grew up round the pitheads, the factories, the mills and the furnaces, many people lived in comparatively small industrial villages and towns. The mortality experience of these areas was often surprisingly good [Wrigley, 1969, p. 175]." In Germany in the late nineteenth century, the crude death rates for the industrial *Kreise* of the *Regierungsbezirke* of Oppeln, Arnsberg, Aachen, and Münster were only slightly higher than that for the surrounding nonindustrial *Kreise*. The industrial *Kreise* for Düsseldorf had a lower crude death rate than those of the other *Kreise*. The differences were, however, small and apparently converging (Haines, 1976, p. 337; Wrigley, 1961, p. 122).

Some additional evidence is given in Table I-15, which gives some correlations between the infant mortality rate (infant deaths per 1000 live births) and the percentage of adult males in mining and metallurgy, the percentage of adult males in agriculture, and the percentage of the population living in urban areas for England and Wales. This was done for a sample of mining

[26] One example may suffice. During the period 1881–1890, the industrial city of Manchester had an expectation of life at birth (both sexes) of 28.78 years. This compared with 43.66 years for all of England and Wales and 51.48 years for selected healthy districts. Cited in Weber (1899, p. 347). See also Wrigley (1969, pp. 173–174).

TABLE I-15 Zero-Order Correlations between Mortality Variables and Indicators of Economic Structure and Urbanization. Registration Districts, England and Wales, 1851, 1861, 1871[a]

	1851	1861	1871
I. Correlation between infant mortality rate and			
1. Percentage adult males in mining and metallurgy			
a. Mining Sample (*N*=61)	(.155)	(.085)	(.221)
b. Random sample (*N*=125)	(.025)	(.073)	.326
2. Percentage adult males in agriculture			
a. Mining sample (*N*=61)	-.648	-.592	-.734
b. Random sample (*N*=125)	-.477	-.365	-.612
3. Percentage urban			
a. Mining sample (*N*=61)	.301	.283	.436
b. Random sample (*N*=125)	.146	.447	.498
II. Correlation between male death rate (ages 25-44) and			
1. Percentage adult males in mining and metallurgy			
a. Mining sample (*N*=61)	--	(.051)	--
2. Percentage adult males in agriculture			
a. Mining sample (*N*=61)	--	.385	--
3. Percentage urban			
a. Mining sample (*N*=61)	--	.368	--

Source: For definition of the sample and variables, see Chapter III.

[a]All numbers in parentheses are not significant at a 5% level (two tail test).

and industrial registration districts (with more than 10% of all adult males in mining and metallurgy) and a random sample of 125 registration districts for 1851, 1861, and 1971. In addition, for the mining sample only, the death rates for males aged 25–44 were correlated with urbanization and labor-force structure for 1861. As may be seen, a higher proportion of economic activity in coal or iron mining or ferrous metallurgy did not result in significantly higher infant mortality (an indicator of overall mortality) or even adult male mortality. The only significant correlation, for the random sample in 1871, may have been so because miners other than coal and iron miners were included at that date. It was, however, urbanization which was significantly and positively correlated with those death rates. A more agricultural environment did have a significantly favorable effect on mortality, but the evidence supports the view that it was urbanization and not industrialization per se (coal mining and ferrous metallurgy in this case) which led to higher mortality.

In conclusion, it is clear that mining and heavy-industrial populations and regions have peculiar demographic characteristics, particularly in the areas of fertility and nuptiality. It remains to be seen how these characteristics relate to social and economic life. Also, a distinction must be made between the general characteristics of mining and industrial populations versus those that are true of a particular group at a particular time and place. This will be clarified in the next chapter, when a model of demographic behavior for mining and industrial populations is elucidated. Demographic differentials and changes over time will both be treated in subsequent chapters, but differentials will be emphasized.

II

A Model of Demographic Behavior for Mining and Heavy-Industrial Populations and Regions

The explanatory model proposed here focuses on the major factors in marriage and fertility decisions as they relate to mining and heavy-industrial populations. It is important to consider both marriage and marital fertility in conjunction, since total fertility is the result of both and since both are affected by many common factors.[1] Migration and mortality also are an integral part of the model and will be discussed as such. Modified, this model should be more generally applicable to other occupational groups, but in this instance the emphasis is on coal miners and metallurgical workers because of their observed high fertility and early marriage.[2]

A number of factors play a role in these differentials in marriage and

[1] Not much will be said concerning illegitimate fertility, because it tended to be less important in mining and heavy-industrial populations and areas. It was of much greater importance, however, for areas with female-dominated labor markets.

[2] The origins of this model stretch back to 1972 and a grant proposal made to National Institutes of Child Health and Human Development, which was subsequently funded (R01-HD-07599) and that has made possible much of this work. A preliminary version was presented to the annual meetings of the Population Association of America in New York City in April, 1974. Subsequent statements of this view appear in Haines (1975, pp. 11–21; 1977a, pp. 32–37; 1977b). Later, it was found that, independently, Professor Dov Friedlander of the Hebrew University had reached a number of the same conclusions working with national and county level data for England and Wales (Friedlander, 1973). This was very encouraging from the viewpoint of the plausibility of the model. There has been increased recent interest in the interactions of industrial labor-force structures and environments with demographic behavior. See, for example, Tilly (1977); Tilly, Scott, and Cohen (1976).

fertility. High marital fertility and earlier and more complete marriage among mining and some metallurgical populations (as well as among other similar occupational groups) can be viewed as the product of socioeconomic and demographic conditions characteristic of miners, iron and steel workers, or of coal or iron areas, as well as due to the other particular circumstances in a given situation. Life styles (as embodied in tastes and costs), potential income outlook, and demographic patterns (particularly sex ratios and possibly mortality) all interact to produce the observed behavior.[3]

Coal mining, and to a lesser extent metallurgy, are not initially urban industries. Although urban agglomerations do eventually grow up around mining and metallurgical nodes, they are not, at first, great administrative, cultural, or commercial centers. In their earlier stages of development, much of the population is drawn from a rural environment. It may be argued that these persons, who were socialized (i.e., whose tastes and preferences were formed) in a rural life style, maintained these tastes (for a desired combination of goods, children, and leisure) in their new situation while simultaneously experiencing the expanded income outlook and opportunities of an industrial wage earner in a growing sector. For example, the Pennsylvania anthracite region was only 15.8% urban in 1850. This rose, however, to 32.7% by 1880 and 59.2% by 1900.[4] The structure of the coal seams themselves often led to the creation of numerous small towns or "patches," rather than large cities. Scranton was a notable exception (Broehl, 1964, pp. 82–85; Roberts, 1904, pp. 145–146). Many of the miners themselves were from rural circumstances, particularly the Irish before 1880 (Broehl, 1964, Chap. 4).[5] For England and Wales in 1851, a sample of 61 mining and metallurgical registration districts had an unweighted average urban percentage of only 22.4% whereas a random sample of 125 registration districts had an unweighted urban percentage of 28.6%.[6] By 1871, however, the average urban percentage in the mining districts was 40% and only 31% in the random sample.[7] For northern France, Ariès noted numerous small industrial villages and towns (Ariès, 1948, pp. 233–240; see also Wrigley, 1969, p. 175).

[3] A similar approach to the economics of fertility is taken by Easterlin (1969, 1978). The latter is an attempt to reconcile the theoretical economic approach, exemplified by the work of Becker (1960, 1965) and the more empirical sociological approach which may be seen in, for example, Blake (1968). More recent theoretical treatment of the economics of fertility may be found in the numerous important articles in T. Schultz (1975) and the work of Turchi (1975a,b).

[4] These calculations were based on U.S. census data on populations for minor civil divisions. The anthracite region and the urban definitions are discussed in Chapters IV and V.

[5] Broehl argues, in fact, that the type of violence exhibited in Schuylkill County in the 1860s and 1870s was the characteristic of the peasant origins of the Irish in the early nineteenth century. By 1850, 26.9% of the mining labor force was Irish-born. By 1880, this had increased to 33.9% (based on census samples).

[6] The national average urban percentage was 35.2 in 1851 for England and Wales.

[7] The national average urban percentage in 1871 for England and Wales was 39.7.

Furthermore, many miners and other workers in such an environment experienced a cost situation intermediate between rural and urban. Many had the opportunity to supplement their money incomes with income in kind from produce raised on small farms and garden plots in the semirural areas. An indication of this would be a relatively high incidence of dwarf farms in mining areas. This was indeed the case for the industrial region of Upper Silesia in 1907, where the incidence of farms less than 2 hectares accounted for over 86% of total farms (as opposed to slightly over 52% for the surrounding three agrarian regions) and about 23% of cultivated land (as opposed to 7% for the three predominantly agricultural regions) (Haines, 1978,Chap. 5).[8] The same was true of the coal mining *Kreise* of the Ruhr area[9] in 1895, which had 91% of total farms under 2 hectares (as opposed to 60% for three adjacent, more agricultural, administrative areas)[10] and over 15% of all farm land in farms under 2 hectares (as opposed to an average of 9% for the surrounding three areas) (Meitzen and Grossman, 1901, pp. 112–115). Some evidence from the 1889–1890 Commissioner of Labor Survey (U.S. Commissioner of Labor, 1890, 1891) suggests a higher proportion of families in coal mining had gardens or small farms than did families in other industries. For example, 43.5% of the mining families surveyed in the United States kept a farm or garden, as opposed to only 12.4% in woolens and 11.6% in cottons. Among the European miners interviewed, 25.8% kept gardens; this was 71% for the small Belgian and German samples. Almost 45% of American mining families kept some livestock, as opposed to only 6% in woolens and 12% in cottons. The other heavy industries (pig iron, bar iron, steel, coke, and glass) fell between mining and textiles with respect to the type of secondary agricultural activity.

There is also evidence that miners and metallurgical workers had relatively high incomes and a generally good standard of living. For example, with respect to nineteenth-century England, "most authorities agree that miners enjoyed a relatively high standard of living" and that "against a background of ill-planned industrial conurbation the houses of many miners seemed well-ordered, healthy, and clean (B. Lewis, 1971, pp. 38, 107)." William Cobbett, nineteenth-century economic publicist and agitator, stated: "Their work is terrible to be sure . . . but at any rate they live well [quoted in Lewis, 1971, p. 29]."

Wages in mining and iron work were generally high in Britain and above the national average. Miners also often received free cottages and free coal

[8] The coal mining region in 1907 consisted of *Kreise* Tarnowitz, Beuthen, Zabrze, and Kattowitz and the *Stadtkreise* Beuthen, Königshütte, and Kattowitz. The agricultural regions were all the remaining *Kreise* of *Regierungsbezirk* Oppeln.

[9] *Kreis* Recklinghausen in *Regierungsbezirk* (R.B.) Münster. *Kreise* Hamm, Dortmund, Hörde, Bochum, Gelsenkirchen, Hattingen, Hagen, and Schwelm; and *Stadtkreise* Dortmund, Bochum, Gelsenkirchen, and Hagen in *R.B.* Arnsberg. *Kreise* Mülheim an der Ruhr, Ruhrort, and Essen; and *Stadtkreise* Duisberg and Essen in *R.B.* Düsseldorf.

[10] *Regierungsbezirke* Münster, Minden, and Kassel.

(Bowley, 1900, pp. 96, 101). Evidence presented by Bowley shows that the average money wages of miners and skilled iron workers were among the highest in the nineteenth century. The wages of printers and, occasionally, building craftsmen were at times higher, but those of sailors, agricultural workers, and cotton and woolen textile workers were lower. Laborers' wages were always lower (Bowley, 1900, pp. 96–109, 130–133, especially Appendix I, Table II, p. 133). For France, Ariès states, with respect to the Pas-de-Calais, that "the deficit of manual labor in the new pits permitted higher salaries, a higher level of living. Nevertheless, the essentials of manners and of social structure and morality remained the same [Ariès, 1948, p. 233]." In Germany, the daily wages of miners were for a shorter day (8–9 hours) than most other industrial workers in the nineteenth century and were generally higher per day (Bry, 1960; Desai, 1968, pp. 108–111; Haines, 1978, Tables III-32 and VI-14). Furthermore, miners usually worked more regularly, five to six shifts per week and usually for a full year, unlike some other industrial workers (Meinert, 1956, Übersichte I and II and pp. 124–175). For example, in current German Marks (M), for 1871, coal miners earned average annual incomes of 700 M, compared to 667 M in steel manufacture, 555 M in machine building, 545 M in printing, and 421 M in cotton textiles. By 1900, men in mining were earning 1085 M per year, and iron and steel workers 942 M per year. Cotton and woolen textiles workers were receiving only 660 M. In general, workers in mining, iron and steel manufacture, machine building, nonferrous metals, brewing, glass manufacture, and printing, and some transport workers received the highest wages. Workers in textiles and food processing were a good bit lower. The differentials were fairly consistent over the late nineteenth century (Desai, 1968, Tables A.1 and A.2). The wages of miners and construction workers were a great deal higher than those of agricultural workers in Upper Silesia (Haines, 1976, pp. 352–354). Thus, for Europe, wages in heavy industry were generally high. Overall:

> *Mining and metallurgy, which required substantial strength and skill, paid adult males far more than the textile industry did. . . . The men who built and installed machines, or who puddled iron, . . . required years to learn their trade fully. Their pay was three to six times greater than that of an unskilled laborer* [Stearns, 1967, p. 124].
>
> *Iron puddlers, a particularly well paid group, were "the aristocracy of the proletariat," proud, clannish, set apart by sweat and blood. Few of them lived past forty* [Landes, 1969, p. 218; see also Courthéoux, 1959].

Similarly, for the United States, it was noted that miners in western Maryland had a relatively high standard of living and that many kept a cow and a small garden (Harvey, 1969, pp. 94–97).[11] Although, in his study of

[11] It was remarked by a contemporary that: "The miners live well, and some of them even luxuriously for their class, and spend their money freely, thus making an active demand for all classes of goods." Quoted from the *Coal Trade Journal*, March 14, 1883, in Harvey (1969, p. 95).

the anthracite areas, Roberts stressed the inadequate earnings of miners, he described saving and consumption behavior characteristic of a good and improving standard of living (Roberts, 1904, p. 346, Chaps. 4 and 9; 1901, pp. 108–128). For the Pennsylvania anthracite region, full-time equivalent annual income in coal mining was approximately $240 in about 1850. A comparable annual income for iron and steel workers was $283 at a daily wage of $1.415. Iron puddlers, rollers and roughers, and furnace keepers in Pennsylvania in 1850 made even more: $2.51, $2.52, $1.63, and $1.65, respectively. This compared to a daily wage for common labor in Pennsylvania of $.80 and full-time equivalent earnings of $163 for cotton manufactures ($.815 per day) and $189 for woolens ($.945 per day). Farm laborers earned only $10.82 per month (about $130 per year on a full-time basis), including board. By 1880, Pennsylvania miners earned about $1.91 per day and $441 per year (based on an estimated 213 days worked per year). Iron and steel workers brought in average full-time equivalent earnings of about $433. Common laborers earned only about $1.25 per day (probably about $250 per year if times were good); workers in cottons and woolens received full-time equivalent earnings of $346 and $381, respectively. Farm laborers received only about $175 in Pennsylvania for a full year's work (including board). The same differentials held up through the twentieth century, although coal mining declined somewhat relative to iron and steel manufacture and other heavy industries.[12] Again, overall, wages and incomes in

[12] Wages and full-time incomes are from Lebergott (1964, Tables A-20, 23, 25, 27–29) and from U.S. Department of Labor (1934). Hours of work in Pennsylvania anthracite mining in 1880 was estimated as an average of 1881–1885, from U.S. Bureau of the Census (1960), Series M-129. Full-time equivalent income is simply the daily wage multiplied by the average number of days worked per year. This was assumed to be 200 days in 1850. These incomes were either estimated by Lebergott or obtained by using the average number of working days from Lebergott (1964) or U.S. Bureau of the Census (1960). Some representative male wages for the period around 1900 include:

	Dollars per day
Coal miner (1902, Pennsylvania)	2.20
Catcher (1899, bar mill, Pennsylvania)	3.42
Roller (1898, bar mill, Pennsylvania)	3.86
Puddler (1899, bar mill, Pennsylvania)	3.73
Furnace keeper (1899, blast furnace, Pennsylvania)	2.47
Laborer (1899, Pennsylvania)	1.52
Boiler maker (1900, New York)	2.52
Machinist (1900, Pennsylvania)	2.50
Moulder (1900, Ohio)	2.81
Cotton spinner (1900, Massachusetts)	1.87
Cotton weaver (1900, Massachusetts)	1.37
Carpenter (1900, Pennsylvania)	2.80
Mason (1900, Pennsylvania)	3.00
Farm laborer (1899, Pennsylvania)	1.34

In terms of full-time equivalent annual earnings in 1899 for Pennsylvania, cottons received $360, woolens $371, and iron and steel $558 (Lebergott, 1964, Tables A-20, 27–29; U.S. Department of Labor, 1934).

mining and heavy industry were relatively high, especially vis-à-vis laborers, textile operatives, and farm workers.

Another index of well-being was home ownership. A large number of mining families in the Pennsylvania anthracite fields actually owned land and their own homes (Roberts, 1904, pp. 133–136). In the 1889–1890 Commissioner of Labor Survey, 26.4% of all families with the head employed in coal and iron mining in the United States sample owned their own homes. Of families in iron, steel, and coke manufacture, 19.9% owned their own homes; and 26.6% of families in glass manufacture were homeowners. In contrast, only 10.6% of textile workers owned their dwellings (i.e., 7.9% in cottons and 16.9% in woolens)[13] (U.S. Commissioner of Labor, 1890, 1891).

Not only did miners and metallurgical workers earn relatively good wages and incomes, they were also characterized by an age–earnings profile that peaked relatively early in the working life of the principal family wage earner. This may be seen in Table II-1, which gives average annual earnings of male family heads (who had earned some income during the year) by age and industry of head from the 1889–1890 Commissioner of Labor Survey. Notably, peaks in income usually came early in the life cycle of the family. By the time a miner or an industrial worker had been working only a short time in his 20s, he was not too far from his peak earning capacity. For example, for the United States sample, the estimated peak age of earnings was 36.6 years for nonhomeowners and 33.1 years for homeowners.[14] The

[13] Sample sizes were coal and iron mining (673 families); iron, steel, and coke manufacture (1817 families); glass (1276 families); and textiles (3043 families, of which 2132 were in cottons and 911 in woolens). Average home ownership in Europe (6.6%) was much lower than for the United States (17.6%).

[14] These ages were estimated from regression equations which had as the dependent variable the income of the husband and as independent variables, among other things, age and age-squared of husband. Other independent variables included industry, location, skill level of occupation, nationality of husband, and family size. The relationship between husband's income and age was strongly and significantly quadratic, and the orientation was correct. Income rose, peaked, and then declined as age increased. The relationship estimated in the regression equation was

$$\text{INCHUS} = \beta_1 + \beta_2 X_1 + \beta_3 (X_1)^2 + \sum_{i=2}^{n} \beta_{i+2} X_i,$$

where β_1 is the constant term, X_1 is the age of husband, β_2 is the estimated coefficient for age of husband, β_3 is the estimated coefficient for age of husband squared, and $\sum_{i=2}^{n} \beta_{i+2} X_i$ is the sum of all other variables and estimated coefficients.

A maximum of INCHUS with respect to age (X_1) occurs when

$$\frac{\partial(\text{INCHUS})}{\partial X_1} = 0 \quad \text{and} \quad \frac{\partial^2(\text{INCHUS})}{\partial (X_1)^2} < 0.$$

Since

$$\frac{\partial(\text{INCHUS})}{\partial X_1} = \beta_2 + 2\beta_3 X_1 = 0,$$

age–earnings profiles thus quickly reached a peak and remained at a plateau for a time before declining in old age. It is interesting to speculate as to the causes of this decline among earnings of older workers: lack of unions and seniority privileges; discrimination against older workers because of declining physical ability; greater education and skill levels among younger and more recently educated cohorts of workers (i.e., a "vintage" human capital model); or a reduction in work effort because of greater contributions of children to family income.[15] It is known, however, that age–earnings profiles for blue-collar workers continue to peak early and remain fairly level over a large age range. This is in contrast to the pattern for white-collar workers who experience rising income on average until late middle age (Mincer, 1974; Oppenheimer, 1974). The reason for the early peak among blue-collar manual workers seems to reflect the premium on youthful strength and stamina for mining and industrial work. Although skills were important in many industrial and mining occupations, they could usually be acquired in a reasonably short period of time.

An early peaking earnings profile would tend to encourage early marriage and childbearing because the family could afford to have children earlier and in greater numbers.[16] Ample employment opportunities at an early age with relatively high pay would certainly encourage children to become independent, leave the home more quickly, and eventually to marry early.

Another relevant aspect of Table II-1 is the level of earnings. Coal mining (and even more particularly iron mining) did *not* provide the highest annual incomes. Coal-mining earnings were not above earnings in iron and steel

---

age of maximum income occurs at

$$X_1 = \beta_2/2\beta_3$$

The second-order condition requires

$$\frac{\partial^2(\text{INCHUS})}{\partial(X_1)^2} = 2\beta_3 < 0,$$

which implies $\beta_3 < 0$. This means that X_1 will always be, as expected, positive. To solve for X_1, one merely substitutes the estimated parameters β_2 and β_3 into Eq. (1). Indeed, it turns out that β_3 is always negative as estimated, without any prior constraints.

It is, in addition, interesting to speculate why earnings peaked earlier for homeowners than for nonhomeowners. They may have been homeowners partly because their incomes peaked earlier. The average incomes for male homeowners in the United States sample was $647, while that for male nonhomeowners was $512. The European portion of the sample showed a later peaking age–earnings profile, for example, 41.5 years in the case of nonhomeowners.

[15] These issues are discussed in greater detail in Haines (1979). Later in the life cycle, income from children made up an increasingly important part of total family incomes.

[16] The explanation for the steeper earnings profile for white-collar workers is often a human capital argument, that is, there is a longer delay in realizing the value of a higher level of education. To move from this to earlier marriage and childbearing among blue-collar workers assumes that white-collar workers could not borrow against their future higher earnings. This, in turn, assumes imperfect capital markets, possibly reasonable for personal borrowing even today.

TABLE II-1 Average Annual Earnings by Age of Family Head. Nine Industries. United States and Five European Countries[a] 1889/1890. (Dollars) (Families with Male Heads. Only Heads with Some Income)

		Age of head							
		15-19	20-29	30-39	40-49	50-59	60+	Unknown	Total
United States									
1.	Pig iron	$326	$484	$547	$509	$518	$376	--	$513
	(*N*)	(1)	(184)	(289)	(187)	(74)	(27)	--	(762)
2.	Bar iron	--	623	715	721	643	531	910	686
	(*N*)	--	(96)	(241)	(172)	(86)	(24)	(1)	(620)
3.	Steel	--	641	624	539	449	458	--	578
	(*N*)	--	(29)	(44)	(36)	(24)	(10)	--	(183)
4.	Coke	--	507	498	543	560	359	--	517
	(*N*)	--	(45)	(90)	(75)	(31)	(8)	--	(249)
1-4.	Iron and steel	326	537	607	594	566	440	910	579
	(*N*)	(1)	(354)	(704)	(470)	(215)	(69)	(1)	(1814)
5.	Coal	--	442	431	450	398	305	350	428
	(*N*)	--	(106)	(190)	(120)	(68)	(23)	(1)	(508)
6.	Iron ore	--	305	346	318	342	167	--	323
	(*N*)	--	(50)	(64)	(30)	(16)	(5)	--	(165)
5-6.	Mining	--	398	410	424	387	280	350	402
	(*N*)	--	(156)	(254)	(150)	(84)	(28)	(1)	(673)
7.	Cottons	211	403	445	388	358	312	633	400
	(*N*)	(3)	(373)	(549)	(573)	(317)	(103)	(16)	(1934)
8.	Woolens	--	467	512	510	449	398	851	491
	(*N*)	--	(152)	(293)	(242)	(123)	(50)	(7)	(867)
7-8.	Textiles	211	422	468	424	383	340	699	428
	(*N*)	(3)	(524)	(842)	(815)	(440)	(153)	(23)	(2801)
9.	Glass	--	726	814	784	756	605	--	778
	(*N*)	--	(260)	(519)	(334)	(132)	(26)	--	(1271)
	Total	240	512	582	537	486	384	694	535
	(*N*)	(4)	(1295)	(2319)	(1769)	(871)	(276)	(25)	(6559)
Five European Countries									
1.	Pig iron	--	354	393	327	319	310	--	352
	(*N*)	--	(14)	(30)	(19)	(12)	(2)	--	(77)
2.	Bar iron	--	287	360	355	348	241	333	337
	(*N*)	--	(36)	(80)	(66)	(51)	(17)	(1)	(251)

manufacture or in glass making. Even woolens were above mining for th United States sample, although not for the European sample. This does nc contravene the notion that miners enjoyed a high level of wages and ir come. It means that other heavy industries (e.g., iron and steel, glass) wer often better off, as has already been suggested. As for the high incomes i woolens, the annual incomes given by Lebergott for woolen manufacture were generally higher than for cotton manufactures for the United States i

TABLE II-1 (Continued)

		Age of head							
		15-19	20-29	30-39	40-49	50-59	60+	Unknown	Total
3.	Steel	--	$362	$479	$480	$441	$218	--	$443
	(*N*)	--	(29)	(87)	(49)	(25)	(11)	--	(201)
4.	Coke	$224	298	319	262	303	257	--	285
	(*N*)	(1)	(2)	(8)	(12)	(4)	(1)	--	(28)
1-4.	Iron and steel	224	326	414	386	368	238	$333	375
	(*N*)	(1)	(81)	(205)	(146)	(92)	(31)	(1)	(557)
5.	Coal	--	360	378	351	368	263	--	361
	(*N*)	--	(22)	(77)	(61)	(25)	(9)	--	(194)
6.	Iron ore	--	281	270	244	232	--	--	254
	(*N*)	--	(2)	(6)	(8)	(3)	--	--	(19)
5-6.	Mining	--	353	370	339	353	263	--	351
	(*N*)	--	(24)	(83)	(69)	(28)	(9)	--	(213)
7.	Cottons	--	293	349	313	333	285	217	323
	(*N*)	--	(96)	(203)	(161)	(66)	(25)	(3)	(554)
8.	Woolens	--	255	272	301	285	323	--	281
	(*N*)	--	(60)	(103)	(81)	(69)	(13)	--	(326)
7-8.	Textiles	--	278	323	309	308	298	217	307
	(*N*)	--	(156)	(306)	(242)	(135)	(38)	(3)	(880)
9.	Glass	--	410	606	400	174	128	--	450
	(*N*)	--	(19)	(16)	(11)	(2)	(2)	--	(50)
	Total	224	308	367	340	334	263	246	339
	(*N*)	(1)	(280)	(610)	(468)	(257)	(80)	(4)	(1700)
Britain Only									
1.	Iron and steel	224	377	479	470	432	271	--	445
	(*N*)	(1)	(53)	(142)	(88)	(63)	(13)	--	(360)
2.	Mining	--	360	394	366	394	285	--	376
	(*N*)	--	(22)	(63)	(53)	(21)	(7)	--	(166)
3.	Textiles	--	338	379	372	358	320	--	366
	(*N*)	--	(75)	(185)	(123)	(71)	(16)	--	(470)
4.	Glass	--	399	494	365	--	--	--	423
	(*N*)	--	(14)	(8)	(4)	--	--	--	(26)
	Total	224	359	420	403	393	296	--	397
	(*N*)	(1)	(164)	(398)	(268)	(155)	(36)	--	(1022)

Source: U.S. Commissioner of Labor, *Sixth Annual Report* (1890). *Seventh Annual Report* (1891).

[a]The countries are Great Britain, France, Germany, Belgium, and Switzerland.

1889 ($372 versus $302) and were comparable to those for coal mining ($361). In contrast, however, annual income for a laborer was $292 (assuming he worked 200 days per year) (Lebergott, 1964, Tables A-20, 25, 27, 28). The higher wages for all industries in the Commissioner of Labor Survey in comparison with those in Lebergott may be accounted for by the fact that Table II-1 has earnings for males only, whereas Lebergott's figures are an average for adult males and females and children. Coal-mining wages were, however, higher than textile wages in the European sample and in the more relevant British subsample (which included most of the coal miners).

In sum, it seems that miners and industrial workers did enjoy relatively high wages and that this income arrived relatively early in life. While working conditions for the miner and heavy-industrial worker were often quite abysmal, the level of living outside the mine, factory, or workshop seems to have been reasonably good.[17]

A relative absence of female employment outside the home is also characteristic of mining and some industrial communities. This point, along with related issues of marriage and sex ratios, has been stressed by several authors (Charles and Moshinsky, 1938; Friedlander, 1973; Tilly, 1977; Tilly, Scott, and Cohen, 1976). A low incidence of female labor-force participation outside the home is generally associated with a labor-force structure dominated by male employment. This same labor-force structure also induces differentially higher net male in-migration in the younger adult years (e.g., 15–40), which raises sex ratios.[18] These higher sex ratios favor earlier marriage for females who, in any event, have a low opportunity cost (in terms of income foregone) for marriage and childrearing. The issue of high sex ratios leading to early marriage for women is assigned considerable importance by Wrigley (1961, p. 170) in his discussion of the industrial region of northwest Europe.

There is evidence of this for areas dominated by mining and metallurgy, where resource factors often dictated location distant from factories or workshops employing women. For England and Wales, where female and child labor underground in mines had been prohibited after Lord Shaftesbury's Act of 1842, the mean proportion of females aged 20 and over employed outside the home in 1871 in 63 registration districts with a significant proportion of the adult male labor force in mining and metallurgy was 24.5% as opposed to 30.1% for a random sample of 125 registration districts.[19] These means were significantly different at an .001 level of probability. At the same date there was a −.50 zero-order correlation between the percentage of adult male employment in minerals work (i.e., mining, quarrying, metallurgy) and the percentage of adult females employed outside the home within the mining districts.[20] Similar results were true for 1851 and

[17] Vivid descriptions of working conditions in the mines in England may be found in *Report of Commission of Inquiry into the Employment of Children and Young Persons in Mines and Collieries . . .* (Ashley Commission), First Report (1842), Second Report (1843) in *Parliamentary Papers* (1842/43) Vols. XV–XVII. See also Disraeli (1845), Engels (1958, pp. 274–294), and B. Lewis (1971, pp. 41–53). Numerous parliamentary inquiries in Britain took evidence on employment in mines and factories in the nineteenth century. On mining in the United States anthracite region see Roberts (1901, Chaps. II, V, VI, VIII) and also Roberts (1904). For miners, "although underground work was dangerous and extremely arduous, the miner enjoyed a relatively high standard of living [B. Lewis, 1971, p. 28]." On puddlers, see Courthéoux (1959).

[18] Males per 100 females by age.

[19] These samples are discussed in greater detail in Chapter III.

[20] This correlation was significantly different from zero at a .001 level of probability.

1861. Charles and Moshinsky commented for the early twentieth century in England and Wales: "In mining districts there are practically no avenues of employment opportunities for women, whereas in textile districts the bulk of the work is carried on by women [Charles and Moshinsky, 1938, p. 143]."

For the anthracite region of Pennsylvania, female labor-force participation was relatively low (5.1 and 15.2% of females aged 15 and over in 1880 and 1900, respectively). This compares with a national average for white females of all ages of 12.1% in 1890 and 20.0% in 1900 (Lebergott, 1964, Table A-11; Oppenheimer, 1970, p. 8). Labor-force participation for wives in the anthracite region was even lower—less than 1% in 1870, 1880, and 1900. The 1889–1890 Commissioner of Labor Survey reported only 1.8 and .5% of all families in mining in the United States and Europe, respectively, having income from wives. The corresponding figures for iron and steel were 1.3 and .5%, and for cottons and woolens 6.2 and 17.6%, respectively (U.S. Commissioner of Labor, 1890, 1891). It was stated that in the 1890s in the Maryland coal fields "women and girls attended almost exclusively to household duties and often kept a garden [Harvey, 1969, p. 29]." The censuses of occupation of England and Wales in 1851, Germany in 1882, and the United States in 1890 showed only a very small employment of women in mining and metallurgy. In *Germinal*, Emile Zola portrays a degree of female labor-force participation which was gradually eliminated by marriage and childbearing.

For England and Wales there was a strong positive relationship between the sex ratio (males per 100 females) for the ages 20–29 and the index of proportions married (I_m). The zero-order correlations for 1871 were .727 and .495 for the 63 mining and metallurgical districts and the 125 randomly selected registration districts, respectively. At the same time, there was a strong negative relationship between the sex ratio (at ages 20–29) and the proportion of females employed outside the home. For 1871, the zero-order correlations were −.702 and −.459 for the mining/metallurgical districts and the random sample. In both cases the results were much the same for the censuses of 1851 and 1861. For the Pennsylvania anthracite mining region between 1850 and 1900, sex ratios were uniformly above 100 (indicating a surplus of males) at all dates for the age groups 20–29 and 30–39, reflecting the impact of differential net in-migration.[21] For England and Wales, the sex

[21] Sex ratios (males per 100 females) were

Ages	1850	1860	1870	1880	1900
20–29	118	102	111	103	106
30–39	122	117	114	114	123

These were derived from published census data in 1850 and 1860 and from manuscript samples in 1870, 1880, and 1900. The high variability in these sex ratios from decade to decade is curious and may be attributable to surges in migration flows which led to temporarily large surpluses of young adult males.

ratio (at ages 20–29) averaged 107.2 for the mining sample in 1871 and only 94.0 in the random sample. The ratios for 1851 were 105.2 and 93.6 for the mining and random samples; the differences were significant at an .001 level. For Upper Silesia in 1871, sex ratios for all age groups above age 15 were considerably above 100 in the industrial region, but well below that for the surrounding agricultural areas (Haines, 1978, Table II-9). Finally, quite comparable findings were made by Wrigley (1961, Table 42) in contrasting the high sex ratios and high female proportions married in younger adult years in the mining and heavy-industrial regions with the lower sex ratios and lower proportions married in the agrarian regions, large cities, and textile areas.

Women not usually being employed in mining and heavy industry, would, in the absence of employment opportunities in other industries (textiles, for example), have been available for work on garden plots or small farms or in the domestic handicraft industry, common in many rural or semirural environments. Thus, the type of activity characteristic of the farm could often be continued while the husband worked in the mine or the smelter. Alternatively, boarders could be taken in, and the wife employed in this way. In census samples from the anthracite counties of Pennsylvania, a significant number of households did take in boarders; 19.3% in 1850, 17.3% in 1880, and 12.1% in 1900. In the Commissioner of Labor Survey, 25.9% of the mining households in the United States took in boarders and 25.2% of the households whose head was employed in iron and steel manufacture. Comparable figures for Europe were 14.1% for mining and 21.4% for iron and steel workers.[22]

A further issue is the earning capacity of the child. While in many cases, child labor underground in the mines was forbidden in the nineteenth century (in Great Britain in 1842 and in Germany in 1903), there was still opportunity for boys (and girls) to work on the surface. There was little prohibition of child labor until the very late nineteenth century in factories in most Western European countries and most states of the United States. For example, the Factory Act of 1833 in Britain dealt only with textiles and then only limited hours for children (Cole and Postgate, 1961, pp. 258–259). The Commissioner of Labor Survey indicated that 27.6% of all United States coal-mining families (and 42.3% in Europe) had income from children. Families in iron and steel had 14.0% with income from children in the

[22] For the Commissioner of Labor Survey, these results are based on the number of households reporting income from boarders. Interestingly, the results for the United States on the proportions of families taking in boarders are quite similar to those cited or found by Modell and Hareven in their investigation of boarding and lodging in late nineteenth-century America (Modell and Hareven, 1973, p. 468). For the United States, however, the textile families showed an even higher propensity to take in boarders (36.4%), possibly due to the greater opportunity to do so in more urban environments. For Europe, the proportion of families earning income from boarding was much smaller (16.7%) (U.S. Commissioner of Labor, 1890, 1891).

United States and 37.2% in Europe. Comparable percentages for cotton and woolen textiles were 44.1 and 44.9, respectively; and for glass manufacture, 17.5 and 30.0. These children were probably mostly older, but viewing these industrial wage-earning families in a life-cycle context shows a marked dependence on children's incomes further on in the life cycle (Haines, 1979). Table II-2 indicates for the states of the United States and the five European countries covered by the Commissioner of Labor Survey that, as of 1890, a number did have age limits in manufacturing and mining and also

TABLE II-2 Child Labor and Compulsory Schooling Laws. Twenty-four States of the U.S. and Five European Countries, 1889/1890

	Minimum age for employment[a]			Educational requirements	
State/country	Manufacturing	Mining	Age limit	Literacy required before employment	Minimum attendance during the year
Alabama	--	15	--	--	--
Georgia	--	--	--	--	--
Illinois	--	14	14	*	--
Indiana	12	12, 14	--	--	--
New York	14	--	14	*	*
Ohio	12	12	16	*	*
Pennsylvania	12, 12, 13	12, 12, 12, 14	16	--	*
Tennessee	--	--	--	--	--
Virginia	--	--	--	--	--
West Virginia	--	12	12	*	--
Connecticut	13	--	14	--	*
Maine	12	--	15	--	*
Maryland	--	--	--	--	--
Massachusetts	13	--	13	--	*
New Hampshire	10, 13	--	12	--	*
North Carolina	--	--	--	--	--
Rhode Island	10	--	15	--	*
New Jersey	10, 12, 14	12, 14	15	--	*
Delaware	--	--	--	--	--
Kentucky	--	--	--	--	--
Louisiana	12, 14	--	14	--	*
Mississippi	--	--	--	--	--
South Carolina	--	--	--	--	--
Missouri	--	12	14	*	--
Belgium	--	12, 21	12	--	*
France	--	13	13	--	*
Germany	13	13	12-16	*	*
Great Britain	10	12, 12	14	*	*
Switzerland	--	--	14	--	*

Source: William F. Ogburn, *Progress and Uniformity in Child Labor Legislation* (1912), pp. 71, 75, 132.

U.S. Office of Education, *Annual Report of the U.S. Commissioner of Education, 1886-1887* (1888), p. 1002.

U.S. Commissioner of Labor, *Coal Mine Labor in Europe*, Twelfth Annual Report of the Commissioner of Labor (1905), passim.

[a]Multiple age limits for manufacturing denote several laws in existence. Usually they denote differing age limits for boys and girls (girls alway having the higher limit). For mining, there are multiple age limits affecting employment above and below ground. Below ground employment always had a higher limit.

had some compulsory education laws. But many southern states in the United States had none, and even the laws in the North were slow in coming (Ogburn, 1912). Furthermore, the compulsory education laws were not usually too comprehensive. In England, education was not compulsory up to 1876, and even then only up to age 12 (Cipolla, 1969, pp. 67–70; Cole and Postgate, 1961, pp. 361–364). The continental industrial countries were somewhat more successful in achieving compulsory schooling laws by the mid-nineteenth century, especially Germany, but also France and Belgium (Cipolla, 1969, pp. 70–71; Levasseur, 1897).

Despite these child labor and compulsory education laws, children were still employed in considerable numbers in some areas and industries. The incidence of families in the Commissioner of Labor Survey with earnings from children has already been noted. In the Pennsylvania anthracite region, child labor was quite common, despite a compulsory schooling law dating from 1849. The law only required three consecutive months of school attendance up to age 16, however, and thus children were free to work up to 9 months of the year. In addition, night schools were provided to allow boys to work and attend school simultaneously (Ogburn, 1912, p. 132; Roberts, 1904, pp. 166, 175). Children below age 13 had been forbidden to work in factories in Pennsylvania since 1849, but it was not until 1879 that regulation of employment in mines was specifically legislated.[23] At that time, boys below age 12 were forbidden from working in mines and girls were excluded altogether. Even in 1900, however, Roberts noted the large number of boys, many under 12, who worked in the breakers of the anthracite mines as slatepickers (Roberts, 1901, p. 100; 1904, pp. 174–177). As of 1889, a substantial portion of all underground workers in the anthracite fields were under age 16 (U.S. Bureau of the Census, 1892, p. 402). In the Maryland coalfields, child labor was unregulated until 1902 and existed throughout the nineteenth and early twentieth centuries, although it seems to have gradually disappeared (Harvey, 1969, pp. 48–57). A major feature of coal-mining populations in the north of France was, according to Ariès, the early age at which children were sent to work, usually on the surface, but sometimes underground as well (Ariès, 1948, pp. 235–236). On the other hand, the German census of occupations in 1882 indicated that employment of children in mining and heavy industry was not widespread. In Upper Silesia, only .5% of workers in mining and metallurgy were under age 15. For the Ruhr area, the incidence of child labor in the mines and metal works was only 1.5% of the total work force (Prussia, 1885, pp. 152–155, 192–195, 200–203, 216–219). In Germany, apparently, relatively strictly enforced compulsory education laws kept children aged 6–14 in school a good part of each day and each year, and thus functioned as an efficient child labor

[23] The references are Pennsylvania Code 21 April 1849, P.L. 62 and 11 June 1879, P.L. 142. See also Roberts (1904, p. 175) and Ogburn (1912, Chap. III).

law.[24] In sum, however, child labor remained important in many mining and heavy-industrial areas in the nineteenth century, thus lowering the "cost" of a child and acting as a possible inducement to higher fertility. In addition, children often remained in families longer in urban and industrial environments, thus further enhancing the value of a child to the family. This has been found for such diverse places as Preston (England), Hamilton (Ontario), and Buffalo (New York) (Anderson, 1971, pp. 53–54; 1972, p. 234; Glasco, p. 149, cited in Katz, 1975, p. 260; Katz, 1975, pp. 259–260).

Tastes are another factor governing fertility and nuptiality behavior. Where there was substantial net in-migration to coal fields or new industrial areas, there may still have been little change in cultural environment, reducing the pressure to change tastes. Thus, for example, where the bulk of the migrants came a short distance, as in Upper Silesia, the Ruhr, northern France, and parts of England in the nineteenth century, migrants would have experienced little change in cultural milieu.[25] Even where long-distance migration was important, as later in the Ruhr, other areas of France, and the United States, migrants often tended to remain together in enclaves, which effectively reduced environmental influences on tastes.[26] Those younger people born in the mining or industrial districts (and this became the dominant element over time) acquired tastes and attitudes from their parents that were closer to those in the original environment than in the new one. This included attitudes toward marriage and the desired mix of goods and children. The net effect was to maintain rural attitudes favoring high fertility. At the same time, the socioeconomic structure of mining and heavy-industrial regions afforded the income-earning potential common to industrial wage employment and, to a diminishing degree, perpetuated rural child costs. The isolation of many mining and industrial communities also insulated the population from slow changes in societal norms.[27]

Finally, there is the argument that a higher incidence of morbidity (ill-

[24] As a result, by 1871 Prussia was able to achieve some reasonably high literacy rates, especially in the western areas and German-speaking areas generally (Cipolla, 1969, Table 10). The education laws were not without loopholes, however. If a local school official deemed the level of education of a child to be adequate by age 12, the child could be released from school.

[25] For Upper Silesia, see Schofer (1975, pp. 34–38). For the Ruhr, see Brepohl (1948, 1957); Koellman (1958). For France, see Ariès (1948, Fig. 15). In the case of England and Wales, much of the migration to the industrial areas of the midlands and the north was short distance. For example, see Anderson (1971, pp. 34–41); Redford (1964).

[26] For the Ruhr, see Koellman (1965, pp. 600–601). For the anthracite mining region see Roberts (1904, pp. 48–56). For work on residential concentration of ethnic groups in Philadelphia, see Burstein (1975) and Greenberg (1977).

[27] Some sense of the isolation of mining communities may be found in literary accounts, such as Emile Zola's *Germinal* (1885), Benjamin Disraeli's *Sybil* (1845), Richard Llewellyn's *How Green Was My Valley* (1940), George Orwell's *The Road to Wigan Pier* (1937). A sociological study for British mining communities (Dennis, Henriques, and Slaughter, 1956) reflects this notion strongly.

ness), debility, and mortality in mining and industrial areas or populations led to higher fertility and earlier marriage. Higher infant and child mortality would increase birth rates if, as might be supposed, parents seek to replace lost children. Or there might be a biological mechanism operating through shortened lactation and therefore shorter postpartum sterility (see Taylor, Newman, and Kelly, 1976). Higher adult mortality, particularly among males, would tend to promote earlier marriage and closer spacing of births if parents have some family-size goal in mind and anticipate a higher probability of a truncated life course. If debility is also high, numerous children might be desirable as a form of social insurance against loss of income and retirement. Although it is difficult to demonstrate differential morbidity and debility, mining and heavy-industrial regions and populations did have somewhat higher infant, child, and adult mortality, as was shown in Chapter I. (See also Friedlander, 1973, p. 41.)

The argument based upon a socioeconomic explanation of higher fertility among miners and certain industrial workers (like those in iron and steel) would run as follows. The conditions of work and the relative geographic and social isolation of mining and some industrial populations acted to preserve relatively high fertility norms characteristic of the semirural environment itself or at least to retard changes in tastes resulting from generalized "modernization" of attitudes toward reproduction. Given tastes and norms as relatively constant or changing more slowly than for the overall population, early income potential, relatively high wages, restricted female employment outside the home, possible secondary employment in agriculture or handicrafts, possible child labor, and higher mortality and debility would all have favored higher fertility and, in part, earlier marriage. Those factors would then have been combined with the peculiar circumstances of each individual situation, such as ethnic, racial, or religious composition, degree of urbanization, and level of education or literacy, to produce the final pattern.

Peak income earning potential did indeed arrive at an earlier age for most members of the industrial labor force (see Table II-1). This was in contrast to agriculture, and was especially true when agriculture was established (as in most of England and Wales, Germany, France, Belgium, and the eastern United States in the later nineteenth century) and farm sites (i.e., potential income opportunities) became available only through inheritance or division of holdings.[28] In industrial employment, and especially in coal mining, a young man was at his peak capacity to work in his late teens and early 20s. In coal mining and iron and steel work, the acquisition of some skills was a

[28] For the influence of economic opportunity in agriculture on fertility in the United States, see Forster and Tucker (1972), where it is argued that frontier areas in the antebellum United States had higher fertility rates in large part because more farm sites (i.e., more economic opportunities) were available. See also Easterlin (1971, 1976, 1977) and Leet (1976).

consideration for men working the coal face (hewers), or iron puddlers and rollers, but brute physical strength was still crucial. The net result should have been, and indeed seems to have been, a lower age at marriage and thus a higher proportion married among young males in mining and metallurgy relative to other occupational groups. Census and vital data from Germany, Britain, and the United States presented in Chapter I all pointed to such a phenomenon. (See pages 23–27 and Tables I-8 to I-12.)

By examining the proportions ever married by age group for various administrative districts in France and Germany, Wrigley (1961, Chap. 7) concluded that the higher fertility of the coal-mining and heavy-industrial districts may be partly attributed to earlier *female* age at marriage than in other industrial areas, agricultural regions, and major cities. By assuming distribution of births by age of mother (since age-specific birth data were not available in published form for these areas in this period), and using life tables he had constructed, he further computed net reproduction rates and accounted for the remainder of the fertility differential by actual age-specific reproduction adjusted for mortality. His conclusion was that it "seems doubtful whether there is any connection [for males] between reaching maximum earning power at an early age and early marriage [Wrigley, 1961, p. 170]." These conclusions were based on an apparent "stickiness" over time of proportions of males ever married by age group despite the fact that the economy was rapidly changing and also on the fact that the proportions by age of ever-married males seemed roughly similar for agricultural and nonagricultural areas.

This conclusion may, however, be disputed. Tables I-10 through I-12 indicate that, when labor force is classified by age, sex, and marital status, then coal miners and metallurgical workers did indeed marry earlier than many other occupations. Wrigley used rather large administrative units (the *Regierungsbezirk* in Germany, the department in France, and the province in Belgium) which included many occupational groups, especially agricultural and industrial populations. Thus cross-sectional differentials may be totally obscured, and, if there were trends over time to older marriage among industrial populations as they constituted a growing proportion of the overall population, the proportions ever married may appear "sticky." Finally, it does appear that proportions of females married by age were affected by the economic nature of the area, being highest at the youngest ages (late teens and early 20s) in mining and metallurgical areas and relatively low in agricultural and textile areas (Wrigley, 1961, pp. 142–145). This was, in turn, partly a reflection of the high sex ratio (males per 100 females) in mining areas, which showed a large surplus of males over females in the young adult years, due to sex selectivity of migration. This would have increased marriage probabilities for young adult females, even with all other things constant (like economic opportunity), which they obviously were not. The low sex ratio in agricultural areas was the obverse of the coin, resulting from net out-migration selective of males. Textile areas (like R. B. Aachen in Germany) showed low sex ratios for young adults because of the selective net in-migration of young females seeking employment in the textile industry.[29] The point is that these sex ratios, and hence the proportions of young married females which they engendered, were themselves reflections of economic opportunity, operating through sex selectivity of migration. Thus economic opportunity operated simultaneously to encourage earlier marriage for miners and earlier and more complete marriage for women in mining areas. It also seems to have encouraged higher intramarital fertility (especially since family size decisions are probably a life cycle phenomenon).

The assumption here is that age at marriage is an important determinant of fertility, that factors affecting "exposure to intercourse" are more important than factors affecting "exposure to conception," to use the terminology of Davis and Blake (1956). This is not unreasonable in the nineteenth century, although there is considerable reason to believe that fertility control within marriage—abortion, if not also contraception—was known and used at this time in Europe and America (Himes, 1936, Part 5). Van de Walle points out that "the existence of restrictions to early and general marriage and the use of contraception are essentially different in intent; one is no substitute for the other. . . . Late marriage would in many respects be a method of avoiding or postponing a first birth only [van de Walle, 1968, p. 498]." Some simulation studies by Crafts and Ireland (1976) have indicated for England for the period 1750 and 1850 that changes in age of marriage likely had little impact on movements in overall fertility. Here, however, all other things being roughly constant, earlier marriage may reflect simultaneously superior economic opportunity earlier in the life cycle *and*, because of this, a desire for more children because more can be afforded. Thus early marriage may be a means, at the margin, to alter desired family size. Early marriage of the wife, not the husband, is really the critical variable, though it is generally assumed that an earlier age of marriage for males implies an earlier age at marriage for females. It has been shown that wives of men in mining and metal manufacture had the highest proportion married under age 25 and that wives of skilled and semiskilled workers (the bulk of the miners) also showed a high proportion married among the various socioeconomic groups. (See Table I-9, page 24.) Thus age at marriage, if not the real cause, was a revealing symptom of the higher fertility among miners.

[29] See Wrigley (1961, pp. 146–147). Both *Regierungsbezirke* Aachen and Düsseldorf had large textile industries and showed lower sex ratios for females aged 20–24 than in *Regierungsbezirk* Arnsberg, which was more concentrated in mining and metallurgy. Arnsberg showed higher proportions of females below age 24 ever married, but this was complicated by the fact that married couples in Arnsberg were predominantly Protestant and thus presumably more prone to exercise intramarital fertility restraint than couples in predominantly Roman Catholic Düsseldorf and Aachen.

Another expectation of this hypothesized relationship between occupation and fertility is that mining and metallurgy were frequently located where there were few female employment opportunities outside the home. Following the reasoning of Mincer (1963), it is argued that the contribution of a wife's income to family income has both a price effect and an income effect. A wife's decision to enter the labor force outside the home should have both a positive effect on fertility (i.e., the income effect of greater family income) and a negative effect (i.e., the price effect caused by the fact that bearing children has an opportunity cost represented by the wife's working time foregone and that there is a tradeoff between work and childbearing). According to Mincer, where most work for women is outside the home (as in the population he studied for the United States in the 1950s), the negative price effect should dominate. That is, a higher female labor-force participation outside the home should lead to lower fertility. Where, however, there is considerable employment opportunity in agriculture or in domestic handicraft industry, the income effect should dominate because the wife can stay home and both work and rear her children. (In this case, the opportunity cost of the wife's time in employment outside the home, and hence the "cost" of a child, should be lower.) That female labor-force participation outside the home has a negative effect on fertility has been emphasized by a number of authors[30] and has been the subject of a large number of studies for both developed and less developed countries.[31] For nineteenth-century England, it has been stated by Hewitt that "[T]he diminution of fertility was common to all married women occupied away from the home. . . . [T]he lower fertility of the mother employed away from home was, in part at least, the almost inevitable result of the conflict between motherhood and the claims of her job [Hewitt, 1958, p. 93]." Work by Tilly and others on fertility and female labor-force participation in France and elsewhere in Europe has also stressed the importance of female employment outside the home in reducing fertility (Tilly, 1977; Tilly, Scott, and Cohen, 1976). Jaffe and Azumi (1960, pp. 52–63) found that a woman's participation in the domestic handicraft industry was quite compatible with childrearing and thus favorable to higher fertility. There has been greater emphasis more recently in specifying the relationship between women's

[30] A number of the policy implications are considered or elaborated in Davis (1967, p. 738); Preston (1972); Blake (1965, p. 62).

[31] See, for example, for developed countries, Cain (1966); Cain and Weininger (1973); Sweet (1970, 1973); Oppenheimer (1973); Mincer (1962, 1963); Mott (1972); Ware (1976). This literature has become closely associated with the economic work on the value of time (Becker, 1965). In this vein, see Michael (1973); Gronau (1973, 1976); Ben-Porath (1973); Heckman (1974); Nerlove (1974); Mincer and Polachek (1974); Turchi (1975). Results are not uniformly favorable, however, to the work–fertility tradeoff, once a number of other variables have been controlled. See Terry (1975) and Ware (1976). For less developed countries, see Stycos and Weller (1967); Rosenzweig (1976); McCabe and Rosenzweig (1976); Dixon (1976); Goldstein (1972); Kasarda (1971).

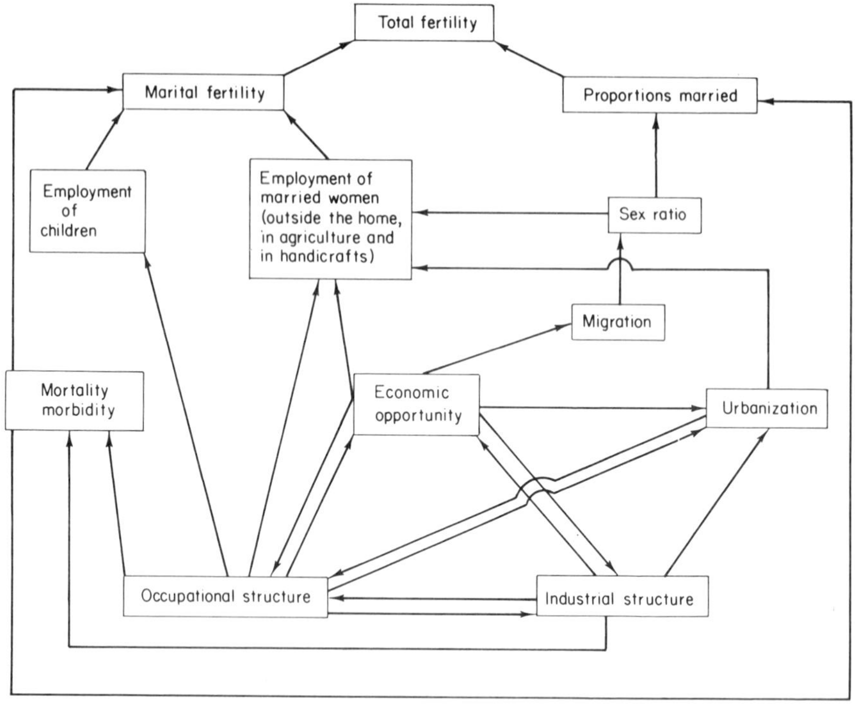

FIGURE II-1 An economic–demographic model of mining and industrial populations. (Economic opportunity includes wages, income, and wealth.)

work and fertility in a simultaneous equations framework (Cain and Dooley, 1976; Gregory, Campbell, and Cheng, 1972; Schultz, 1976), which is an issue which will be dealt with in greater detail later.

These remarks should be qualified by the fact that higher fertility among wives of miners and metallurgical workers may have resulted from *both* the husband's participation in mining or heavy industry and the relative lack of available employment outside the home characteristic of mining and some industrial areas. In this case, there was both an income effect (i.e., a tradeoff between potential family income and number of children, holding tastes and relative prices constant) and a price effect (i.e., the opportunity cost of the wife's time). The latter effect really lowered the "cost" (or relative price) of a child through a lower opportunity cost of the wife's time.[32] Higher husband's income increased the means to have more children. In industries

[32] This discussion of the "cost" of children is rather brief. For a more detailed treatment, see Espenshade (1972); Lindert (1973); Repetto (1976); Mueller (1976). An interesting simulation of life-cycle effects of the alternative cost of children for the agricultural versus the nonagricultural sectors with different fertility and mortality levels is provided by Lorimer (1967).

like mining and metallurgy with relatively high male earnings, this may have more than compensated for the loss of the wife's income.

In sum, then, it is hypothesized that coal mining and some similar occupations in heavy industry (like iron puddling) involved a particular combination of early peaking income–earnings profiles over the life cycle, low levels of female labor-force participation outside the home, and lower child costs that favored higher fertility and earlier and more extensive marriage. In addition, the migration patterns and less urban characteristics of mining and metallurgical communities led to costs, tastes, sex ratios, and marriage patterns conducive to larger families. Finally, higher mortality, morbidity, and debility among miners and industrial workers and higher mortality among their children *may* also have favored earlier marriage and more births both to ensure target family size and to help provide for old age and infirmity among the parents. A diagrammatic representation of the interrelations of the elements of the model is presented in Figure II-1. These features of mining and industrial populations, as they interacted with other, more particular, socioeconomic dimensions and as they changed over time, will be examined in the following chapters.

III

Evidence from Aggregate Data: England and Wales, Prussia

One approach to testing some of the hypotheses suggested by the discussion in Chapter II is to analyze small geographic areas with high concentrations of population associated with coal mining and ferrous metallurgy. A series of cross-sectional studies of these small areal units is undertaken in order to test whether, among other things, the proportion of the male labor force in mining and metallurgy made any difference in fertility levels. This was done for England and Wales in 1851, 1861, and 1871 and for Prussia in 1882, 1895, and 1907.

The regions in England and Wales and in Prussia were based on the smallest administrative units for which both vital statistics and adequate labor-force data could be obtained. This turned out to be the registration district in England and Wales and the *Kreis* in Prussia. The districts and *Kreise* were then selected by the proportion of male population in coal mining and ferrous metallurgy. In the case of England and Wales, districts were selected which had more than 10% of the male population aged 20 and over in coal mining and iron smelting. In addition, for comparative purposes, a random sample of 125 districts was taken at all dates studied. In the case of Prussia, *Kreise* with more than 10% of the male labor force in mining and metallurgy were chosen. For Prussia the analysis was confined to the major industrial areas of the Ruhr, Saar, and Upper Silesia, so that a few *Kreise* were excluded.[1] Whenever subdivisions of registration districts or

[1] These were relatively small, isolated coal-mining *Kreise*, such as Waldenberg and Neurode in Lower Silesia.

Kreise were made, these were taken as separate units of observation. The results were based on the most recent occupational census prior to 1914 which contained sufficient detail for small administrative units. These were the census of 1861 for England and Wales and the *Berufszählung* (occupational census) of 1907 for Germany. The reason for taking separate samples for mining and metallurgical districts is that areas with a significant proportion of the population in these industries constitute a rare or special occurrence. It is thus appropriate to sample completely these special districts in order to make comparisons with national averages (or in the case of England and Wales, a national sample of districts). Ten or more percent of males in mining and metallurgy certainly does not constitute an economically homogeneous population, but it does indicate a labor market strongly influenced or even dominated by the type of structure created by heavy industry. More importantly, it allows a sample which can demonstrate differences in conditions and behavior *within* mining areas. It must be remembered, however, that a test of the hypotheses advanced above can only imperfectly be studied using data for small, albeit more homogeneous, geographical areas.

ENGLAND AND WALES, 1851, 1861, AND 1871

The period chosen for this series of cross-sectional studies was dictated by the availability of sufficiently detailed published statistics to allow an adequate treatment at the registration district level. The censuses of 1851, 1861, and 1871 were the only ones for which sufficient detail was available on occupational structure. The census of 1841 lacked occupational data and sufficient accompanying vital statistics. The censuses of 1881 and later years lacked occupational data for registration districts. The sample, thus restricted to the period 1851–1871, unfortunately precedes the decline in period fertility, although cohort fertility was probably already declining (Habakkuk, 1972, pp. 54–55).

Table III-1 provides information on the variables used. The principal sources were, as indicated, the censuses of 1841 through 1871 and the *Annual Reports of the Registrar General* from 1841 through 1872. Most of the data were accepted without correction except, notably, birth statistics. Following the work of Glass (1951) and Teitelbaum (1974), births were adjusted for each district on the basis of the correction factor for its county. The exception was births used in computing infant mortality rates, since infant deaths were probably underreported as well as births. Although several adjustments were tried to correct for underreporting of infant

TABLE III-1 Regression Variables for Selected Districts in England and Wales: 1851, 1861, 1871[a]

Variable	Definition
I_f	Index of overall fertility[b] (1851, 1861, 1871)
I_g	Index of marital fertility[b] (1861, 1871)
I_m	Index of proportions married[b] (1861, 1871)
I_h	Index of illegitimate fertility (1861, 1871)
MFR	General marital fertility ratio (legitimate births per 1000 married women 15-49) (1851).
MM	a. Percentage of males 20+ in mining and metallurgy (1851, 1861) b. Percentage of males 20+ in minerals employment (1871)
FOH	Percentage of females 20+ employed outside the home[c] (1851, 1861, 1871)
PE	Percentage of males 20+ in primary employment (farming and animal husbandry) (1851, 1861, 1871)
IMR	Infant mortality rate (infant deaths per 1000 live births per annum) (1848/1850, 1858/1860, 1868/1870).
URM	Percentage of population in principal towns (1951, 1861, 1871)
RNM	Rate of residual net migration in the previous decade (per 1000 per annum) (1841/1850, 1851/1860, 1861/1870)
SXR	Sex ratio, ages 20-29 (males 20-29 per 100 females 20-29) (1851, 1861, 1871)

Source: Registrar General, *Census of 1841, 1851, 1861, and 1871: England and Wales,* passim. Registrar General, *Annual Reports of the Registrar General, 1841 through 1872,* passim. Births were adjusted by county level adjustment figures furnished by Michael Teitelbaum. See Michael Teitelbaum, "Birth Under-Registration in the Constituent counties of England and Wales: 1841-1910," *Population Studies,* Vol. 28, No. 2 (July, 1974), pp. 329-343.

[a]For the rates I_f, I_g, I_h, and MFR, births are taken as three year averages around the central date. For IMR, births and infant deaths are lagged 2 years.

[b]For definitions of I_f, I_g, and I_m see Ansley J. Coale, "Factors Associated With the Development of Low Fertility: An Historic Summary," United Nations, *World Population Conference: 1965,* Vol. II (New York: 1967), pp. 205-209.

[c]Females employed outside the home for 1851 and 1861 was arrived at by taking the total female population aged 20 and over and subtracting women classified as keeping house, pensioners, agricultural workers, and certain selected occupations (for 1851 and 1861 only) which could be identified as in the home (such as keeping a store or tavern in the home, or a washerwoman), or for which a woman was identified as the wife of an occupied male (e.g., a butcher's wife or an innkeeper's wife). There was little basis for discriminating domestic handicraft industry. For 1871, females employed outside the home is total female population 20+ less pensioners, women classed as keeping house, and women in agricultural employment.

deaths,[2] it was felt safest simply to divide uncorrected infant deaths by uncorrected live-births to obtain the infant mortality rate.

The dependent variables used were Coale's indices of overall fertility (I_f), marital fertility (I_g), and proportions married (I_m). These indices are really a form of indirect standardization of birth rates using the highest observed fertility schedule, that of married Hutterite women in the United States in the 1920s, as the standard schedule. In addition, the index of illegitimate fertility (I_h) was also calculated (Coale, 1967; for definitions see Appendix Table III-1). For the computation of I_g, I_m, and I_h, population by age, sex, and marital status is required. This was not available in 1851 and so the General Marital Fertility Ratio (MFR) was computed as a substitute for I_g.

Among the independent variables, it should be noted that the average infant mortality rate was lagged 3 years to account for the fact that fertility is expected to adjust to infant mortality with a lag of 2 to 4 years (T. P. Schultz, 1969, pp. 160–161.) Some labor-force structure variables (percentage of adult males in mining and metallurgy, percentage of adult males in primary employment, and percentage of adult females employed outside the home) are included, as well as some additional demographic variables (percentage of population in principal towns, rate of net migration in the previous decade, and the sex ratio for ages 20–29).

Means of the variables from Table III-1 for the two samples for the three dates are given in Table III-2. In addition, tests of the statistical significance of the differences of the means of each variable between the samples were made.[3] This table confirms a number of notions about mining areas[4] relative to the national sample of districts. First, the mining areas had, at all three dates, significantly higher overall fertility, marital fertility, proportions married, and even illegitimate fertility. Second, the mining areas, while less agricultural than the national sample, still had a substantial proportion of the male labor force in agriculture (PE). Third, extrahousehold female labor-force participation (FOH) was significantly lower at all three dates in the mining areas. Fourth, the degree of urbanization (URB) was initially lower than that in the national sample (1851) but moved to being more urban by 1871. Fifth, the mining areas consistently showed much lower net

[2] Several assumptions about the share of unreported births which were also unreported infant deaths were considered, ranging from 0 to 75%. All were arbitrary and some led to strange results. Some regressions between child and infant mortality were attempted in an effort to try to use the better reported child deaths to estimate infant deaths. The results were also not encouraging and so were discarded.

[3] This test is strictly a test of the differences of means from two independently distributed populations. The assumption of independence is not completely held since several districts appear in both samples. It is only a modest number (14 in 1851 and 1861 and 9 in 1871) and their removal from the random sample actually *increases* the differences and reduces the variances, thus making the differences even more significant.

[4] Henceforth, for convenience, the sample of mining and metallurgical counties will be called the mining sample.

TABLE III-2 Mean Values of Regression Variables: Registration Districts, England and Wales, 1851, 1861, 1871

	1851			1861			1871		
Variable[a]	Mining sample	Random sample	Significance of difference[b]	Mining sample	Random sample	Significance of difference[b]	Mining sample	Random sample	Significance of difference[b]
I_f	.422	.364	***	.433	.369	***	.452	.378	***
I_g	NA[d]	NA		.716	.683	***	.738	.698	***
MFR (per 1000)	260.8	245.6	***	NC[e]	NC		NC	NC	
I_m	NA	NA		.563	.502	***	.576	.507	***
I_h	NA	NA		.069	.054	***	.066	.050	***
MM (%)	20.7	2.2	***	24.5	3.1	***	39.9	12.5	***
PE (%)	21.1	41.2	***	18.6	39.3	***	13.4	32.6	***
FOH (%)	21.7	26.5	***	22.3	26.3	***	24.5	30.1	***
IMR (per 1000 live births)	150.6	137.3	***	149.7	137.5	***	154.3	135.6	***
URB (%)	22.4	28.6	*	27.3	27.0	n.s.[c]	40.0	31.0	**
RNM (per 1000 population)	-.28	18.7	***	1.17	5.92	***	.79	5.68	***
SXR (per 100)	105.2	93.6	***	101.4	92.3	***	107.2	94.0	***

[a]For definitions of variables and sources, see Table III-1.

[b]Based on a test of significance of the difference of two means drawn from independently distributed populations.

[c]n.s. = Not significant at a 10% level.

[d]NA = Not available.

[e]NC = Not calculated.

*$p < .1$.

**$p < .05$.

***$p < .01$.

out-migration than the national sample, pointing to greater economic opportunity.[5] Finally, the sex ratio, as expected, was much higher in the mining areas, reflecting differential in-migration of males. Thus mining areas could be characterized as having higher marital fertility, higher levels of nuptiality, higher infant mortality, higher sex ratios, more in-migration and lower levels of extrahousehold female employment relative to the national sample. In addition, there was much more homogeneity among the mining areas with respect to their fertility and nuptiality. The coefficients of variability[6] were consistently smaller for the mining sample, indicating lesser dispersion around the higher means. This may be seen in Table III-3.

Since the period considered here was immediately prior to the decline in period fertility rates in Britain (dating from the mid-1870s), it is of interest to note differences in the fertility measures over time. It is surprising that, despite corrections for underregistration, I_f was rising for both the mining and the random samples from 1851 to 1861 and from 1861 to 1871. In only one case, however, was this increase significant (in the mining sample for 1861–1871). Marital fertility (I_g), on the other hand, showed significant increases in both samples for 1861–1871. Proportions married (I_m) increased slightly over the decade 1861–1871, and concurrently, illegitimate fertility declined. The changes were, with one weak exception, however, insignificant. It does not seem unusual that increased incidence of marriage should be accompanied by declining illegitimate fertility, but that the decline in period fertility rates was immediately preceded by declines in age of marriage and increasing proportions married is notable.[7] It also appears that cohort fertility was already declining when marriage incidence was increasing (Habakkuk, 1972, pp. 54–55).

The expected relationships of the independent variables to the dependent variables were as follows:

1. Percentage of males in mining and metallurgy (MM)—expected to be positively related to I_f, I_m, and GFR and possibly positively related to I_g and MFR.
2. Percentage of males in agricultural employment (PE)—expected to be positively related to I_f, I_m, I_g, and GFR, and MFR on the grounds that agriculture is more compatible with larger families because of the economic role of families and the higher value of children.
3. Percentage of females in employment outside the home—expected to be negatively related to I_f, I_g, I_m, GFR, and MFR.

[5] Positive RNM indicates net out-migration.

[6] Sample standard deviation divided by the mean.

[7] I_m is really a standardized measure of proportions married but indirectly takes marriage age into account. Falling mean age at marriage was observed directly in the 1850s and 1860s, times of economic prosperity. It subsequently began to rise in the less prosperous times after the 1870s (see Habakkuk, 1972, pp. 54–56).

TABLE III-3 Means, Standard Deviation, Coefficients of Variability, and Significance Tests of Differences of Means: Measures of Fertility and Nuptuality: Coal Mining Registration Districts and a Random Sample of 125 Registration Districts: England and Wales, 1851, 1861, 1871

	I_f		I_g		I_m		I_h		GFR		MFR	
	Coal mining	Random sample	Coal mining	Random sample	Coal mining	Random sample	Coal mining	Random sample	Coal mining	Random sample	Coal mining	Random sample
A. *1851*												
M	.42203	.36370	--	--	--	--	--	--	161.69	138.60	260.76	245.58
Sample *SD*	.04552	.05090	--	--	--	--	--	--	18.717	19.446	20.150	26.841
Z-statistic[a]	(7.89)***		--		--		--		(7.80)***		(4.34)***	
Coefficient of variability[b]	.108	.140	--	--	--	--	--	--	.116	.140	.077	.109
B. *1861*												
M	.43310	.36933	.71569	.68270	.56308	.50198	.06908	.05373	--	--	--	--
Sample *SD*	.05009	.05245	.04344	.05236	.05596	.05748	.02502	.01963	--	--	--	--
Z-statistic	(8.03)***		(4.98)***		(6.93)***		(4.10)***		--		--	
Coefficient of variability	.116	.142	.061	.077	.099	.114	.362	.365	--	--	--	--
C. *1871*												
M	.45254	.37787	.73790	.69778	.57559	.50682	.06622	.05010	--	--	--	--
Sample *SD*	.04923	.05359	.03655	.04478	.05793	.06712	.01935	.01960	--	--	--	--
Z-statistic	(9.90)***		(5.24)***		(7.28)***		(5.18)***		--		--	
Coefficient of variability	.109	.142	.050	.064	.101	.132	.292	.391	--	--	--	--
D. *1851/1861*												
Z-statistic[c]	(-1.27)	(-0.86)	--		--		--		--		--	
E. *1861-1871*												
Z-statistic[c]	(-2.18)**	(-1.274)	(-2.80)***	(-2.16)**	(-1.22)	(-.62)	(-.71)	(1.32)*	--		--	

[a]This statistic is the test of significance of the difference of two means drawn from independently distributed populations. In this case it tests whether the coal mining sample mean is significantly different from the random sample mean.

[b]Coefficient of variability = $\frac{\text{Sample Standard Deviation}}{\text{Mean}}$

[c]This statistic is the test of the differences in means between 1851 and 1861 and between 1861 and 1871 within the coal mining sample and within the random sample.

*$p < .1$.

**$p < .05$.

***$p < .01$.

4. Infant mortality rate (IMR)—expected to be positively related to I_f, I_g, GFR, and MFR on the assumption that it is surviving children and not births that parents desire. Also a biological mechanism may shorten birth intervals with greater infant mortality through interruption of lactation. A lag of 3 years is built in, as previously mentioned. For example, infant mortality for 1848–1850 is related to fertility for 1850–1852 (T. P. Schultz, 1969, pp. 160–161, 1976b; Taylor, Newman, & Kelly, 1976).

5. Percentage of population in principal towns (URB)—expected to be negatively related to fertility and nuptiality, assuming that urban areas are associated with higher child costs and perhaps more modern "attitudes." There is some doubt on this point, however, since for urbanized heavy-industrial areas in the nineteenth-century continental Europe, higher fertility was found relative to surrounding agrarian areas (Wrigley, 1961, Chap. 7).

6. Rate of net migration in the previous decade (RNM)—expected to be positively related to I_f, I_g, I_m, GFR, and MFR (when a positive value of RNM indicates net in-migration) on the grounds that migration flows reflect differential economic opportunity.

7. Sex ratio: males 20–29 per 100 females 20–29 (SXR)—a higher age-specific sex ratio should encourage more complete marriage (and hence be positively related to I_m) and thus favor higher overall fertility (I_f and GFR). The effect on marital fertility (I_g and MFR) should be small but perhaps positive if a higher sex ratio reflects greater opportunities and incomes for males relative to females and there is some measure of fertility control within marriage.

It should be noted that the available data do not permit testing of all the hypothetical relations involved with occupational fertility differentials. This is especially true for child costs and benefits and also for relative income-earnings profiles. It is hoped, however, that the inclusion of the variables MM and PE should take account of some of these factors, though not testing for their specific effects.

Ordinary least squares (OLS) regressions were applied to both the mining sample and the random sample at all three dates. The various fertility and nuptiality variables were, in turn, taken as independent variables. Initially a simple linear equation was used, and two alternative specifications were tried, one excluding and one including the sex ratio.[8]

The results for the mining sample are presented in Table III-4 and for random sample in Table III-5. The coefficients in parentheses are those not significant at least at a 10% level. Also presented are the adjusted R-squared

[8] The reason for this decision was the high degree of correlation between the sex ratio (SXR) and the percentage of females employed outside the home (FOH), which tended to increase the standard errors of both coefficients and reduce significance levels for FOH. It was desirable to see how FOH performed in the absence of SXR.

TABLE III-4 OLS Regression Equations: Coal Mining Districts: England and Wales, 1851, 1861, 1871. Overall Fertility, Marital Fertility and Nuptiality[a]

Dependent variables	Independent variables									
	Constant	MM	PE	FOH	IMR	URB	RNM	SXR	R^2_{adj}	*F*-ratio
A. *1851*										
1. I_f	.4617	(.0002)[b]	-.0019	-.0009	(.0002)	-.0002	(-.0006)	NI[c]	.328	5.887
2. I_f	.3133	(-.0005)	-.0023	(-.0001)	(-.0000)	-.0004	(.0005)	.0017	.413	7.026
3. MFR	234.7	(-.2356)	-1.0424	(-.1919)	-.1898	-.1968	-.4042	NI	.213	3.708
4. MFR	256.0	(-.5644)	-1.2317	(.1541)	-.2832	(-.1174)	(-.1024)	.8009	.304	4.750
B. *1861*										
5. I_f	.3834	.0016	-.0011	-.0009	.0004	-.0004	-.0009	NI	.547	13.074
6. I_f	.2209	.0009	-.0012	(.0001)	(.0003)	-.0004	(-.0006)	.0017	.601	13.917
7. I_g	.8044	.0009	(-.0007)	(-.0001)	-.0006	-.0004	(-.0005)	NI	.127	2.453
8. I_g	.7901	(.0008)	(-.0007)	(.0000)	-.0006	-.0004	(-.0004)	(.0002)	.111	(2.070)
9. I_m	.4499	.0014	-.0011	-.0015	.0010	-.0003	-.0008	NI	.578	14.715
10. I_m	.2439	(.0005)	-.0013	(-.0003)	.0008	-.0004	(-.0005)	.0022	.649	16.839
C. *1871*										
11. I_f	.2981	.0017	(-.0001)	-.0018	.0009	(-.0002)	(.0000)	NI	.699	24.995
12. I_f	.2105	.0014	(-.0000)	-.0013	.0009	(-.0001)	(-.0004)	.0008	.713	23.002
13. I_g	.6807	(.0006)	(-.0003)	(-.0001)	(.0003)	(-.0001)	(.0002)	NI	.041	(1.443)
14. I_g	.8028	.0010	(-.0004)	(-.0008)	(.0003)	(-.0002)	(-.0004)	-.0011	.092	(1.900)
15. I_m	.4761	.0013	(-.0008)	-.0026	.0008	(-.0002)	(-.0002)	NI	.621	17.961
16. I_m	.2407	(.0004)	(-.0007)	-.0013	.0009	(-.0000)	.0008	.0021	.716	23.333

[a] *N* = 125; for a definition of variables, see Table III-1.

[b] Figures in parentheses are coefficients not significant at least at the 10% level (using a one-tailed test).

[c] NI = not included.

TABLE III-5 OLS Regression Equations: Random Sample of 125 Registration Districts: England and Wales, 1851, 1861, 1871. Overall Fertility, Marital Fertility, and Nuptiality[a]

Dependent variables	Independent variables									
	Constant	MM	PE	FOH	IMR	URB	RNM	SXR	R^2_{adj}	*F*-ratio
A. *1851*										
1. I_f	.2742	.0030	.0006	(-.0004)[b]	.0005	-.0006	-.0009	NI[c]	.413	15.516
2. I_f	.1364	.0025	.0007	(.0002)	.0004	-.0003	-.0008	.0014	.504	18.972
3. MFR	241.3	.6962	(.0955)	(.0359)	(-.0419)	-.3003	-.6436	NI	.254	8.020
4. MFR	211.6	(.5825)	(.1001)	(.1655)	(-.0595)	-.2537	-.6254	.2968	.263	7.330
B. *1861*										
5. I_f	.2958	.0037	.0010	-.0009	.0004	-.0002	-.0005	NI	.451	18.007
6. I_f	.2272	.0033	.0006	(-.0004)	.0003	-.0002	(.0004)	.0008	.544	22.135
7. I_g	.6821	.0030	.0011	(-.0003)	-.0002	(-.0002)	(-.0005)	NI	.396	14.577
8. I_g	.6484	.0028	.0006	(-.0000)	-.0003	(-.0002)	(-.0001)	.0004	.415	13.562
9. I_m	.4289	.0025	.0003	-.0011	.0007	(-.0002)	(-.0004)	NI	.248	7.821
10. I_m	.3618	.0021	(-.0001)	-.0007	.0006	(-.0002)	(.0005)	.0008	.319	9.301
C. *1871*										
11. I_f	.3085	.0008	.0007	-.0018	.0007	(.0001)	(-.0006)	NI	.204	6.313
12. I_f	.1105	.0007	.0011	(-.0006)	.0007	(.0002)	(-.0002)	.0015	.348	10.461
13. I_g	.6510	.0018	.0014	(.0005)	-.0003	(.0003)	(-.0005)	NI	.197	6.065
14. I_g	.6160	.0018	.0015	(.0007)	-.0003	.0003	-.0004	(.0003)	.197	5.338
15. I_m	.4986	(-.0006)	(-.0007)	-.0031	.0010	(-.0001)	(-.0004)	NI	.250	7.871
16. I_m	.2524	(-.0009)	(.0002)	-.0015	.0011	(-.0001)	(.0000)	.0018	.392	12.398

[a] N = 125; for a definition of variables, see Table III-1.

[b] Figures in parentheses are coefficients not significant at least at the 10% level (using a one-tailed test).

[c] NI = not included.

values and F-ratios. The results confirm some prior expectations about the effects of the designated independent variables on fertility and nuptiality, at least for areas. The proportion of males in mining and metallurgy was, when significant, positively related to fertility and marriage. In other words, controlling for the effects of the other variables, the marginal effect of a larger proportion of miners in the population was to increase both marital fertility and proportions married in an area.[9] The effect was clearly stronger in the random sample (with 13 of 16 coefficients significant) than in the mining sample (with only 8 of 16 coefficients significant), indicating, relative to all areas of the country, that the higher fertility and earlier marriage of the mining and metallurgical districts stood in much greater contrast.

For the percentage of adult males in primary employment (PE), a contrasting result appears. For the mining sample, a higher proportion of persons in farming and animal husbandry led to lower fertility and later marriage whereas the reverse was true for the random sample. Clearly, the fertility of the agricultural population was high relative to the national average but lower relative to the average for districts with numerous miners and metal workers. The effect for the mining sample diminished over time, however, so that by 1871 all the coefficients for PE were insignificant.

It was earlier hypothesized that extrahousehold female employment (FOH) would result in lower fertility and marriage. Those coefficients in Tables III-4 and III-5 which were significant were indeed negative but a substantial proportion of all coefficients (in 19 out of 32 equations) were insignificant.[10] It is notable, however, that *both* marriage and marital fertility were usually negatively associated with this variable. Related to this is the closely negatively intercorrelated variable of the sex ratio (SXR) for young adults (aged 20–29). This variable was strongly positively associated with overall fertility, marital fertility, and marriage. Female employment and the sex ratio often reflect the simultaneous effect of the same thing, differential male employment opportunity, and so interact. In those equations in which both variables were present, the sex ratio generally performed much better than female employment, perhaps indicating a stronger association of fertility and marriage with sex imbalances among young adults than with actual employment of females. The mechanisms through which the sex ratio acted were both higher marital fertility and higher proportions married. The effect on marital fertility was, however, weaker—as indicated by the lower coefficients in the I_g equations which even become insignificant in 1871.

[9] A question may arise as to why the proportion of adult males employed in mining and metallurgy is included at all on the right-hand side of the regression equation. The answer is that it is of interest to see what effect varying *proportions* of miners and metal workers in the labor force have on fertility and marriage. It is also important to control for those varying proportions in the labor force when examining the effects of other social demographic, and economic variables.

[10] A nonlinear specification of the OLS equations resulted in much better performance of this variable, with 30 out of 36 coefficients significant, suggesting nonlinearity.

Of the other independent variables considered, the lagged infant mortality rate (IMR) was positively related to overall fertility and proportions married. The latter relationship is rather puzzling. It might have been the case that people married earlier in response to a higher recognized environmental risk of infant death, but it is more likely that a high level of infant mortality was caused by a low age of marriage. Since infant mortality is higher for young women relative to those in their mid-20s (United Nations, 1973, p. 127) and since a high I_m usually implies higher proportions married below age 25, there might be some basis for a positive relation between proportions married and infant mortality. The relationship of infant mortality to marital fertility was, when significant, negative—which is very puzzling, since this relation would be expected to have been most strongly positive. It would seem more logical that marital fertility would adjust, even in a regime of natural fertility, to high infant mortality. But such seemed not the case in mid-nineteenth century Britain.

The urbanization variable had the expected negative effect on overall and marital fertility in 1851 and 1861 and on marriage as well in 1871. The relationship appeared to weaken over time and even turned positive for marital fertility for the random sample in 1871. It is possible that newer norms, increased female labor-force participation, and rising child costs associated with urbanization early operated to depress fertility and marriage but that this altered over time. Perhaps, by 1871, a greater proportion of urban population in most districts reflected greater economic opportunity.

The rate of net migration (RNM) was mostly insignificant after 1851 with the significant coefficients showing mostly negative signs (i.e., the expected ones). A higher degree of out-migration would thus be associated with lower fertility and marriage because high net out-migration can be a proxy for poor economic opportunities which should tend to depress both fertility and marriage. It was, however, generally a weak variable.

Overall, the previously mentioned equations provide some support for several of the hypotheses advanced regarding factors specific to mining areas which might tend to promote fertility and marriage. A higher proportion of males in mining and metallurgy was associated with higher levels of fertility and marriage in an area. A higher sex ratio, more infant mortality, and a lower level of extrahousehold female employment were features characteristic of mining areas relative to the national average of districts and all tended to increase fertility and nuptiality. In addition, for 1851, the fact that mining districts were relatively less urban exercised a positive influence on marriage and fertility. By 1871, when the mining districts had become more urban, the effects of urbanization had become insignificant. These results are supported by the regressions run for the mining samples.

In general, the two sets of equations (from the mining and the random samples) were rather similar at the three dates in terms of the direction and often the significance of the coefficients. The levels of the coefficients were usually different and a few coefficients, like the proportion of males in mining and metallurgy and in primary employment, showed noticeable differences. It is of some interest, then, that many of the same overall relationships held both for the national district sample and for the special subset of the mining districts.

The overall equations were modestly successful in explaining overall variation, as measured by the R-squared values adjusted for degrees of freedom. The group of socioeconomic and demographic variables used explained between 20 and 50% of overall variation in marriage and fertility for the random sample and up to 70% for the mining sample. The R-squared values and the F-ratios (measuring the joint significance of all the variables) tended to become higher in both samples for overall fertility and proportions married, as opposed to marital fertility. This was most dramatic for the mining sample, where the R-squared values rose for overall fertility between 1851 and 1871 and proportions married between 1861 and 1871 but fell for marital fertility between 1851 and 1871. The equations for marital fertility in the 1871 mining equations actually had insignificant F-statistics, indicating that the independent variables lacked any significant explanatory power. Since $I_f \cong I_g \cdot I_m$, it is clear that for both samples, variations in marriage, rather than marital fertility, became increasingly important in accounting for variation in overall fertility.[11] This is confirmed by the coefficients of variability which were lower for marital fertility than for overall fertility or the index of proportions married and also declined over time for marital fertility but not for the other measures (see Table III-3). Although there *were* differences in marital fertility, and although the *level* of marital fertility was significantly higher in the mining areas (see Table III-2), control of overall period fertility for areas was still largely through marriage. Viewed from another perspective, it appears that on the very eve of the decline in marital fertility in Britain (dating from the 1870s), marital fertility was becoming increasingly *less* important in explaining variations in overall fertility. The socioeconomic and demographic factors which might be expected to influence fertility control within marriage were, instead of becoming more important, becoming less so. This certainly presents a challenging issue whose resolution depends, in part, on work done for the period after 1870–1872.

Before concluding this section, it should be pointed out that a number of estimation problems surround the application of ordinary least squares with a simple linear specification in this case. First, it is not clear that the relationship has been properly specified. To assess the importance of this problem, a nonlinear specification was estimated. The form selected tried to account for expected nonlinearities, especially in percentage variables

[11] The precise relationship is $I_f = I_g \cdot I_m + I_h \cdot (1\text{-}I_m)$, but since I_h is quite small in this case, $I_f \cong I_g \cdot I_m$ is a good approximation. This may be better viewed as $\ln I_f \cong \ln I_g + \ln I_m$, where logarithms make the relationship additive.

which are upper and lower bounded. The transformed equations were estimated in the form:

$$\ln I_f = \beta_1 + \beta_2/\text{MM} + \beta_3/\text{PE} + \beta_4/\text{FOH} + \beta_5 \text{ IMR} + \beta_6/\text{URB} + \beta_7\text{RNM} + \beta_8\text{SXR} + E,$$

where $\ln I_f$ is the natural logarithm of I_f, β_1 is the constant term, β_i for i = 2–8 are in coefficients and E is the error term. A small positive number (.5%) was added to MM, PE, FOH, and URB to avoid cases with division by zero. Similar equations were estimated with $\ln I_g$, $\ln I_m$, and ln MFR as dependent variables. The results of this alternative specification are not presented because a comparison between the exponential–reciprocal form and the linear form showed that the simple linear model performed quite well. The transformed equations usually gave slightly higher adjusted R-squared values. One variable, the percentage of females employed outside the home (FOH) was greatly improved by the transformation becoming significant in 30 to 36 equations. This strongly suggests that it was nonlinear in its relationship to fertility and nuptiality. The urban percentage became even less significant in the transformed case, indicating that the initial specification of URB was probably correct. The other variables showed about the same patterns.

A further type of specification error arises if important independent variables are missing. If these missing variables are in any way correlated with the regressors in equation, then biased coefficients and erroneous significance tests may result (Johnston, 1972, pp. 168–169). The problem is certainly serious, but there is no way to correct for it. If the missing variables are known, however, and if their correlations with other independent variables are also known, then the direction of the biases can be inferred. At present, it is best just to bear in mind the qualification that not all desired variables (e.g., educational levels, religious or ethnic composition) could be included. A third problem which arises is multicollinearity between the independent variables. This is a problem of experimental design and is tolerable as long as the t-values are not lowered a great deal. One instance of this was the high correlation between the sex ratio (SXR) and extrahousehold female employment (FOH). The inclusion of SXR usually caused FOH to become insignificant, so equations were specified both with and without SXR to examine the significance of FOH.

Finally, there is a serious problem with simultaneous equation bias (Johnston, 1972, pp. 341–352) for at least two independent variables, female employment and infant mortality. As an example, low fertility may be a cause as well as an effect of high extrahousehold female employment. That is, women may be in the labor force *because* they have few children as well as the reverse. Similarly, high fertility may be a cause as well as an effect of high infant mortality because higher-order births experience higher mortality (Wray, 1971, pp. 409–418). The result of such a situation is biased coefficients, which may lead to erroneous *t*-statistics. The solution is to specify and estimate a simultaneous equations system. This was done for 1861 and 1871 for both samples using two-stage least squares (TSLS). The system was estimated for 1861 in the following form:[12]

$$\begin{aligned} I_f &= \mathrm{f}(\mathrm{MM, PE, FOH, IMR, RNM, SXR}) \\ \mathrm{FOH} &= \mathrm{g}(I_f, \mathrm{URB, SXR}) \\ \mathrm{IMR} &= \mathrm{h}(I_f, \mathrm{MED}), \end{aligned}$$

where MED is medical personnel per 10,000 population. A similar system for 1871 had to be estimated without the infant mortality equation because data were unavailable to calculate MED.

The results (presented in Tables III-6 and III-7) generally indicate that the coefficients of female employment and infant mortality estimated by OLS were downwardly biased, thus causing them to be rejected as insignificant too often. The problem with TSLS equations is that *t*-statistics are usually lowered by using this procedure (i.e., the estimates have higher standard errors) and that *t*-statistics, *F*-ratios, and *R*-squared values do not have the same interpretation as for OLS except for rather large samples. The results of OLS estimates for relatively small samples may be biased but are often efficient (i.e., have small standard errors). Given the fact that TSLS reveals that OLS downwardly biases both female employment and infant mortality, it appears that the OLS estimates are reasonable and that these coefficients may simply be found insignificant too often. This is encouraging from the standpoint of the original model. The other results in the fertility equation are quite consistent with the results of the original linear model. The female labor-supply equation also gives good outcomes. More women worked outside the home in districts which were more urban, had lower fertility, and which had lower sex ratios. All these are the expected relationships. It might be argued that it is the employment of *married* women and not total women which is more relevant. This would have been really true for the marital fertility equations only (I_g and MFR). At any rate, labor-force data for registration districts were not available by sex and marital status, so this refinement could not be made.

Looking at historical differences in fertility and marriage among different occupational groups in England and Wales and concentrating on coal-mining populations, it was found that coal miners have had higher fertility and earlier and more complete marriage than most other occupational groups. These differentials existed in the nineteenth century and persisted into the twentieth. A comparison of a sample of mining areas with a random

[12] It should be noted that urbanization is now specified as affecting fertility through female employment and not as acting directly. Here URB is the instrumental variable necessary to estimate the FOH equation. The variable MED is also the instrument in the IMR equation.

TABLE III-6 Two-Stage Least Squares Regression Equations: Coal Mining Districts: England and Wales, 1861 and 1871. Overall Fertility

Dependent Variables		Independent Variables										
A. *1861* (*N* = 61)												
I_f	=	-2.582	+	.0053MM	+	.0177PE	-	.0136FOH	+	.0193IMR	-	.0078RNM
		(12.613)[a]		(.0192)		(.0766)		(.0481)		(.0738)		(.0316)
		+.0004SXR										
		(.0193)										
FOH	=	75.531	-	61.104I_f	+	.0943URB		.8109SXR				
		(10.938)		(40.436)		(.0450)		(.1411)				
IMR	=	74.324	+	159.038I_f	+	.4005MED						
		(35.951)		(72.769)		(.5157)						
B. *1871* (*N* = 63)												
I_f	=	.4540	=	.0004MM	-	.0005PE	-	.0054FOH	+	.0012IMR	-	.0007RNM
		(.4749)		(.0019)		(.0016)		(.0074)		(.0006)		(.0007)
		+.0006SXR										
		(.0027)										
FOH	=	72.269	-	3.572I_f	+	.0562URB	-	.4509SXR				
		(9.734)		(32.491)		(.0333)		(.0905)				

[a]Figures in parentheses are standard errors of the coefficients.

TABLE III-7 Two-Stage Least Squares Regression Equations: Random Sample of 125 Registration Districts: England and Wales, 1861 and 1871. Overall Fertility

Dependent variable		Independent variables							
A. *1861* (N = 125)									
I_f	=	-.2451	+	.0096MM	+	.0041PE	-	.0157FOH	+ .0018IMR
		(1.062)[a]		(.0131)		(.0071)		(.0347)	(.0043)
		+.0004RNM	+	.0028SXR					
		(.0021)		(.0042)					
FOH	=	54.319	-	72.2351I_f	+	.1074URB	-	.0460SXR	
		(10.634)		(33.242)		(.0319)		(.0456)	
IMR	=	137.407	+	21.224I_f	+	.2880MED			
		(45.062)		(104.958)		(.2988)			
B. *1871* (N = 125)									
I_f	=	-.1880	+	.0019MM	+	.0027PE	-	.0051FOH	+ .0004IMR
		(.5504)		(.0026)		(.0032)		(.0101)	(.0007)
		+.0013RNM	+	.0027SXR					
		(.0020)		(.0023)					
FOH	=	53.082	-	22.510I_f	+	.1619URB	-	.2073SXR	
		(9.360)		(35.957)		(.0250)		(.0707)	

[a] Figures in parentheses are standard errors of the coefficients.

sample of districts for 1851, 1861, and 1871 revealed higher average overall fertility, marital fertility, and proportions married in the mining areas than in the random sample.

It was hypothesized that a number of factors favorable to fertility acted on mining populations. Those include males reaching peak earning capacity at a relatively early age, relatively lower child costs in mining areas, frequent lack of employment opportunities for women, higher infant mortality and adult male debility and morbidity, and a taste and cost structure more rural than urban in the earlier stages of development. These factors combined to create earlier and more complete marriage for both males and females in mining and in mining areas and also higher marital fertility. Net in-migration selective of males in many mining areas led to sex ratios further favoring earlier marriage for females. Analysis of the mining and random samples yielded support for the hypotheses concerning female employment, infant mortality, the sex ratio, and urbanization for mining and heavy-industrial areas.[13]

The period under consideration preceded the decline in period fertility rates (after the mid-1870s), and there is some evidence for areas at this time that marriage differentials were much more important in explaining fertility differentials. This was particularly true for the mining districts by 1871, which may indicate that marriage long remained more important in controlling fertility in more distinctly working-class areas. There was virtually no change in period fertility measures and proportions married over this period. Further, there was little evidence of structural change with respect to the determinants of fertility and marriage in the mining areas. Joint F-tests for the mining equations of 1851 relative to 1861 and of 1861 relative to 1871 were insignificant even at a 5% level.[14] The same tests for the random sample did indicate significant differences in the coefficients over time, however. The later fertility decline among mining populations might be connected to this lag in structural change, although work with individual data must be carried out.

PRUSSIA, 1882, 1895, 1907

An analysis parallel to that for registration districts in England and Wales was conducted for Prussia *Kreise* which had more than 10% of the male

[13] No support was found for the adult morbidity hypothesis, using adult male death rates as an independent variable. It was assumed that adult male mortality might be a proxy for adult male morbidity and debility. But this assumption was probably not valid, and so the original hypothesis remains a viable one.

[14] For a description of this test of significance between two different sets of regression coefficients, see Chow (1960).

labor force in mining and metallurgy.[15] No random sample was done in this case, however. These cross-sectional analyses were made, each one related to the three pre-World War I occupational censuses (1882, 1895, 1907). Table III-8 provides a listing of the variables, their definitions, and sources. Not all the same variables could be used at each date because of a lack of data at the *Kreis* level. In particular, only the General Fertility Ratio and, for 1907, the General Marital Fertility Ratio, were used as dependent variables. The indices I_f, I_g, and I_m could not be calculated for *Kreise* because census data cross-classified by age, sex, and marital status were unavailable in sufficient detail. The percentage of males in primary employment was not used because of problems of collinearity. Two additional variables were utilized for the Prussian *Kreise*: the percentage of the population over age 10 which was illiterate (LIT) and the percentage of the population which was Roman Catholic (RC).

The average values from the sample of the mining and metallurgical *Kreise*[16] are compared to national averages for Germany in Table III-9. The results are again encouraging for many of the original hypotheses. General fertility and, in 1907, marital fertility were significantly higher in the mining sample, which had, of course, markedly higher proportions of the labor force in mining and metallurgy than for the nation as a whole. The mining sample had a higher sex ratio in the adult years than for Germany overall, its proportion of females employed outside the home was significantly lower, and it exhibited net in-migration while Germany as a whole had slight net out-migration. Unlike the British case, these industrial areas had lower infant mortality than the national average. This is partly because these industrial areas were not located in or near the highest areas of infant mortality in Germany, which included rural provinces in East Elbian Prussia and in southern Bavaria (Knodel, 1974, pp. 163–174). The level of infant mortality in these industrial *Kreise*, compared to that of adjacent rural areas, was comparable or higher. (For Upper Silesia, see Haines, 1976, pp. 343–345). Also the Prussian mining *Kreise* were already considerably more urban than Germany in 1882.[17] Finally, these *Kreise* had a higher proportion of Roman Catholics, which was probably merely fortuitous. They were also slightly (though insignificantly) more illiterate in 1871.

The results from the regression analysis for these Prussian *Kreise* are given

[15] There were 19 *Kreise* in Ruhr, Saar, and Upper Silesian regions which were chosen in 1882. By 1895, through subdivision, the number had risen to 26. It had risen still further, to 28, by 1907 but the sample at that date was reduced back to 19 by aggregation in order to alleviate collinearity problems caused by redivision of areas which were quite similar.

[16] The sample of *Kreise* will henceforth also be called the mining sample.

[17] This may have reflected, in part, the more strictly demographic definition used in Germany, all *Gemeinden* with a population of 2000 or more, which set a rather low limit for the level of urbanization.

TABLE III-8 Regression Variables for Selected *Kreise* in Prussia, 1882, 1895, 1907[a]

GFR	General fertility ratio (*a*. Live births per 1000 women 14-49 per annum [1875 related to 1882]; *b*. Live births per 1000 women 15-49 [1895 and 1910 related to 1907])
MFR	General marital fertility ratio (legitimate live births per 1000 married women aged 15-45 [1910 related to 1907])
RC	Percentage of population Roman Catholic (1880 related to 1882; 1895; 1910 related to 1907)
IMR	Infant mortality rate (infant deaths per 1000 live births per annum) (1875/1877 related to 1882; 1891/1895; 1906/1910 related to 1907)
URB	Percentage of population in incorporated areas over 2000 population (1875 related to 1882; 1895; 1910 related to 1907)
MM	Percentage of total labor force in mining and metallurgy (1882, 1895, 1907)
LIT	Percentage of population above age 10 illiterate (1871) (for the 1882 analysis only)
FOH	Percentage of females employed outside the home[b] (*a*. Percentage of females 14+ employed outside the home, 1882/1885; *b*. Percentage of females 15-59 employed outside the home, 1907/1910)
RNM	Rate of net migration for the preceding intercensal quinquennium (per 1000 population per annum) (*a*. 1891/1895 for 1895; and *b*. 1906/1910 for 1907)
SXR	Sex ratio (Males per 100 females) (*a*. Ages 20-49 for 1875 and 1895 and *b*. Ages 21-45 for 1910)

Sources: Occupational Censuses: 1882: Prussia, Statistisches Landesamt, *Preussische Statistik*, Bd. 76, Teil I (1885)
1895: Germany, Statistisches Reichsamt, *Statistik des deutschen Reichs*, Neue Folge, Bd. 109 (1898)
1907: Germany, Statistisches Reichsamt, *Statistik des deutschen Reichs* Neue Folge, Bd. 209 (1910)

Population Censuses: Prussia, Preussische Statistik, Bd. 30 (1875), Bd. 39 (1877), Bd. 66 (1883), Bd. 96 (1888), Bd. 121 (1893), Bd 148 (1897/1898), Bd. 206 (1908), Bd. 234 (1913). For 1871, 1875, 1880, 1885, 1890, 1895, 1905, and 1910.

Vital Statistics: Prussia: *Preussische Statistik*, Bd. 36, 42, 45 48, 123, 127, 134, 138, 143, 149, 155, 207, 213, 220, 224, 229, 233, 23

Urbanization: 1875: Germany, Statistisches Reichsamt, *Statistik des deutschen Reichs*, Bd. 57 (1883).
1895 and 1910: Germany, Statistisches Reichsamt, *Vierteljahreshefte zu Statistik des deutschen Reichs* (1902), I; (1912), IV.

[a]For all vital rates, births and deaths are taken as a 5 year average around the central data.

[b]Females employed outside the home consists of total female labor force (excluding unpaid family workers) exclusive of pensioners and women employed in agriculture. There was no basis for distinguishing domestic handicraft employment.

in Table III-10. Only a simple linear untransformed specification is pr sented, since it performed so well. For each date, two equations we estimated, one with and one without the sex ratio, just as in the British cas Overall, inclusion or exclusion of the sex ratio seems to have caused only few changes. Among those *Kreise* that had a significant proportion of t male labor force in mining, the variable representing percentage of ma

TABLE III-9 Mean Values of Regression Variables: Germany and Mining and Metullurgical Kreise of Prussia: 1882, 1895, 1907.

Variable	1882 Mining sample	1882 Germany	1882 Significance of difference[a]	1895 Mining sample	1895 Germany	1895 Significance of difference[a]	1907 Mining sample	1907 Germany	1907 Significance of difference[a]
GFR (per 1000)	198.2	153.5	***	189.8	144.6	***	173.3	117.5	***
MFR (per 1000)	--	--		--	--	--	327.8	223.3	***
RC (%)	71.0	35.9	***	66.4	36.0	***	71.8	36.7	***
IMR (per 1000 live births)	176.8	231.7	***	170.8	220.6	***	160.2	169.9	n.s.
URB (%)	59.7	39.0	***	69.1	50.2	***	78.4	60.0	***
MM (%)	31.4	2.4	***	30.4	2.7	***	33.7	3.6	***
LIT (%)	16.8	12.5[b]	n.s.	--	--	--	---	---	--
FOH (%)	8.0	10.2	**	--	--	--	12.1	19.1	***
RNM (per 1000 population)	--	--		5.4	-1.9	***	3.5	-0.5	n.s.
SXR (per 100)	106.2	95.2	**	106.8	95.8	***	111.6	99.3	***

Source: See notes to Table III-8. Also, *Statistishes Jahrbuch für das deutsche Reich*, various volumes.

[a]Based on the test of the difference of a mean from a given point (i.e., the national rate, ratio or percentage).

[b]Prussia

* $p < .1$.
** $p < .05$.
*** $p < .01$.
n.s. = not significant at a 10% level.

labor force in mining and metallurgy (MM) had the expected positive sign and was highly significant at all three dates (always at least at a 1% level of statistical significance). For the variable of female labor-force participation outside the home (FOH), which was available only for 1882 and 1907, the signs were all in the expected negative direction and the coefficients were significant in "explaining" variations in general fertility and for one of the marital fertility equations for 1907. Infant mortality was an insignificant variable in accounting for fertility in mining areas except in 1895, but, for general fertility, the signs were the expected positive ones. In all cases, the regressions gave quite high adjusted R-squared magnitudes and every equation was jointly significant at the 1% level, despite the fact that the number of observations was relatively small (19 in 1882, 26 in 1895, and 19 in 1907). For these Prussian mining *Kreise* in 1907, the regressions were slightly more successful in explaining general fertility than marital fertility, though the effect was not really as dramatic as for England and Wales in 1861 and 1871.

Urbanization was, in this case, measured by a more strictly demographic definition: the proportion of total population in incorporated areas over 2000 population. The results of this variable proved ambiguous, however. In 1882, urbanization was significantly and positively related to fertility, while in 1907 it was significantly and negatively related to fertility in the equations

TABLE III-10 OLS Regression Equations: Prussia, 1882, 1895, 1907. Selected *Kreise*[a]

		Constant	RC[b]	IMR	MM	URB	LIT	FOH	SXR	RNM	R^2_{adj}	F-
A. *1882*												
1.	GFR	179.9	-.3963	(.0009)[c]	.7382	.5610	.6264	-2.636	NI[d]	NI	.830	15[illegible]
2.	GFR	151.1	-.3571	(.0110)	.6407	.4675	.7079	-2.213	(.2741)	NI	.820	12[illegible]
B. *1895*												
1.	GFR	122.9	(-.0756)	.2718	.9535	(-.1147)	NI	NI	NI	.8194	.671	11[illegible]
2.	GFR	51.7	(-.0273)	.3831	.9132	(-.1964)	NI	NI	(.5550)	(.4778)	.679	9[illegible]
C. *1907*												
1.	GFR	137.1	(.2385)	(.2101)	.9962	-.3169	NI	-2.073	NI	.9298	.840	1[illegible]
2.	GFR	208.6	(.2354)	(.1334)	1.021	(-.0486)	NI	-2.366	(-.7207)	1.2226	.858	16[illegible]
3.	MFR	321.8	1.4200	(-.2671)	1.664	-1.067	NI	-2.063	NI	(-.1941)	.765	10[illegible]
4.	MFR	487.3	1.4129	(-.4447)	1.792	(-.4456)	NI	(-2.742)	(-1.668)	(.4836)	.784	10[illegible]

[a]For 1882 and 1907, *N* = 19. For 1895, *N* = 26.

[b]For a definition of variables, see Table III-8.

[c]Figures in parentheses are coefficients not significant at least at a 10% level (using a one-tailed

[d]NI = not included.

without the sex ratio. This may have reflected a shift from cities being the locus of more economic opportunity (in the 1870s and 1880s) and thus raising fertility, to cities being the leaders in the fertility decline (after 1900). The fact that urban areas were leaders in the decline has been noted for Germany by Knodel (1974, pp. 89–110). The idea that urbanization afforded more employment opportunities outside the home for women is suggested by positive zero-order correlations between urbanization and extrahousehold female labor-force participation (.450 in 1882 and .316 in 1907). There is, however, an indication that mining, in Germany at least, did tend to be concentrated in urban areas. The zero-order correlations between urbanization (URB) and proportion of males in mining and metallurgy (MM) were positive and significant and had values of .758 in 1882, .573 in 1895, and .503 in 1907. This probably reflects the definition of urbanization which included relatively small incorporated areas (2000 and over). Mining communities could quickly have reached the defined status of urban areas and would thus be counted as such, though they were still semirural.

Net migration (RNM), where the coefficient was significant (i.e., for the general fertility in 1895 and 1907), points to the hypothesis that in-migrants were responding to economic opportunity and were, therefore, likely to increase fertility in the area of destination. The lack of a significant coefficient for marital fertility in 1907 may indicate that the effect of migrants is to increase earlier and more complete marriage rather than increase marital fertility. This seems plausible for heavy net in-migration areas which had considerable mining and smelting activity. This phenomenon was observed by Wrigley for Arnsberg in Germany (Wrigley, 1961, pp. 143–145).

The proportion of the population Roman Catholic (RC) was included because in Germany there appears to have been some difference of demographic behavior according to religious belief (Wrigley, 1961, pp. 148–150). The supposition is that higher proportions of Roman Catholics (relative to Protestants) would lead to higher marital fertility (if not general fertility) because of the pronatalist attitudes of the Roman Catholic Church and the prohibition of most contraception practices. In 1882, however, just the opposite appears to have been the case: General fertility was higher in more heavily Protestant areas. The more heavily Protestant Ruhr had high fertility relative to more Catholic areas like the Saarland, Upper Silesia, and Aachen. In 1907, on the other hand, the variable RC was significant and positive for marital fertility but insignificant for general fertility. This is closer to the expected pattern, which might have begun to assert itself as the fertility decline began. There is, however, no way to ascertain if this were true in 1882 or 1895 because refined marital fertility ratios were not available for these dates.

The sex ratio (SXR), when added to the equations, did not perform particularly well as an independent variable. It was uniformly insignificant and even gave unexpectedly negative signs in 1907. One feature of the sex ratio was, however, that it was strongly positively correlated with the level of urbanization. The zero order correlations between SXR and URB were .779 in 1882, .730 in 1895, and .811 in 1907. This high degree of collinearity may have helped to obscure and weaken the relation of the sex ratio in general fertility, which, in any event, was weakening over time. The zero-order correlation between SXR and GFR was quite strong and significant in 1882 (.794), but it then declined to .409 in 1895 and .124 in 1907. In all cases the relationship was, however, positive, as expected.

As in the British case, the same caveats about the variables and relationships apply. In particular, this is yet another case which should be specified in a simultaneous equations framework. Such a system was specified for 1907 in the form:

$$\begin{aligned} \text{GFR} &= f(\text{RC, IMR, MM, FOH, RNM, SXR}) \\ \text{FOH} &= g(\text{GFR, URB, SXR}) \\ \text{IMR} &= h(\text{GFR, MED}), \end{aligned}$$

where MED, as before, was medical personnel per 10,000 inhabitants. The results again indicated that the coefficients for female employment outside the home were generally downwardly biased in the OLS equations, which strengthens the case for the hypothesized relationship between female employment and fertility.

Summarizing the Prussian results, the consistent positive relation between the proportion of the male labor force in mining and metallurgy and fertility was substantiated. Extrahousehold female labor-force participation had a depressing effect on fertility once the effects of urbanization and the extent of mining activity were taken into account. The level of urbanization had an initially positive relation to fertility, but this eventually turned negative. The sex ratio seemed to have little effect on general fertility, but this was probably due to the high correlation with urbanization. There was a higher sex ratio in the more urban areas, again substantiating the roles of economic opportunity and migration. Many of these findings, except for the results on urbanization in 1882, were similar to those for England and Wales.

CONCLUSIONS

This study of data for small areas with high concentrations of population in mining and metallurgy does furnish some support for a number of the hypotheses advanced in Chapter II. Based on cross-sectional regression analysis of registration districts for England and Wales (1851, 1861, and 1871) and *Kreise* for Prussia (1882, 1895, 1907), it was found that the proportion of adult males in mining and metallurgy was consistently positively related to fertility (and, in the British case, marriage) and that the proportion of females employed outside the home was usually negatively related to fertility and marriage. The sex ratio was generally positively associated with fertility and nuptiality, but the relationship was clearer for England and Wales. The mining and metallurgical districts had higher average fertility and proportions married than the national average (or average of districts in the British case) and also had significantly higher sex ratios among adults, higher net in-migration, lower levels of female employment, and rapidly growing levels of urbanization. All these accord with the expectations about mining and heavy-industrial areas which would tend to influence fertility and marriage.

There are problems with using only data on geographic areas, not the least of which is the "ecological fallacy." What may be true for areas may not be the same for individuals within those areas. This is less the case for smaller, more homogeneous districts, but remains nonetheless. In order to circumvent, in part, this problem and to obtain a closer look at particular mining and industrial populations, the remainder of the book will be devoted to four case studies: the Pennsylvania anthracite region, 1850–1900; Durham and Easington in England, 1851–1871; Merthyr-Tydfil in South Wales, 1851–1871; and the U.S. Commissioner of Labor Survey of working-class families in nine industries for 1889–1890.

APPENDIX. COALE'S INDICES OF OVERALL FERTILITY, MARITAL FERTILITY, AND PROPORTIONS MARRIED

Standard Schedule:	Age groups (*i*)	Births per married Hutterite woman, 1921-1930. (F_i)
	15-19	.300
	20-24	.550
	25-29	.502
	30-24	.447
	35-39	.406
	40-44	.222
	45-49	.061

I_f = index of overall fertility

$$= \frac{B_t}{\Sigma F_i w_i}$$

I_h = index of illegitimate fertility

$$\frac{B_t^I}{\Sigma F_i u_i}$$

I_g = index of marital fertility

$$= \frac{B_t^L}{\Sigma F_i m_i}$$

I_m = index of proportions married

$$= \frac{\Sigma F_i m_i}{\Sigma F_i w_i}$$

$$I_f = I_g \cdot I_m + I_h (1 - I_m)$$

B_t = total births at time *t* in the population studied

B_t^L = legitimate births at time *t* in the population studied

B_t^I = illegitimate births at time *t* in the population studied

w_i = total women in the ith age group in the population studied (using five year age groupings)

m_i = total married women in the ith age group in the population studied (using five year age groupings)

u_i = total unmarried women in the ith age group in the population studied (using five year age groupings)

F_i = births per woman in the "standard" population in the ith age interval

Source: Ansley J. Coale, "Factors Associated with the Development of Low Fertility: An Historic Summary," United Nations, *World Population Conference: 1965*, Vol. II (New York: United Nations, 1967), pp. 205-209.

IV

The Pennsylvania Anthracite Region, 1850–1900

INTRODUCTION AND BACKGROUND

The focus of this chapter is the anthracite coal mining region of eastern Pennsylvania. This particular area was chosen because of its early development, high degree of concentration of coal production and labor force, relatively large size, and contrasts between different elements of the population—the native and foreign born, rural and urban, agricultural and nonagricultural, mining and other occupational groups. It also embodied the nonurban yet industrial character of mining employment early in the development of the industry. The location of the coalfields and some of the major places within them may be seen in Figure IV-1.

For purposes of convenience, only the four major producing counties were selected: Lackawanna/Luzerne, Schuylkill, and Northumberland.[1] For 1900, the largely rural counties of Susquehanna, Wayne, and Wyoming were included to increase the representation of agricultural populations. As Table IV-1 indicates, the bulk of the anthracite coal population and labor force in Pennsylvania was centered largely in these four counties. As of 1889–1890, they produced 92.9% of Pennsylvania's anthracite and had 93.4% of anthracite-mining labor force in the state. They were also quite large, having 65.2% of all the coal mining workers in Pennsylvania at that

[1] There were actually only three counties up to 1878, when Lackawanna County (which includes the city of Scranton) was created from the northern part of Luzerne County.

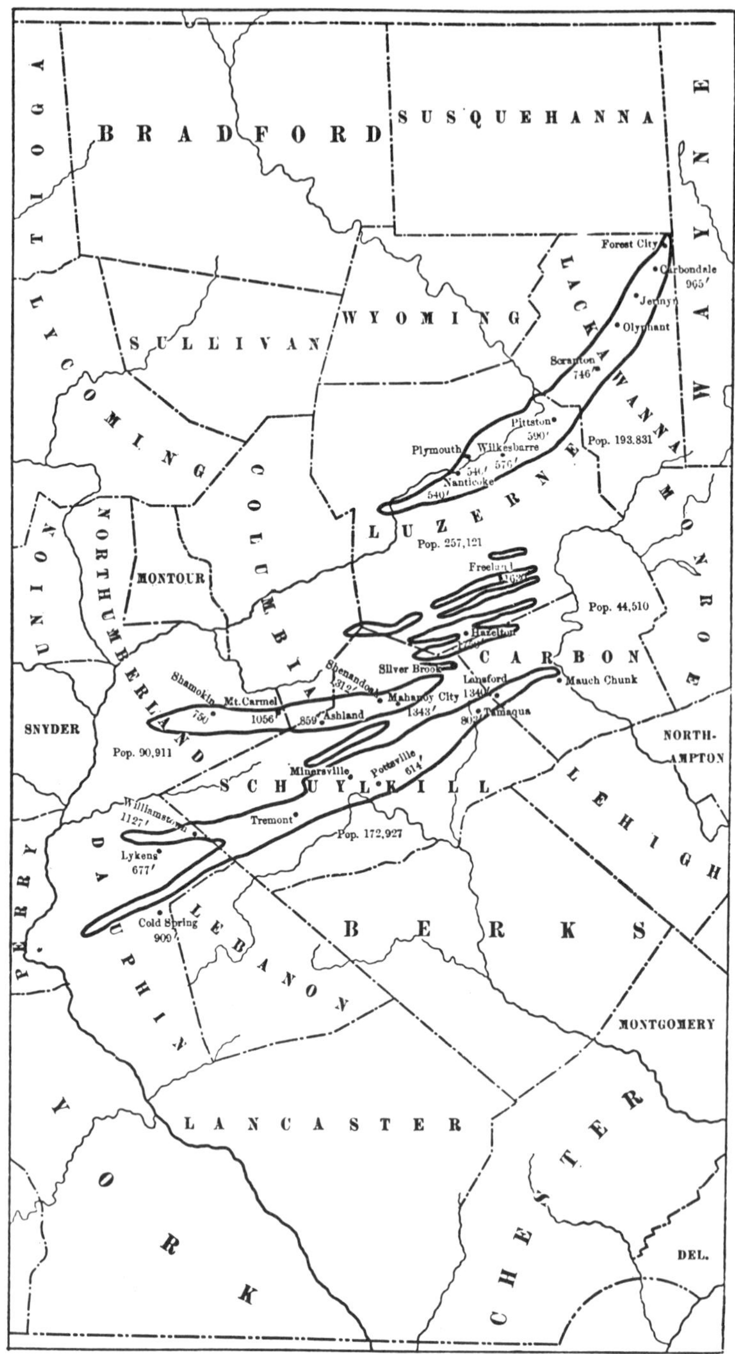

FIGURE IV-1 The anthracite coalfields of eastern Pennsylvania, ca. 1900. (From Roberts, 1904, page 2.)

	Total coal output (1889)	Percentage of total (1889)	Persons employed (1889)	Percentage of total (1889)	Total population (1890)	Persons employed as percentage of total population	Employed below ground[a] (1884)	Males 21+ (1890)	Employed below ground as percentage of male population 21+
I. *Anthracite*									
Susquehanna and Sullivan	351,842	.85	884	.71	51,713	1.71	494	15,311	3.23
Lackawanna	8,939,621	21.98	25,388	20.44	142,088	17.86	15,962	38,847	41.09
Luzerne	16,607,177	40.84	46,821	37.70	201,203	23.27	26,490	55,045	48.12
Carbon	1,210,973	2.98	3,206	2.58	38,624	8.30	1,363	10,440	13.06
Schuylkill	9,052,619	22.26	20,892	24.87	154,163	20.04	17,700	41,224	42.94
Columbia	628,395	1.54	2,531	2.04	36,832	6.87	1,367	9,557	14.30
Northumberland	3,176,740	7.81	12,879	10.36	74,698	17.24	7,924	19,851	39.92
Dauphin	697,485	1.71	2,322	1.86	96,977	2.39	1,452	26,563	5.47
Total	40,665,152	100.00	124,203	100.00	796,298	15.60	72,752	216,838	33.55
II. *Bituminous*									
Allegheny	4,717,431	13.04	9,386	17.47	551,959	1.70	8,172	158,396	5.16
Cambria	1,751,664	4.84	2,761	5.14	66,375	4.16	2,429	18,127	13.40
Clarion	596,589	1.65	943	1.76	36,802	2.56	783	8,728	8.97
Clearfield	5,224,506	14.44	7,715	14.36	69,565	11.09	6,717	18,003	37.31
Elk	614,113	1.70	1,183	2.20	22,239	5.32	937	7,055	13.28
Fayette	5,897,254	16.30	6,569	12.23	80,006	8.21	5,656	21,536	26.26
Jefferson	2,896,487	8.01	3,720	6.92	44,005	8.45	3,228	11,746	27.48
Mercer	575,751	1.59	1,095	2.04	55,744	1.96	871	14,682	5.93
Tioga	1,036,175	2.86	2,400	4.47	52,313	4.59	1,843	14,833	12.42
Washington	2,364,901	6.54	3,977	7.40	71,155	5.59	3,566	19,799	18.01
Westmoreland	7,631,124	21.10	9,068	16.88	112,819	8.04	7,699	31,119	24.74
Others[b]	2,868,094	7.93	4,895	9.11	599,721	.82	4,108	—	—
Total	36,174,089	100.00	53,712	100.00	1,762,703	3.05	46,009	—	—

Source: U.S. Dept. of the Interior, Census Office, *Eleventh Census of the United States, 1890*, "Report of the Population of the United States," Vol. I, Part I (Wash., D.C.: GPO, 1892), Table 79. "Report on Mineral Industries in the United States, 1889," (Wash., D.C.: GPO, 1892), pp. 399-407.

[a] Excluding boys under 16.

[b] 17 counties each producing less than 500,000 tone in 1889.

date. A glance at the bituminous coal-mining areas reveals a greater dispersion of population and labor force. Furthermore, these areas experienced a somewhat later development, not really growing significantly until after the Civil War. In fact, even in 1890, Pennsylvania anthracite production employed 39.6% of all coal miners in the United States, while Pennsylvania bituminous mining employed only about 17% (calculated from U.S. Bureau of the Census, 1975, Series M-107 and M-130). Finally, as again apparent from Table IV-1, the proportion of total and adult male populations that were engaged in mining was relatively higher in the anthracite region. Thus, it seems logical to concentrate on the anthracite counties.

The Pennsylvania anthracite region was indeed the focus of early and extremely rapid development. It was producing over 55.3% of the total coal output in the United States during the period 1846–1850 (U.S. Bureau of the Census, 1975, Series M-93 and M-123).[2] Much of the early growth was concentrated in Schuylkill County in the southern end of the region, long a bastion of free-wheeling private enterprise. The opening of the Schuylkill navigation to Pottsville in 1825 was the key to cheap transportation of the bulky output to Philadelphia and other eastern markets (Yearly, 1962, Part One).[3]

> *Villages and towns appeared literally overnight. The number of buildings in Pottsville increased sixfold from 1826 to 1829. The population—heavily weighted with Philadelphians—multiplied itself to twenty-seven times its original size in roughly the same period, and between 1829 and 1844 it very nearly doubled itself. Port Carbon with just a single family in 1829 had nine hundred and twelve people a year later, and essentially the same pattern of development held for Minersville, Llewellyn, New Castle, Middleport, Paterson, St. Clair, and Tamaqua. Into these places, as locally compiled censuses show, came a vital, predominantly white population "in no mood for trifling". . . . It was composed of immense crowds of adventurers, along with an assortment of ex-farmers, townsmen, laborers, clerks, anxious to play their cards right . . . make their killing . . .* [and] *ready to engage in the "laudable business of penetrating the bowels of the earth."*
>
> *Waves of land speculation kept these desperate populations moving and, as a consequence, during the years subsequent to their founding, coal communities in many cases grew neither swiftly nor steadily* [Reprinted with permission from C. K. Yearly, Jr., *Enterprise and Anthracite: Economics and Democracy in Schuylkill County*, 1820–1875, page 31. Copyright © 1962 by The Johns Hopkins University Press].

The focus of coal production gradually moved north into Luzerne and what was to become Lackawanna County. This can easily be traced in population growth. In the decade of the 1840s, Schuylkill County grew at an

[2] "In 1850 the anthracite product of Pennsylvania was nearly two-thirds of the coal production of the country [64.2%] [Parker, 1905, p. 668]."

[3] An analytical study of the early development of the anthracite industry (1820–1865), using production-function techniques, may be found in Schaefer (1977).

exponential rate of 7.37% per annum while Lackawanna/Luzerne County grew at only 2.42% (which was below the national average of 3.07%). By the 1860s, however, Schuylkill County grew at only 2.63% per year while Lackawanna/Luzerne was increasing at the rate of 5.78% per annum. The reason for this was quite clear—the development of the railroads (Hunter, 1951a, pp. 186–187, 1951b, pp. 464–465; Yearly, 1962). The Lackawanna and Lehigh Valley railroads developed the northern fields; and, eventually, the southern fields fell into the hands of the Philadelphia and Reading[4] (Roberts, 1901, pp. 62–69). The domination of the industry by large transportation companies resulted in a demise of competition (Yearly, 1962, pp. 197–217) and the formation of a rather successful cartel (Jones, 1914) to regulate prices and production. It may also have been partly responsible for the Molly McGuires and other labor unrest (Broehl, 1964, Chap. 13). But, it did not appear to retard growth.

Despite the more rapid growth of bituminous coal production than of anthracite (bituminous production had grown to 75.5% of total national coal production by 1896–1900), the anthracite region continued extremely rapid development over the later nineteenth century. As may be seen in Table IV-2, average annual production grew from 3,851,600 tons during 1846–1850 to 55,625,400 tons for 1896–1900, an average growth rate of 5.34% per annum. Between 1870 and 1896–1900, employment grew from 35,600 to an average of 145,639, a growth rate of 5.12% per year. One reason for the roughly parallel growth in output and employment after 1870 was the relative stagnation in gross worker productivity (i.e., output per worker per year). This was, however, partly due to fewer hours worked per year, since after 1886–1890, output per man-hour began to rise.

The rapid rise of the northern fields can easily be seen in the development of the city of Scranton. In 1840 there was virtually nothing there. Only farmland covered what was to become a major metropolitan area. Then, in 1840, George W. and Seldon Scranton founded the Lackawanna Iron and Coal Company. The city was not named and incorporated until 1851, but by 1860 it had 9223 inhabitants and was already the second largest urban area in the anthracite region, close behind Pottsville (9444 persons). It reached 102,026 by 1900 and was the 39th largest city in the United States, experiencing an average growth rate of 6.01% between 1860 and 1900. It was touted for its "newness and its roughness—its helter skelter way of doing things—its ups and downs—its push and enterprise—its rapid growth and busy hum—its work-a-day dress—its grime and smut and business air [*Scranton Daily Times*, 14 July 1873. Cited in Berthoff, 1965, p. 262]." And yet the more urban character of Scranton, Wilkes-Barre, and Pottsville was not really

[4] In 1848, in the Schuylkill region, there were over 120 operators with 161 collieries. By 1870 over 75% of the mines had been acquired by the Philadelphia and Reading (Roberts, 1901, pp. 18–19).

TABLE IV-2 Production and Employment in the Pennsylvania Anthracite Coal Industry, 1840-1900

Period	Production		Employment		Productivity	
	Total production (000 short tons)	Average value per ton (F.O.B. mine dollars)	Average workers on active days	Average days worked	Output per worker per year (tons)	Output per man hour (tons)
1841/1845	1822.6	NA[a]	NA	NA	-	-
1846/1850	3851.6	NA	NA	NA	-	-
1851/1855	7030.8	NA	NA	NA	-	-
1856/1860	9492.4	NA	NA	NA	-	-
1861/1865	11,560.4	NA	NA	NA	-	-
1866/1870	17,571.6	NA	35,600[b]	NA	560.6[a]	-
1871/1875	23,442.8	NA	50,760.0	NA	461.8	-
1876/1880	25,800.2	1.47[c]	68,700.0	NA	375.5	-
1881/1885	36,198.2	1.96	90,209.8	213.4	401.3	1.880
1886/1890	43,951.8	1.75	116,291.0	203.2	377.9	1.860
1891/1895	53,405.2	1.51	132,572.8	196.8	402.8	2.047
1896/1900	55,625.4	1.47	145,638.6	163.0	381.9	2.343
Census years						
1850	4,327	NA	NA	NA	-	-
1860	10,984	NA	NA	NA	-	-
1870	19,958	NA	35,600	NA	560.6	-
1880	28,650	1.47	73,373	NA	390.5	-
1890	46,469	1.43	126,000	200	368.8	1.844
1900	57,368	1.49	144,206	166	397.8	2.396

Source: U.S. Bureau of the Census, *Historical Statistics of the United States, Colonial Times to 1970* (Washington, D.C.: G.P.O., 1975), Series M123, 126, 130, 134.

[a]NA = Not available.

[b]1870 only.

[c]1880 only.

characteristic of most of the region. The geography and geology led to many small mining towns, or "patches," with picturesque names: Mauch Chunk, Shamokin, Shenandoah, Tamaqua, Nanticoke, Oil City, Mahanoy. Many would grow to sizable places, but many started, and long remained, as isolated small industrial villages and towns.

The choice of the time period for study, 1850–1900, was dictated by the availability and usefulness of the census manuscripts necessary to conduct an analysis. Prior to 1850, the census manuscripts did not provide full information on each individual enumerated (U.S. Bureau of the Census, 1973b; Wright and Hunt, 1900). After 1900, no census manuscripts have been made available for public use.[5]

Table IV-3 presents selected characteristics of the region. As is evident, population increased substantially, from 140,057 in 1850 to 714,790 in 1900.[6] Although the growth rate declined over time, the average growth between 1850 and 1900 was 3.26% per annum. (This compares with a national average of 2.37%.) Accompanying this was an increase in the urban percentage after 1860.[7] Like other mining areas, the anthracite region began as only modestly urban, and the urban share increased dramatically in the later stages of development. Similarly there was a substantial decline in farming and a rise in nonagricultural activity among the adult male population after 1850. The share of farming is almost certainly understated for 1850 and 1860, since the category "Laborer" undoubtedly contained some agricultural workers who were not more explicitly designated.[8] The increase in mining and service employments[9] was clear, as was the expansion of the class of laborers and the relative decline of farming.

A distinguishing feature of the anthracite region was its ethnic diversity, strongly reflecting the successive waves of immigration to the United States. "Welsh and English miners, Irish laborers, and Germans of various occupations entered the region at the start of mining in the 1820's, and continued to come, along with Italians, Poles, Slovaks, and other Eastern Europeans—colloquially 'Hungarians'—after 1870 [Berthoff, 1965, p. 266]." As Table IV-3 points out, 20 to 25% of the total population was actually foreign born. The proportion remained roughly steady, ranging from 21.0% in 1850 to

[5] No census manuscripts are available for 1890, since these were almost entirely burned accidentally in 1921.

[6] This excludes the additional counties, Susquehanna, Wayne, and Wyoming, added to the 1900 sample.

[7] The decline in the urban percentage between 1850 and 1860 was due to a more rapid growth of areas designated nonurban relative to urban areas. Urban areas are defined in footnote *c* of Table IV-3. The general selection criteria were size and demonstrably urban identity (such as the designation city).

[8] The instructions to the census enumerators concerning occupation were not exceptionally precise until 1870 (see Wright and Hunt, 1900, pp. 152, 158–159).

[9] Service occupations are found in the category "Mercantile, Food, Lodging, Transport" and, in part, in "Professional and Other."

TABLE IV-3 Selected Characteristics of the Pennsylvania Anthracite Region, 1850-1900[a]

		1850	1860	1870	1880	1900
1.	Total population	140,057	208,676	318,787	405,431	714,790
2.	Average annual growth rate from previous census	4.08%	3.99%	4.24%	2.40%	2.84%
3.	Child-woman ratio[b]	758.50	764.10	700.00	629.00	567.80
4.	Percent urban[c]	15.82%	13.66%	28.02%	32.69%	59.24%
5.	Percent foreign-born	21.05%	25.24%	27.71%	23.67%	23.18%
	a. Percent Irish	10.54	12.52	12.06	10.29	3.55
	b. Percent British	6.61	6.42	10.08	8.01	5.61
	c. Percent other	3.90	6.30	5.57	5.36	14.01
	d. (Percent Slavic)					(9.43)
6.	Percent of males 15+					
	a. Farming	17.65%	18.66%	12.94%	11.98%	10.64%
	b. Laborers	28.14	25.58	24.14	33.99	19.08
	c. Mining	10.97	14.90	21.12	28.24	29.02
	d. Manufacturing, crafts construction	18.25	17.37	17.62	12.85	14.58
	e. Mercantile, food, lodging, transport	8.34	10.99	12.83	13.90	15.66
	f. Professional and other	3.58	4.31	4.53	8.45	9.50

Source: Samples of enumerators' manuscripts. U.S. Bureau of the Census, *U.S. Census of Population 1850...1860...1870...1880...1900.*

[a] Lackawanna/Luzerne, Schuylkill, and Northumberland counties for 1850-1880.

[b] Children aged 0-4 per 1000 women aged 15-49.

[c] Urban areas were taken as follows: (a) 1850. Luzerne County (Carbondale Borough, Pittston, Wilkes-Barre Borough and Township). Schuylkill County (Pottsville Borough). (b) 1860. Luzerne County (Carbondale, Scranton, Wilkes-Barre, Pittston). Schuylkill County (Pottsville). (c) 1870. Luzerne County (Hazel Township, Hazelton Borough, Pittston Borough, Wilkes-Barre Township and City, Carbondale City, Scranton City). Schuylkill County (Pottsville Borough). (d) 1880. Lackawanna County (Carbondale City, Scranton City). Luzerne County (Hazel Township, Hazelton Borough, Pittston Borough, Wilkes-Barre City and Township). Schuylkill County (Mahanoy City Borough, Pottsville Borough, and Shenandoah Borough). Northumberland County (Shamokin Borough). (e) 1900. Lackawanna County (Carbondale City, Scranton City, Dunmore Borough, Olyphant Borough). Luzerne County (Hazel Township, Hazelton City, Nanticoke Borough, Newport Township, Pittston City and Township, Plains Township, Plymouth Borough and Township, Wilkes-Barre City and Township). Schuylkill County (Ashland Borough, Mahanoy Township, Mahony City Borough, Pottsville Borough, Shenandoah Borough, Tamaqua Borough, West Mahanoy).

27.7% in 1870. Some areas were much more heavily populated by immigrants. Scranton, for example, in 1870, had fully 45% of its population born outside the United States. The anthracite region had almost twice the proportion of foreign born found in the United States, that being 9.7% in 1850 and 13.6% for 1900 (U.S. Bureau of the Census, 1975, Series A-2, 105, 107, 112–114). The ethnic composition did indeed change from one which was primarily Anglo-Irish (up to 1880) to one which was dominated by Slavic and Italian immigrants. By 1900, over 45% of all foreign born were of Slavic or Italian origins. It was also true that the image of the "melting pot" was not particularly appropriate for this region. Berthoff has documented a "vertical division of local society into ethnic fragments," each striving to maintain separate identity and location. Scranton's "Little England" became an Italian community after 1880, and the borough of Shenandoah moved from being a stronghold of Welsh migrants in the 1860s to being a "great Polish city" by 1882 (Berthoff, 1965, p. 269). Local groups and societies reflected this ethnic separation, having titles like the Hibernians, Polish Alliance, Caledonians, Slovak Union, Sons of St. George, Grütli Verein, and Mazzini Society. The various groups were observed to be "clannish and the best places at their disposal are given to their friends [Berthoff, 1965, p. 268, quoting a letter in the Delaware, Lackawanna and Western Railroad company papers]." This ethnic separation, which has never disappeared, was important in preserving customs, mores, and tastes characteristic of the area of origin in the place of destination.[10] This exercised an influence, albeit difficult to measure, on demographic behavior.

THE SAMPLE

In order to investigate more closely age-specific and differential fertility, as well as nuptiality, mortality, and migration, the enumerators' manuscripts of the U.S. censuses of population from 1850 to 1900 were sampled. The types of data available from the census manuscripts are presented in Table IV-4. It is quite obvious that many of the questions posed in Chapter II cannot be answered with such data, but quite a number can. In particular, the importance of marital fertility decline versus changes in marriage patterns and the age pattern of fertility decline for various groups in the economy can also be assessed. Fertility and nuptiality differentials and their changes over time can be analyzed. Finally, migration patterns and even differential mortality can, to a certain extent, be studied.

The census schedules were systematically sampled with a random starting point for each county. Individuals were sampled by household and were

[10] An example of the strong preservation of norms among migrants has been documented for the Italians of Buffalo. See McLaughlin (1971).

TABLE IV-4 Information Available on Individuals from the U.S. Census Enumerators' Manuscripts 1850-1880, 1900

Demographic characteristics	1850	1860	1870	1880	1900
Name	x	x	x	x	x
Age	x	x	x	x	x
Sex	x	x	x	x	x
Color or race	x	x	x	x	x
Relationship to head of family or household				x	x
Married in past year	x	x	x	x	
Marital status				x	x
Number of years married					x
Social characteristics					
Free or slave	x	x			
Infirmities and handicaps	x	x	x	x	x
Education					
Literacy	x	x	x	x	x
School attendance	x	x	x	x	x
Place of birth	x	x	x	x	x
Place of birth of parents			x	x	x
Citizenship			x		x
Eligibility to vote			x		
Year of immigration					x
Can speak English					x
Number of children ever born					x
Number of children surviving					x
Farm residence					x
Economic characteristics					
Occupation	x	x	x	x	x
Duration of unemployment				x	x
Value of real estate	x	x	x		
Value of personal estate		x	x		

Source: U.S. Bureau of the Census, *Population and Housing Inquiries in U.S. Decennial Censuses, 1790-1970*, Working Paper No. 39 (Washington, D.C.: G.P.O., 1973), pp. 5-9.

later aggregated into families and households. The family, defined as any conjugal unit or any parent–child unit, was the basis for the fertility analysis. One exception to this rule was that boarders were classified each as a separate family (unless there was a conjugal unit or parent–child unit among the boarders in a household, in which case that was considered a family unit).[11] The household was the coresident unit of enumeration and, in the majority of cases, coincided with the family. This process of assignment of individuals to families and households was quite straightforward for 1880 and 1900, where information on relationship to head of household and marital status could be combined with data on name, age, sex, occupation, and order of enumeration. For the censuses of 1850, 1860, and 1870, however, information on relationship to head of household and marital

[11] Servants were kept with the primary family in each household except when there was a conjugal unit or a parent–child unit among the servants. This was then considered a separate family.

status was lacking and so family and household relationships had to be inferred from name, age, sex, order of enumeration, and place of birth. The number of ambiguous cases fortunately proved to be quite small.[12] The published aggregate data and the sample data were compared for such things as age and sex distribution and place of birth. The agreement was quite close, pointing to a good approximation of the parent population by the sample.[13]

METHODS

Census samples are well suited to the application of the body of techniques known as own-children methods, so-called because they rest on the assignment of children to their mothers in family groups. The method was originally developed for application to fertility measurement by Grabill and Cho (1965) and was extensively applied by them to U.S. census data (Cho, Grabill, and Bogue, 1970). Subsequently, the obvious advantages of these methods for estimating fertility in developing countries which take periodic census but which lack adequate vital registration have prompted much wider application, particularly by Lee-Jay Cho and his associates at the East–West Population Center. (See, for example, Cho, 1971, 1973; Aris, 1976; Arnold, Phananiramai, Retherford, and Cho, 1976; Arretx, 1976; Engracia, 1976; Poedjastoeti, 1976; Retherford and Cho, 1974.) These same advantages make the method especially appropriate for historical demographic work on the United States, for which census samples may be generated but where vital statistics are lacking or are inadequate in coverage or detail.

Another group of methods, which may also be subsumed in the own-children category, are those pertaining to indirect mortality estimation, especially for infant and child mortality. Stemming from the original work of Brass (1975; Brass and Coale, 1968; United Nations, 1967), techniques are available to estimate childhood mortality from data on children ever

[12] It would have been desirable to have had roughly equal sample sizes at all dates, but the way the samples were originally taken mitigated against this outcome. The exact sample sizes are

	1850	1860	1870	1880	1900
Individuals	11,238	9,872	8,862	7,606	11,131
Families	3,027	2,658	2,437	1,922	3,031
Households	1,906	1,822	1,537	1,453	2,289
Percentage of total population sampled	8.02	4.73	2.78	1.88	1.39

[13] A series of chi-square tests were applied to the sample for such dimensions as age and sex distributions and place-of-birth data. The tests revealed generally insignificant differences between the sample and the actual distributions.

born (parity) and children surviving (child survivorship) to adult women. These methods have been refined (Sullivan, 1972; Trussell, 1975) and have been modified to allow the age distribution of surviving own children to be used (Cho, 1973; Preston, 1976; Feeney, 1976.) It is even possible, with the proper census questions, to estimate adult mortality as well. (For a summary, see Hill and Trussell, 1977.) Since the fertility estimation procedures require mortality estimates, both groups of techniques will be applied in calculating age-specific fertility in the anthracite counties.

FERTILITY, MORTALITY, AND MARRIAGE, 1850–1900

Differential Fertility, 1850–1900

The only published materials usable for fertility measures are United States population census data cross-classified by age and sex, and these were given only in sufficient detail prior to 1860 to allow the computation of child–woman ratios at the county level.[14] Table IV-5 gives child–woman ratios (children 0–4 per 1000 women aged 15–49) for the censuses of 1850 and 1860 for selected counties of Pennsylvania. The first three counties (Lackawanna/Luzerne, Schuylkill, and Northumberland) were major anthracite producers. The next five (Wayne, Wyoming, Monroe, Carbon, and Dauphin) were surrounding counties with some mining (especially in Dauphin and Carbon), but were mostly agricultural in 1850 and 1860. Dauphin County, however, contained the city of Harrisburg. The next six counties (Allegheny, Cambria, Clearfield, Fayette, Jefferson, and Westmoreland) later became important bituminous coal producers but were at this time mostly agricultural. Allegheny contained the cities of Pittsburgh and Allegheny, which constituted 42.5% of its total population in 1860. Philadelphia, of course, was Pennsylvania's largest city, and the second largest city in the United States at this time.

The remaining six counties (Delaware, Bucks, Berks, Montgomery, Chester, and Lancaster) were older, settled agricultural counties surrounding Philadelphia, although they too contained several larger urban areas (Reading, Lancaster, Norristown). The contrast is informative. The coal-mining counties did have high fertility (as measured by child–woman ratios) relative to the state average and especially relative to the urban counties (Allegheny and Philadelphia) and the settled agrarian counties around Philadelphia. But fertility in the mining counties was at about the same level as in some of the more rural and remote agricultural counties (e.g., Cambria, Clearfield, Jefferson) and even some rural counties nearby (Monroe). It is thus not clear whether the relatively high fertility of Lackawanna/Luzerne, Schuyl-

[14] There is no record of any population census ever having been taken for Pennsylvania other than the U.S. census (see Dubester, 1948).

TABLE IV-5 Child-Woman Ratios for Selected Counties in Pennsylvania, 1850 and 1860, (White Population)

Counties	1850 Child-Woman ratio[a]	1850 Percent of state average	1860 Child-Woman ratio[a]	1860 Percent of state average
Lackawanna/Luzerne	739.64	121	758.42	124
Schuylkill	811.43	133	808.48	132
Northumberland	669.93	110	651.63	106
Wayne	667.14	109	681.37	111
Wyoming	690.87	113	659.59	108
Monroe	783.06	128	763.75	125
Carbon	804.42	132	865.96	141
Dauphin	630.71	103	603.65	98
Allegheney	603.86	99	665.83	109
Cambria	678.73	111	824.47	134
Clearfield	871.85	143	819.07	134
Fayette	675.64	111	607.22	99
Jefferson	832.58	136	847.38	138
Westmoreland	626.49	103	649.77	106
Philadelphia	456.04	75	485.26	79
Delaware	487.53	80	500.13	82
Bucks	537.73	88	535.63	87
Berks	685.20	112	655.16	107
Montgomery	551.49	90	552.36	90
Chester	540.21	88	531.89	87
Lancaster	591.30	97	633.02	103
Pennsylvania	610.69	---	612.66	---

Source: U.S. Bureau of the Census, *Seventh Census of the United States: 1850*, Vol. I (Washington, D.C.: 1854), pp. 154-155. *Eighth Census of the United States: 1860*, Vol. I (Washington, D.C.: 1864), pp. 406 and 408.

[a] Children 0-4 per 1000 women aged 15-49.

kill, and Carbon counties was due to the mining population or the agricultural population of this less densely settled area. Northumberland County in the mining area showed a somewhat lower fertility. (The lower fertility of Dauphin County, also in the mining area, was probably due, in part, to the presence of Harrisburg.)

Time trends in child–woman ratios for the anthracite counties are given in Table IV-6 which shows a steady decline throughout the nineteenth century in all the areas concerned.[15] Notably, the anthracite region had

[15] The only exception was a slight upturn between 1850 and 1860 for the measure using children 0–4 per 1000 women aged 15–49. This might have been, in part, a function of the relatively heavy infant and child mortality from a cholera epidemic in the year just prior to the census of 1850.

TABLE IV-6 Child-Woman Ratios: Pennsylvania Anthracite Mining Counties, Pennsylvania, and the United States, 1800-1900. (White Population Only)

Year	Children 0-9 per 1000 women 16-44[a]			Children 0-4 per 1000 women 15-49		
	Anthracite counties[b]	Pennsylvania	United States	Anthracite counties[b]	Pennsylvania	United States
1800	2221	1881	1844	-----	-----	-----
1810	2099	1841	1824	-----	-----	-----
1820	2171	1748	1735	-----	-----	-----
1830	1741	1536	1586	870.2	751.1	781.0
1840	1647	1456	1514	832.8	720.6	743.6
1850	1580	1322	1335	758.5	610.7	613.3
1860	1698	1293	1308	764.1	612.7	627.0
1870	1484	1191	1268	700.0	556.0	589.7
1880	1393	1130	1184	629.0	506.7	537.4
1890[c]	----[d]	1003	1072	-----[d]	438.5	473.2
1900	1197	992	1043	567.8	447.7	465.1

Source: (1) Anthracite counties: (a) 1800-1860: U.S. Bureau of the Census. *U.S. Census of Population 1800...1810...1820*...1830...1840...1850... *1860*. (b) 1870-1900. Samples of manuscript enumerators' schedules.

(2) Pennsylvania and United States: *U.S. Censuses of Population, 1800-1900.*

[a] Age structure distributions were adjusted for 1830 and 1860 to obtain women aged 16-44. Age distributions thereafter were estimated from manuscript census samples or calculated directly from published data.

[b] For 1800 and 1810 the territories of the counties of Luzerne and Northumberland were included as then constituted. For 1820, territories of Luzerne, Schuylkill, and Northumberland counties were included as currently organized. After 1840, the only major boundary change was the separation of Lackawanna county from Luzerne county in 1878. For 1900, the anthracite counties are supplemented by Wayne, Wyoming, and Susquehanna counties.

[c] Age at nearest birthday rather than age of last birthday was asked in 1890.

[d] Not available.

considerably higher fertility as measured by this rather crude census measure. In the later part of the nineteenth century, which is the time frame considered here, the fertility decline in the anthracite counties was slightly less than that for Pennsylvania (25.7% versus 26.9%) between 1860 and 1900. The decline in the anthracite region was, however, virtually identical to that for the entire United States (25.8%). This allowed fertility in the anthracite region to remain roughly 25% above the Pennsylvania average and 22% above the national mean.

To understand differential fertility and the process of decline, however, more detailed information is clearly required. To treat the issue of differential fertility, it was decided to use age-specific marital child–woman ratios (own children aged 0–4 per married woman by age). This expresses surviving births per surviving mother from an average point of 2½ years before the census date. Thus, it is net of mortality, especially infant and child mortality, which makes it somewhat more valuable as a measure of effective fertility than of current actual births. Married women were used because the context of the analysis was the family.

There are, of course, problems with this measure, including underenumeration of young children relative to adult women and age misstatement for both women and children. A study by Coale and Zelnik of age heaping and completeness of enumeration for the U.S. censuses since 1880 reveals that there was substantial age misstatement in the census of 1880 and probably in earlier censuses as well. Further, there was more underenumeration among children than among adult women of childbearing age (Coale and Zelnik, 1963, pp. 6–7, 179–180). Some perusal of the age distributions of the sample populations here also indicates age heaping.[16] The problem of age heaping is solved somewhat by using grouped age data (e.g., ages 0–4, 5–9, etc.), but the preferences for ages ending in zero and five means that each age group will receive some incorrect members of the lower end (except the group 0–4) and lose some at the upper end. These may not balance. The problem of underenumeration is more serious and, while corrections can be applied to group data, they are difficult to estimate. Furthermore, family data used for analysis below cannot be so adjusted. Nothing is done at this point to correct the data. It must, however, be borne in mind that the child–woman ratios used here are probably somewhat understated. A final problem in the analysis of fertility from census data is children who are absent from the home or who have left home. This is likely to be minimized for very young children and is a reason why children aged 0–4 per woman by age was used in preference to some measure like total children present for married women aged 34–44. On the positive side, one of the obvious virtues of this measure, and of own-children methods in general, is that fertility (and mortality) can be cross-classified by any census dimension available which includes, for married women, both their own attributes and those of their husbands and families. This permits quite detailed studies of both differential fertility and fertility decline and is quite appropriate in a historical context where an increasing number of census manuscript samples are becoming available.[17]

Table IV-7 presents these child–woman ratios for all women aged 15–49 for the four counties at the censuses of 1850 through 1900.[18] They are cross-classified by a number of other variables, including occupation of family head, literacy[19] of spouse and family head, nativity of parents, resi-

[16] Computation of Meyer's blended index to detect age heaping also gave significant indication of it.

[17] For an example of an early application of these techniques see Hareven and Vinovskis (1975).

[18] The 1900 sample also includes some families from Susquehanna, Wayne, and Wyoming Counties.

[19] Illiteracy was defined in the 1850 and 1860 censuses as persons age 20 and over unable to read and write. For 1870, 1880, and 1900 it was persons age 10 and over who could not read or write.

TABLE IV-7 Children 0-4 per 1000 Married Women 15-49 Classified by Occupation and Literacy of Family Head, Literacy and Labor Force Activity of Spouse, Nativity of Head and Spouse, and Residence and Wealth of Family. Lackawanna/Luzerne, Schuylkill, and Northumberland Counties, Pennsylvania, 1850-1900. (Families with both Husband and Wife Present)

	1850	N^b	1860	N^b	1870	N^b	1880	N^b	1900[a]	N^b
I. *Occupation of family head*										
a. Farmers	1190.9	330	1035.7	252	993.6	156	859.5	121	766.1	171
b. Laborers	1090.9	374	1187.7	341	1169.9	259	977.5	267	919.0	247
c. Miners	1219.7	223	1125.8	279	1067.5	326	1205.9	306	1117.2	512
d. Manufacturing, etc.	1100.3	329	1203.9	304	1106.9	262	798.8	164	815.9	277
e. Mercantile, etc.	1120.3	133	1039.1	172	1022.9	175	924.5	159	819.9	311
f. Professional and other	1008.3	113	871.4	70	878.8	66	615.4	39	518.9	106
II. *Nativity of parents*										
a. Both native	1123.2	958	1060.0	683	984.3	573	881.9	391	812.7	897
b. One foreign-born	1318.2	88	1224.1	116	1264.0	125	1200.0	140	934.5	229
c. Both foreign-born	1113.0	460	1203.2	620	1116.2	551	1035.8	525	1048.5	495
III. *Literacy of spouse*										
a. Illiterate	1186.8	182	1209.0	268	1093.8	373	960.2	226	1023.8	252
b. Literate	1125.3	1317	1142.0	1106	1061.7	875	986.7	830	882.6	1346
IV. *Literacy of family head*										
a. Illiterate	1175.1	297	1107.3	177	1081.5	270	1090.9	165	1041.0	195
b. Literate	1152.0	1158	1143.3	1235	1070.7	976	962.9	889	885.5	1415
V. *Residence*										
a. Rural	1152.6	1186	1164.8	1189	1067.0	925	1004.0	742	904.9	778
b. Urban	1053.1	320	987.0	230	1080.2	324	926.8	314	900.7	846
VI. *Wealth*										
a. 0-500	1122.0	1098	1179.3	948	1098.0	714	—	—	—	—
b. 501-1000	1241.1	141	1080.6	124	1071.4	112	—	—	—	—
c. 1001-2000	1214.9	121	1126.8	142	1121.2	132	—	—	—	—
d. 2001-5000	967.7	93	1078.9	114	1062.2	159	—	—	—	—
e. 5000 +	1132.1	53	846.2	91	878.8	132	—	—	—	—
VII. *Does spouse work?*										
a. Not working	—	—	1138.9	1397	1076.1	1235	981.0	1050	909.9	1609
b. Working	—	—	909.1	22	500.0	6	000.0	2	153.8	13
VIII. *Total*	1130.5	1506	1136.0	1419	1070.5	1249	981.1	1056	902.7	1624

Source: Samples of census enumerators' schedules.
[a]For 1900, the sample also includes Susquehanna, Wayne, and Wyoming Counties.
[b]The number of cases in each category (e.g., Occupation, Nativity, etc.) may not add up to the total

nce (rural or urban),[20] wealth,[21] and economic activity of the spouse.[22] The tios here point to the highest fertility among miners relative to the other cupational groups, with the exception of the year 1870. The first rank of ining populations is altered, however, when these ratios are standardized the overall age structure of married women at each date. In Table IV-8, e actual age-specific child–woman ratios were standardized to the age ucture of married women at each date (Part A) and in 1880 (Part B).[23] The st ranking of miners was lost for 1850, 1860, and 1870, while the ranking of rmers and farm laborers rose. Miners maintained their dominant position 1880 and 1900. The younger age structure of miners' wives relative to ose of farmers played a role in raising their overall child–woman ratios. ne actual age-specific ratios (not shown) point to few differentials in 1850. me statistical tests on the differences between age-specific child–woman tios in 1850 revealed only a few significant differences between occupa- nal groups at the same age.[24] Farmers were more often higher and ofessionals more often lower.

After some rather considerable fluctuations over time, by 1900 miners' ves definitely had higher child–woman ratios than all other occupational oups. Since infant and child mortality was likely not below average for milies in coal mining, the ratios in Tables IV-7 and IV-8 probably under- ate the true differentials in age-specific fertility. The differentials remain spite standardization (Table IV-8) showing that they were not caused to y large extent by more favorable age structure among miners' spouses. rmers and farm laborers, formerly having had ratios close to or above ose of miners, had now dropped well below miners and even below the pulation average. The overall child–woman ratios for farmers were only .3% of those for miners in 1880 (and 76.3% for standardized ratios). They d also dropped to 86.3% of the population average (91.7% for stan- rdized ratios) in 1880 as opposed to 105.3% (and 111.8%) in 1850. The ofessional group remained the group with fewest young children present.

[20] For a definition of urban areas, see the footnotes to Table IV-3.

[21] Wealth was the value of real estate only in 1850, but included the value of personal and l estate in 1860 and 1870. In 1880 and 1900, no question on wealth was asked.

[22] This was done only for 1860, 1870, 1880, and 1900 since the 1850 census did not consis- ntly ask for female occupations unless the female was head of household.

[23] Actually, the age distribution of family spouses was used at each date, but this did not eatly differ from the actual distribution of married women in the 1880 and 1900 censuses ich included data on marital status.

[24] The differences between average numbers of children 0–4 were tested among all six cupational groupings for each of the eight age groups. Tests were only made for the ferences within each age group, not between them. Of the 120 possible tests, only 21 were nificant. Five showed that farmers were significantly higher than certain other groupings at e same age, and 7 showed that professionals were significantly lower. Miners were signif- ntly different from other groups in only 7 out of 40 cases, and 3 of these related to farmers d professionals.

TABLE IV-8 Standardized Marital Child-Woman Ratios[a] Classified by Occupation of Family Head, Nativity and Literacy of Head and Spouse, and Residence and Wealth of Family. Lackawanna/Luzerne, Schuylkill, and Northumberland Counties, Pennsylvania, 1850-1880, 1900. (Families with Husband and Wife Present)[b]

	A[c]					B[e]				
	1850	1860	1870	1880	1900[d]	1850	1860	1870	1880	1900[d]
I. *Occupation of family head*										
a. Farmers	1272.2	1080.7	1087.0	900.7	883.0	1225.2	1055.6	1041.8	900.7	879.1
b. Laborers	1113.5	1193.7	1174.8	976.3	886.8	1067.2	1159.2	1123.8	976.3	873.4
c. Miners	1198.9	1174.6	1037.0	1180.5	1063.5	1162.7	1108.8	991.5	1180.5	1038.2
d. Manufacturing, etc.	1098.1	1201.2	1084.1	816.4	839.1	1056.6	1152.7	1043.2	816.4	824.7
e. Mercantile, etc.	1103.5	982.9	1015.4	889.5	800.6	1036.8	937.6	965.4	889.5	796.7
f. Professional and other	934.5	800.2	863.9	622.5	525.1	868.3	749.0	855.6	622.5	514.2
II. *Nativity of parents*										
a. Both native	1141.3	1079.8	997.6	831.3	806.8	1091.6	1036.7	955.9	831.3	795.7
b. One foreign-born	1235.0	1174.8	1195.5	1109.2	975.2	1180.1	1129.5	1140.0	1109.2	956.2
c. Both foreign-born	1098.6	1187.0	1107.7	1166.9	1023.4	1060.1	1143.8	1064.2	1166.9	1004.5
III. *Literacy of spouse*										
a. Illiterate	1203.3	1098.9	1110.7	1064.4	1002.5	1158.0	1056.1	1074.4	1064.4	983.8
b. Literate	1151.1	1063.5	1063.9	969.0	882.9	1102.6	1008.0	1016.9	969.0	869.3
IV. *Literacy of family head*										
a. Illiterate	1217.8	1068.8	1082.0	1172.2	1006.0	1173.5	1020.5	1039.3	1172.2	981.9
b. Literate	941.2	1070.0	1070.9	953.0	885.9	1101.8	1015.9	1026.0	953.0	872.4
V. *Residence*										
a. Rural	1161.1	1171.0	1085.0	1002.9	915.0	1115.1	1125.9	1036.4	1002.9	901.9
b. Urban	1061.6	990.4	1000.0	939.6	888.6	1012.7	940.7	1011.5	939.6	871.4
VI. *Wealth*										
a. 0-500	1112.7	1056.8	1079.4	——	——	1064.7	1000.9	1033.9	——	——
b. 501-1000	1238.9	970.0	1024.4	——	——	1179.6	929.4	977.8	——	——
c. 1001-2000	1220.6	1268.2	1140.2	——	——	1171.2	1246.3	1100.7	——	——
d. 2001-5000	1180.5	1211.9	1143.4	——	——	1157.6	1158.5	1102.1	——	——
e. 5000 +	1271.4	949.7	944.9	——	——	1172.6	892.1	904.4	——	——
VII. *Total*	1130.5	1136.0	1070.5	984.0	901.3	1093.3	1092.7	1070.5	984.0	901.3

Source: Sample of manuscript census enumerators' schedules.

[a]Children 0-4 per 1000 married women 15-49.

[b]Numbers of cases for each cell may be found in Table IV-7.

[c]Standardized to the overall age structure of married women at each date.

[d]For 1900, the sample also includes Susquehanna, Wayne, and Wyoming Counties.

All other occupational groups had dropped behind miners by 1880. A set of significance tests on the combinations of differences between the ratios for occupational groups suggests that the leading position of coal miners was statistically significant.[25] In 1900, the differentials by occupation of family head showed that the dominant position of miners continued. Overall, the higher fertility of miners' wives is strongly supported for 1880 and 1900 but not for 1850.

To account for the lower fertility among miners' wives in 1850, it must be remembered that the anthracite region was still fairly agrarian in 1850, that the fertility of farm wives was high relative to that of other occupational groups (see Tables IV-7 and IV-8, Section I), that a majority of miners and their wives were foreign born, and that, at this date, foreign-born families had significantly lower fertility than families with both parents native born. (See Table IV-8, Section II.) Many of the miners in 1850 were of English, Scottish, or Welsh origins, and this group had the lowest age-specific child–woman ratios among all nativity categories.[26] In the 1850 sample, 52.7% of all miners and mine workers were British born, and 88.0 % were foreign born in general, while, on the other hand, farmers and farm laborers were overwhelmingly native in origin (96.9%).

By 1880 the situation had changed. Miners had higher child–woman ratios, whether overall or standardized, relative to all other occupational groups. This occurred despite the altered ethnic composition of the group (only 57.6% foreign born in 1880 relative to 88.0% in 1850) *and* the declining fertility of native-born relative to foreign-born persons, which had been taking place steadily since 1850. Statistically, the differences between native- and foreign-born fertility ratios were significant. The decline of native-born fertility can be most clearly seen in Panel B of Table IV-8 where the child–woman ratios for families with both parents native born declined steadily from 1850. These ratios were standardized to the age structure of all married women in 1880 so the decline was not due to changing age structure. On the other hand, these standardized ratios for families with both parents foreign born actually increased between 1850 and 1880. The contaminating influence of infant and child mortality might tend to cause the ratios to rise over time if mortality of children was improving relative to that of adult women over time, but, as is shown subsequently, even compensating for this factor still leaves an increase in foreign-born fertility between 1850 and 1880. The situation in 1880 also prevailed in 1900, despite declines in the fertility of miners' wives and of the foreign born. Overall, fertility

[25] Of the 38 actual cases which could give tests of other groups relative to miners (there were two empty cells), 15 (or 39.5%) were significant. In contrast, of the remaining 73 actual cases, only 15 (or 20.5%) were significant.

[26] The nativity categories used were Pennsylvania born, other U.S. born, British (English, Scottish, Welsh), Irish, German, other. For 1900, categories for Italian and Slavic were added.

grouped by husband's occupation showed declines between 1850 or 1860 and 1900, with some widening of differentials. For example, miners–mine workers and laborers showed declines of 8.4% and 22.6%, respectively, between peak fertility and 1900. At the other extreme, professionals showed a decline of 48.5% between 1850 and 1900. This is a pattern similar to that in Britain in the late nineteenth and early twentieth centuries when class fertility differentials (measured by occupational groupings) widened before they narrowed. The higher-status groups experienced declines earlier and more rapidly (Innes, 1938). Parity data, available from the 1900 census and presented earlier in Chapter I (Table I-5, page 18), also showed higher fertility among older wives (i.e., wives aged 35–44 and 45–54) of miners and mine workers relative to wives in other occupational groups.

A number of the other variables in Table IV-7 by which child–woman ratios were classified showed notable trends and differentials over time. As observed before, native-born fertility was, after 1860, below foreign-born, and the relative differential tended to widen over time. Whereas the ratio of average children aged 0–4 per woman in families with one or both of the parents foreign born to the average for native parents was 1.14 in 1860, it had risen to 1.25 by 1900. In contrast, the rural–urban differential was small, although, with the exception of 1870, rural fertility was generally higher. This is perhaps due to the peculiar nature of coal mining, which kept the mining population in smaller places, closer to workable locations in the coal seams. This would tend to increase the representation in rural areas of nonagricultural population and, hence, reduce the contrast between rural and urban characteristics.

Along the other dimensions presented in Table IV-7, illiterate parents generally had higher fertility than parents who were literate, although literacy is a relatively poor index of education. This accords with what has generally been found for a number of developing countries (see Holsinger and Kasarda, 1976, pp. 156ff; Hawthorn, 1970, pp. 102–103), and it is notable that fertility declined more rapidly among literate than illiterate parents. (For wives, marital fertility declined 22.7% between 1860 and 1900 among literate wives and only 15.3% among illiterate wives.) The child–woman ratios classified by wealth showed little pattern in the cross-section and only mild decline up to 1870. Finally, working wives showed lower fertility than nonworking wives and both showed a downward trend after 1860. A striking feature of this particular dimension was the small number of wives who actually worked. In 1860, of *all* families with both husband and wife present, only 1.7% had working wives; and this was a high year. In 1870, 1880, and 1900 the percentages were .9, .4, and .8, respectively. This confirms the earlier prediction about the lack of employment of married women in mining areas. Because the absolute numbers of wives working was so small in the samples, this dimension was dropped from the multivariate analysis which follows.

As mentioned before, the marital child–woman ratios in Table IV-7 were ffected by changes in the age structure of married women over time and by ifferences in age structure across groups. Table IV-8 corrects for this with ge-standardized child–woman ratios. The results are really a series of eighted averages of the actual age-specific marital child–woman ratios, ith the weights in Panel B remaining the same throughout. Thus abstracting from the effects of age structure, Panel B indicates that the patterns of ecline remained and that, although the differentials were altered somehat, the basic picture was unchanged. The percentage declines from 1850 or 1860, if that was the peak) are given in Table IV-9. Fertility in urban reas was not consistently below rural fertility. Native-born fertility was, fter 1850, below foreign-born and declined more rapidly (27.1% between

TABLE IV-9 Relative Declines in Overall and Age-Standardized Marital Child-Woman Ratios. Pennsylvania Anthracite Counties, 1850-1900[a]

	Percentage decline from 1850[b] to 1900	
	Marital child-woman ratios	Standardized marital child-woman ratios[c]
I. Occupation of family head		
a. Farmers	35.7	28.2
b. Laborers	22.6	24.6
c. Miners	8.4	10.7
d. Manufacturing, etc.	32.2	28.4
e. Mercantile, etc.	26.8	23.2
f. Professional and other	48.5	40.8
II. Nativity of parents		
a. Both native	27.6	27.1
b. One foreign-born	29.1	19.0
c. Both foreign-born	12.9	12.9
III. Literacy of spouse		
a. Illiterate	15.3	15.0
b. Literate	22.7	21.2
IV. Literacy of family head		
a. Illiterate	11.4	16.3
b. Literate	23.1	20.8
V. Residence		
a. Rural	22.3	19.9
b. Urban	14.5	14.0
VI. Total	20.5	17.6

[a] Lackawanna/Luzerne, Schuylkill, and Northumberland counties for 1850-1880. For 1900 Susquehanna, Wayne, and Wyoming counties were added.

[b] From 1860 if that was higher than 1850.

[c] Standardized to the age structure of all married women in 1880.

1850 and 1900 as opposed to 19.0% where one parent was foreign born and 12.2% where both parents were foreign born). The fertility of illiterate parents remained higher and declined more slowly than that of literate parents. For example, standardized fertility of illiterate spouses declined only 17.2% between 1850 and 1900, but 21.2% for literate spouses. The declines for farmers and professionals were reduced but were still above average. And rural fertility declined faster than urban. Overall, changes in age structure accounted for only about 14% of the decline in the unstandardized marital child–woman ratio between 1860 and 1900. The major part was actual decline in age-specific marital child–woman ratios. In summary, over this period, standardized native-born fertility declined by more than foreign-born, rural by more than urban, fertility of literate parents by more than that of illiterate parents, and farmers, professionals, and manufacturing–craft–construction personnel by more than laborers and miners. All groups, however, experienced some declines. Also some expectations concerning mining populations and areas have been confirmed, especially the higher fertility among miners' wives and the lower fertility among working wives in mining areas.

Up to this point, trends and differentials in marital fertility have been discussed only along individual dimensions, such as residence, nativity, literacy, labor-force activity, or occupation. It would be convenient, however, to treat them simultaneously and assess the impact of one dimension or variable on fertility while controlling for the effect of the others. Since one approach to this problem, increasingly detailed cross-classifications, quickly runs into very small cell sizes, multiple regression analysis has been applied. Table IV-10 presents ordinary least squares (OLS) regressions using families from the censuses of 1850 through 1900 as the units of observation. The number of children aged 0–4 was used as the dependent variable, and only families with both the husband and wife present and with wife aged 15–54 were chosen. Panel II of Table IV-10 gives the magnitudes of the coefficients estimated by OLS and their level of significance, while Panel IV provides β-coefficients in an effort to assess the importance of each coefficient.[27] The variable for wealth was included only for the censuses of 1850, 1860, and 1870. Female labor-force participation was not included because of the extremely small numbers of employed wives in the sample.

In general, the most important variables were the age of spouse and the age of spouse squared. This particular nonlinearity was included because fertility is clearly parabolic with respect to age of woman. The negative on the "age of spouse squared" coefficient indicates the proper orientation (i.e.

[27] The β-coefficient is defined as the regression coefficient multiplied by the ratio of the standard error of the particular independent variable to the standard error of that dependent variable. It represents the amount of change in the dependent variable induced by a standardized change ceteris paribus of a particular independent variable.

TABLE IV-10 Regression Equations with Number of Children 0-4 as the Dependent Variable for Lackawanna/[illegible], and Northumberland Counties, Pennsylvania, 1850-1900. (Families with Both Husband and Wife Present, Women Aged 15-54)

	1850		1860		1870		1880		1900	
I. *Dependent variable*										
Children 0-4										
II. *Independent variables:*										
1. Constant	-1.6529	NC[a]	-1.5385	NC	-1.3975	NC	-.4212	NC	-.7816	NC
2. Literacy of spouse	.0571	n.s.[b]	.0437	n.s.	.0477	n.s.	.0525	n.s.	.0507	n.s.
3. Farmer	.2226	**	.2133	*	.1838	n.s.	.2215	n.s.	.2988	***
4. Laborer	.0610	n.s.	.2772	**	.1839	n.s.	.2244	n.s.	.3088	***
5. Miner	.2203	**	.2611	**	.0835	n.s.	.4179	***	.4710	***
6. Manufacturing, etc.	.0904	n.s.	.3222	***	.1461	n.s.	.1231	n.s.	.2622	***
7. Mercantile, etc.	.0929	n.s.	.1527	n.s.	.0660	n.s.	.2052	n.s.	.2395	**
8. Age of spouse	.1886	***	.1782	***	.1878	***	.1187	***	.1248	***
9. Age of spouse squared	-.0031	***	-.0030	***	-.0032	***	-.0022	***	-.0022	***
10. Wealth	-.0000	n.s.	-.0000	n.s.	-.0000	n.s.	NI[c]	NI	NI	NI
11. Native-born spouse	.0167	n.s.	-.0500	n.s.	-.2774	***	-.2792	***	-.1826	***
12. British-born spouse	-.2037	*	-.0742	n.s.	-.3391	***	-.2113	**	-.1798	**
13. Irish-born spouse	.0457	n.s.	.0452	n.s.	-.1019	n.s.	-.1328	n.s.	-.1049	n.s.
14. Residence	-.0671	n.s.	-.2109	***	-.0587	n.s.	-.1002	**	-.0873	**
III. *Other information*										
1. *N*	1615		1521		1348		1138		1695	
2. R^2 adjusted	.185		.180		.212		.193		.211	
3. *F* -ratio	29.166	***	26.647	***	28.929	***	23.595	***	38.760	***

β-Coefficients

	1850	1860	1870	1880	1900
IV. *Independent variables:*					
1. Constant	NC	NC	NC	NC	NC
2. Literacy of spouse	(.0264)[d]	(.0190)[d]	(.0203)[d]	(.0198)[d]	(.0201)[d]
3. Farmer	.1027	.0881	(.0659)	(.0760)	.1012
4. Laborer	(.0288)	.1249	(.0794)	(.1019)	.1211
5. Miner	.0844	.1091	.0384	.1965	.2350
6. Manufacturing, etc.	(.0405)	.1392	(.0625)	(.0469)	.1059
7. Mercantile, etc.	(.0286)	(.0517)	(.0238)	(.0770)	.1009
8. Age of spouse	1.9055	1.6938	1.8191	1.1593	1.2425
9. Age of spouse squared	-2.2207	-2.0186	-2.1950	-1.5352	-1.6191
10. Wealth	(-.0089)	(-.0003)	(-.0015)	NI	NI
11. Native-born spouse	(.0085)	(-.0263)	-.1460	-.1442	-.0940
12. British-born spouse	-.0644	(-.0234)	-.1274	-.0772	-.0548
13. Irish-born spouse	(.0182)	(.0202)	(-.0446)	(-.0546)	(-.0246)
14. Residence	(-.0300)	-.0819	-.0269	-.0482	-.0470

Source: Sample of manuscript census enumerators' schedules.

**p* < .1.
***p* < .01.
****p* < .05.

[a] NC = Not computed.
[b] n.s. = Not significant at least at a 10% level.
[c] NI = Not included.
[d] Figures in parentheses are β-coefficients not significant at least at a 10% level.

concave from below). In terms of a number of the factors mentioned earlier, education of the wife, as measured by literacy, had a depressing effect on fertility,[28] although the effect was consistently insignificant. Urban residence also had a negative impact on fertility, but the effect was significant only in 1860, 1880, and 1900.[29] The nativity of spouse demonstrated a relatively strong relationship to fertility. After 1850, the fact that a wife was native born predicted lower fertility for her, and this relationship became stronger and more significant over time. This is illustrated by the β-coefficient which became larger over time (at least up to 1880). The fact that the spouse was British born also had a depressing and increasingly significant effect over time, while the relationship for an Irish spouse was first positive, then negative, but never significant. Wealth showed a relatively unimportant negative impact on childbearing, but occupation showed some interesting relations.[30] The fact that the husband was engaged in mining had the most powerful and influential impact on fertility. The coefficients were significant with only one exception (1870) while the β-coefficients for miners were largest in 1880 and 1900 and second highest (behind that for farmers) in 1850. In other words, in 1880 and 1900 the head of the family being in mining was more likely to produce higher fertility than membership in any other occupational category—holding age, residence, literacy, and ethnicity constant.

Each equation was jointly significant (as measured by the F-ratio) and each explained about 20% of the variation in the number of children aged 0–4 per married woman. This particularly dependent variable, however, creates problems for the application of OLS regression. It is not continuous (i.e., it takes on only a maximum of five or six values) and is upper and lower bounded. Such limited-value dependent variables cause standard errors for the coefficients and, hence, hypothesis tests, to be incorrect and may lead to predicted values outside the boundaries of the variable. (See, for example, Goldberger, 1964, pp. 249–250; Nerlove and Press, 1973, pp. 1–9; Theil, 1971, pp. 628–636.) While the problem of incorrect standard errors has been shown to be less important in large data sets (Ashenfelter, 1969), the problems remain. One method of circumventing these difficulties is to apply a logit formulation, which uses iterative procedures to approximate the least-squares solution. The dependent variable has, in this case, a natural ordering that allows the technique to be applied. The method should produce

[28] Literacy was a dummy variable coded 0 = literate; 1 = illiterate. Thus, a positive sign indicates a depressing effect of literacy on fertility.

[29] Residence was also a dummy variable coded 0 = rural; 1 = urban. A negative sign thus points to a negative influence of urban residence on current fertility.

[30] The consistently positive signs for all occupation dummy variables implies that the omitted dummy variable, that for "Professional and other," had a large negative impact on fertility. At least one dummy variable must be omitted from any group in a regression equation in order to avoid perfect collinearity in the matrix of observations.

unbiased coefficients with standard errors such that the ratio of the coefficient to its standard error has the *t*-distribution.[31]

The results from the multinomial logit estimations are presented in Table IV-11. It is very encouraging that the results are quite similar to those given by the OLS equations in Table IV-10. One additional variable was added in 1900: whether the spouse was Slavic born. This had a slightly positive but insignificant effect on fertility. Perhaps the main result of the application of this logit model has been to show that OLS regression is indeed quite robust in the face of these departures from the assumptions of the general linear model.

An alternative, and in many ways more convenient, method of analysis, multiple classification analysis (MCA) was also applied.[32] This technique actually gives an adjusted child–woman ratio for each subcategory of a given predictor variable (e.g., "miners and mine workers" as a category of the predictor variable "occupation of family head"). This adjusted mean is in fact the category mean adjusted for the effects of other predictor variables. One of the advantages of this technique is that it allows coefficients for all the dummy variables to be estimated.

Results are presented only for the censuses of 1850 and 1900 in Tables IV-12 and IV-13. The categories are slightly different from those in Table IV-10, particularly with respect to nativity. Age squared was also not included. In this analysis, predictor variables must all be arranged into categories, rather than be allowed to remain in "continuous" form (e.g., age of spouse and wealth). The averages for each subcategory of the predictor categories are given in the second column. These are simply the child–woman ratios for women 15–54 classified by each category. The adjusted means (fourth column) are the child–woman ratios in each subcategory adjusted for the effect of all the other predictors. The ϵ^2 is the proportion of total variation "explained" by the whole predictor while the β^2 is a measure of the variation "explained" by the adjusted predictor. F-ratios give the statistical significance of the whole analysis (overall F-ratio) for each predictor (F-ratio for predictor). Finally, an overall measure of proportion of variation explained is given by the adjusted R-squared value (R^2_{adj}).

[31] The computer package from which this logit procedure was taken is the GLIM package. (For a brief description, see Nelder and Wedderburn, 1972.) A binomial error structure was assumed.

[32] It should be emphasized that this technique is also vulnerable to the problem of a limited value dependent variable. It also has other difficulties, particularly if interaction effects are present but not specified. If interaction effects are omitted, then, among other things, the percentage of variation "explained" will be biased downward. It does have the advantage of being insensitive to nonlinearities in the data (Andrews *et al.*, 1973, pp. 24–32). Multiple classification analysis and multiple regression are really very similar in the nature of the estimation methods. It is really the convenience of the result which should dictate the choice between one or the other.

TABLE IV-11 Multinomial Logit Regression Equations with Number of Children Aged 0-4 as the Dependent Variable for the Pennsylvania Anthracite Region, 1850-1900

	1850		1860		1870		1880		1900	
	Coefficient	*t*-ratio	Coefficient	*t*-ratio	Coefficient	*t*-ratio	Coefficient	*t*-ratio	Coefficient	*t*-ratio
I. *Dependent Variable*										
Children 0-4										
II. *Independent Variables*										
1. Constant	-5.794	-10.690 ***	-6.074	-9.844 ***	-7.677	-11.921 ***	-6.010	-9.246 ***	-7.671	-13.068 ***
2. Literacy of spouse	-.02844	-.369 n.s.[a]	.0678	.812 n.s.	.0235	.303 n.s.	.0522	.561 n.s.	.0964	.964 n.s.
3. Farmer	.3130	2.464 **	.3364	2.102 **	.2006	1.096 n.s.	.4336	1.740 *	.4197	2.607 **
4. Laborer	.1097	.864 n.s.	.3896	2.450 **	.1612	.932 n.s.	.4646	1.994 **	.3938	2.697 **
5. Miner	.3078	2.152 **	.3844	2.288 **	.0206	.118 n.s.	.6907	2.952 ***	.5977	4.331 ***
6. Manufacturing, etc.	.1344	1.067 n.s.	.4940	3.146 ***	.1264	.744 n.s.	.3033	1.259 n.s.	.3220	2.221 **
7. Mercantile, etc.	.1459	0.992 n.s.	.2611	1.554 n.s.	.0220	.125 n.s.	.4224	1.768 *	.2461	1.709 *
8. Age of spouse	.3422	10.694 ***	.3546	9.933 ***	.4926	12.795 ***	.3436	9.138 ***	.4459	12.560 ***
9. Age of spouse squared	-.0058	-12.094 ***	-.0060	11.304 ***	-.0082	-13.936 ***	-.0060	-10.492 ***	-.0077	-14.022 ***
10. Wealth	-.00003	-.265 n.s.	-.0000	-.111 n.s.	-.0000	-.193 n.s.	NI	NI	NI	NI
11. Native-born spouse	-.0026	-.020 n.s.	-.0856	-.823 n.s.	-.3625	-3.208 ***	-.4118	-3.050 ***	-.2575	-2.077 **
12. British-born spouse	-.3083	-1.903 *	-.1245	-.915 n.s.	-.4478	-3.245 ***	-.2974	-1.906 *	-.2586	-1.626 n.s.
13. Irish-born spouse	.03189	.226 n.s.	-.1843	-.163 n.s.	-.1058	-.833 n.s.	-.1758	-1.188 n.s.	-.0934	-.510 n.s.
14. Slavic-born spouse	NI[b]	NI	NI	NI	NI	NI	NI	NI	.0329	.242
15. Residence	-.0792	-1.031 n.s.	-.2751	-3.126 ***	-.1182	-1.481 n.s.	-.1373	-1.708 *	-.1116	-1.760 *
III. *Other Information*										
1. *N*	1615		1521		1348		1138		1695	

*$p < .1$ **$p < .05$ ***$p < .01$

[a]n.s. = Not significant at least at a 10% level.

[b][illegible]

TABLE IV-12 Multiple Classification Analysis--Ratios of Children Aged 0-4 per Married Woman Aged 15-54 by Selected Predictor Categories, Lackawanna, Luzerne, Schuylkill, and Northumberland Counties, Pennsylvania, 1850. (Married Women with Husbands Present)[a]

Predictor category	Category means	Number of cases	Adjusted means	ε^2	β^2	F-ratio for predictor
I. *Nativity*				.003	.002	2.066
1. Both parents native	1.0476	1030	1.0549			
2. One parent foreign	1.2447	94	1.2352			
3. Both parents foreign	1.0469	490	1.0333			
II. *Occupation of family head*				.005	.005	1.522
1. Farmer/farm laborer	1.0533	375	1.1347			
2. Laborer	1.0301	399	1.0463			
3. Miner/mine worker	1.1732	231	1.1043			
4. Manufacturing/crafts/ construction	1.0576	347	1.0133			
5. Mercantile/lodging/ transport/servant	1.1094	128	1.0823			
6. Professional/other	.9179	134	.9012			
III. *Literacy of Spouse*				.017	.006	13.626***
1. Illiterate	1.0859	326	1.1138			
2. Literate	1.0784	1238	1.0589			
3. Does not apply	.4000	50	.7001			
IV. *Residence*				.002	.0004	3.295
1. Rural	1.0804	1269	1.0687			
2. Urban	.9797	345	1.0225			
V. *Wealth*				.006	.002	1.805
1. $0-500	1.0568	1004	1.0335			
2. 501-1000	1.1382	152	1.1201			
3. 1001-2000	1.1513	152	1.1228			
4. 2001-5000	1.0882	136	1.1312			
5. 5001-10,000	.8519	108	1.0199			
6. 10,000 and over	.9677	62	1.0721			
VI. *Age of spouse*				.192	.187	54.508***
1. 15-19	.4667	60	.7962			
2. 20-24	1.1539	247	1.1558			
3. 25-29	1.4368	332	1.4346			
4. 30-34	1.3378	302	1.3222			
5. 35-39	1.1565	262	1.1401			
6. 40-44	.8391	174	.8218			
7. 45-49	.4609	128	.4302			
8. 50-54	.0642	109	.0309			

Source: Sample of census enumerators' manuscripts.

[a]Overall mean = 1.0589; N = 1614; overall F-ratio = 18.594***; R^2adjusted = .194.

**$p < .05$.

***$p < .01$.

ε^2 = Proportion of total variation from the overall mean "explained" by category;

β^2 = Variation "explained" by adjusted categories.

As should be expected, the adjusted R-squared value was about the same as for the regression equations (20%), and the multiple classification analyses for both 1850 and 1900 were also jointly significant (as measured by the overall F-ratio). The individual predictors, with the exception of the age of spouse, had rather low ϵ^2 and β^2 statistics and thus explained only a small portion of total variation. Besides age of spouse, only literacy of spouse was significant in 1850. For 1900, on the other hand, occupation of family head, nativity, and literacy of spouse were significant. As to the patterns of rela-

TABLE IV-13 Multiple Classification Analysis -- Ratios of Children Aged 0-4 per Married Woman Aged 15-54 by Selected Predictor Categories, Lackawanna, Luzerne, Schuylkill, Northumberland, Susquehanna, Wayne, and Wyoming Counties, Pennsylvania, 1900. (Married Women with Husbands Present)[a, b, c]

Predictor/Category	Category means	Number of cases	Adjusted means	ε^2	β^2	*F*-Ratio for predictor
I. *Nativity*				.008	.006	7.203***
1. Both parents native	.7565	949	.7626			
2. One parent foreign	.8594	249	.9058			
3. Both parents foreign	.9412	544	.9095			
II. *Occupation of Family Head*				.029	.011	10.271***
1. Farmer/farm laborer	.6615	195	.8493			
2. Laborer	.8505	281	.8209			
3. Miner/mine worker	1.0385	520	.9514			
4. Manufacturing/crafts/ construction	.7366	372	.7557			
5. Mercantile/lodging/ transport servant	.7687	268	.7814			
6. Professional/other	.5283	106	.5888			
III. *Literacy of spouse*				.003	.001	3.006**
1. Illiterate	.9250	280	.8132			
2. Literate	.8122	1459	.8320			
IV. *Residence*				.000	.001	.008
1. Rural	.8309	834	.8626			
2. Urban	.8271	908	.7980			
V. *Age of spouse*				.216	.216	68.343***
1. 15-19	.5000	42	.4710			
2. 20-24	1.0667	224	1.0609			
3. 25-29	1.2452	310	1.2568			
4. 30-34	1.1408	341	1.1355			
5. 35-39	.9725	291	.9676			
6. 40-44	.4605	215	.4599			
7. 45-49	.1389	180	.1580			
8. 50-54	.0144	139	.0064			

** $p < .05$

*** $p < .01$.

[a] Overall mean = .8289: N = 1742. Overall F-Ratio = 31.760***; R^2 = .238; R^2adjusted = .231.

[b] ε^2 = Proportion of variation from the overall mean "explained" by category.

[c] β^2 = Variation "explained" by adjusted categories.

tionships, the relatively high fertility of the native born in 1850 was confirmed, as was the dramatic alteration by 1900. The high fertility among farmers, once the effects of other variables were taken into account, was notable. Residence showed a higher fertility for rural relative to urban populations in both 1850 and 1900, but the differences were insignificant. Literacy gave higher fertility among illiterate spouses in 1850, but, in 1900, once the effects of other variables were controlled, literate spouses were more fertile.

For the consideration of occupation and fertility, it is notable that the unadjusted category means (child–woman ratios) placed miners and mine workers at the top rank of the six occupational groups in both 1850 and 1900. When taking account of age of wife, ethnicity, rural–urban residence, literacy of wife, and, in 1850, wealth, miners and mine workers dropped to second place in 1850, but in 1900 remained in first place. The rankings are as follows (from highest to lowest):

1850

Unadjusted	*Adjusted*
Miners, etc.	Farmers, etc.
Mercantile, etc.	Miners, etc.
Manufacturing, etc.	Mercantile, etc.
Farmers, etc.	Laborers
Laborers	Manufacturing, etc.
Professional and other	Professional and other

1900

Unadjusted	*Adjusted*
Miners, etc.	Miners, etc.
Laborers	Farmers, etc.
Mercantile, etc.	Laborers
Manufacturing, etc.	Mercantile, etc.
Farmers, etc.	Manufacturing, etc.
Professional and other	Professional and other

In all cases, the absolute value of the child–woman ratio for miners' families decreased "holding all other things constant" (i.e., for adjusted means). But the rank (relative value) was high in relation to the overall child–woman ratio and to the ratios for other occupational categories. Among other notable features of this analysis were the consistently low rankings achieved by the category "Professional and other" and the much higher ranking of farmers and farm laborers once the means were "adjusted" for the effects of other variables. For the other variables, it is notable that the regular pattern of age-specific child–woman ratios was little altered by "adjusting" for the effects of the other predictors considered here. (This is clear from comparing the unadjusted and adjusted means for the categories within age of spouse). There was also no regular pattern of convergence or divergence of the adjusted compared to the unadjusted child–woman ratios. Sometimes the adjusted ratios moved closer together and sometimes farther apart. In contrast to the regression results, the occupational subcategories from multiple classification, other than "Professional and other," did not have uniformly positive effects on child–woman ratios, when the effects of other variables were controlled.

The fact that occupation and nativity (which, as mentioned, was closely associated with occupation) became significant predictors in 1900 supports the hypothesis that a more typical pattern of occupational fertility differentials, reinforced by ethnic fertility differentials, had appeared by 1900. The particularly high fertility of native-born farmers was no longer the case in 1900 as it had been in 1850, and the factors influencing high fertility among miners came more fully into play. The distinctive pattern of 1900 had, in fact, already appeared by 1880, although the results are not presented here

Fertility Decline, Marriage, Mortality, and Migration, 1850—1900

Since the data available also permit some detailed discussion of fertility decline, it would seem useful to deal with that very important issue. The prolonged and steady fertility decline in the United States in the nineteenth century has received considerable attention. A number of studies have approached it from a descriptive demographic point of view. (See, for example, Grabill, Kiser, and Whelpton, 1958, pp. 12–24; Taeuber and Taeuber, 1958, Chap. 13; Thompson and Whelpton, 1933, Chap. VIII) while others have used a methodological perspective (Coale and Zelnik 1963). There has been substantial interest in rural fertility decline, particularly for the antebellum period (Yasuba, 1962; Forster and Tucker, 1972 Easterlin, 1971, 1976, 1977; Easterlin, Alter, and Condran, 1978; Leet, 1976 Potter, 1965). The emphasis in these studies has been on the relationship of fertility to land availability, inheritance, the costs and benefits of children and relative economic deprivation (see also Lindert, 1978). All of these authors (with the exception of Potter) have found land availability (a measured by several density ratios or by farm size) to be extremely importan in predicting fertility differentials at any point in time, whereas the degree o urbanization or industrialization, or the percentage of foreign born, wa found to be relatively unimportant. More recently, Vinovskis (1976a), ha suggested that literacy was an important, and unfortunately neglected factor in accounting for interstate fertility differentials for 1850 and 1860 fo states other than the American West. He also has pointed out that the degree of urbanization and the sex ratio were important and significan predictors. In the case of urbanization, while it was relatively less importan early in the nineteenth century in explaining fertility differentials, it tended to grow in importance over time.

Somewhat less attention has been paid to fertility in urban, industria America in the later nineteenth century. This was perhaps due to the fac that events in the latter part of the century conformed more to the conventional view of the demographic transition (Notestein, 1953; see also Coale 1974) in which urbanization and industrialization play an important role Nonetheless, it remains true that the sustained decline in fertility, which began at least in 1800, continued unabated after 1860 (see Table IV-6) and that this decline came increasingly from urban and industrial populations

One important study in this area was that of Okun (1958), who examined the roles of a number of factors relating to the decline of white birth ratios in the United States between 1870 and 1950. In general, he found that the proportion and age composition of women in childbearing ages and the proportion of foreign-born women among white women of childbearing age were unimportant in accounting for the decline. Further, the redistribution of the white population from rural to urban areas also accounted for only a small part of the reduction in fertility. The resulting conclusion was that "changes in the [white] birth ratio are ascribable primarily to changes in the reproductive pattern of persons living in fixed environmental subdivisions—rural and urban, rural–farm and rural non-farm, large city and small [Okun, 1958, p. 15]."

Given the continued fertility decline that occurred after 1860, increasing urbanization and continuing industrialization, and the rapidly changing ethnic and occupational composition of the population, it would seem appropriate to analyze demographic change in urban, industrial America.

Fertility decline can be viewed from two perspectives, period rates and cohort fertility. In this section, most attention will be paid to the former, although there is some evidence on the latter. Two main dimensions of differential fertility will be emphasized: rural–urban and native–foreign born. This is because these two dimensions can be readily discussed in terms of both overall and marital fertility and because they are of intrinsic interest themselves for mining and industrial areas.[33]

Some insight into the process of fertility decline by cohorts is available from the 1900 census, which asked questions on children ever born, children surviving, and number of years married. Table IV-14 presents average parities by age for total women and married women with husband present, and by marital duration for all married women. The increasing parities of women of completed or nearly completed fertility experience confirm the results provided by the child–woman ratios. There is, however, a tendency for very old women to understate true parity and so the results for women older than, say, 60 (i.e., born before 1840) or having been married more than about 40 years (i.e., married before 1860) are less certain. Also, the smaller cell sizes for women of advanced ages or marital durations also contribute to large sampling variation. Nonetheless, the results confirm the pattern of decline and also show that, as Okun noted for the whole United States, declines were taking place within both rural and urban areas and also among both native- and foreign-born populations. Completed family size was always higher among the foreign born relative to the native born and was often, though not consistently, higher among rural than among urban women. In addition, the higher fertility in the anthracite counties relative to the whole United States is confirmed by results tabulated from the 1910 U.S.

[33] Occupational-fertility differentials, especially those pertaining to husbands' occupation, are a marital-fertility phenomenon.

TABLE IV-14 Average Number of Children Ever Born for Total Women, Married Women, and Married Women with Husbands Present, Classified by Nativity and Residence. Seven Pennsylvania Counties,[a] 1900

Year of birth/age	Total women		Native-born women		Foreign-born women		Rural women		Urban women	
	Average children ever born	N^b	Average children ever born	N^b	Average children ever born	N^b	Average children ever born	N^b	Average children ever born	N^b
Total women										
1881-1885 (15-19)	.064	514	.060	449	.094	64	.065	246	.063	268
1876-1880 (20-24)	.666	494	.569	376	.975	118	.845	219	.524	275
1871-1875 (25-29)	1.788	453	1.559	340	2.478	113	1.913	196	1.693	257
1866-1870 (30-34)	3.144	422	2.627	268	4.045	154	3.281	185	3.038	237
1861-1865 (35-39)	4.284	355	3.556	232	5.658	123	4.060	167	4.484	188
1856-1860 (40-44)	4.451	264	4.049	182	5.342	82	4.264	125	4.619	139
1851-1855 (45-49)	5.134	216	4.401	147	6.696	69	5.196	107	5.073	109
1846-1850 (50-54)	5.534	204	4.950	121	6.386	83	5.631	103	5.436	101
1841-1845 (55-59)	5.621	132	4.854	82	6.880	50	5.681	72	5.550	60
1836-1840 (60-64)	5.540	87	4.511	45	6.643	42	5.525	40	5.553	47
1831-1835 (65-69)	5.978	89	5.510	51	6.605	38	5.023	43	6.870	46
1830 and earlier (70+)	5.387	106	5.453	64	5.286	42	5.406	64	5.357	42
Married women with husbands present										
1881-1885 (15-19)	.683	41	.793	29	.417	12	.684	19	.682	22
1876-1880 (20-24)	1.439	223	1.403	149	1.514	74	1.589	112	1.288	111
1871-1875 (25-29)	2.468	310	2.296	213	2.845	97	2.479	142	2.458	168
1866-1870 (30-34)	3.749	347	3.373	204	4.287	143	3.893	159	3.628	188
1861-1865 (35-39)	4.884	292	4.229	179	5.920	113	4.601	143	5.154	149
1856-1860 (40-44)	5.000	215	4.559	143	5.875	72	4.713	108	5.290	107
1851-1855 (45-49)	5.376	178	4.750	124	6.815	54	5.516	91	5.230	87
1846-1850 (50-54)	6.221	140	5.837	86	6.833	54	6.145	69	6.296	71
1841-1845 (55-59)	6.057	88	5.472	53	6.943	35	6.432	44	5.682	44
1836-1840 (60-64)	6.000	47	5.308	26	6.857	21	6.200	25	5.773	22
1831-1835 (65-69)	6.111	36	5.381	21	7.133	15	5.444	18	6.778	18
1830 and earlier (70+)	5.846	26	5.824	17	5.889	9	5.263	19	7.429	7
Year and duration of marriage (married women)										
1896-1900 (0-4)	.945	328	.948	231	.938	97	1.000	146	.901	182
1891-1895 (5-9)	2.497	400	2.304	260	2.857	140	2.528	193	2.469	207
1886-1890 (10-14)	4.122	328	3.670	206	4.885	122	4.149	154	4.098	174
1881-1885 (15-19)	5.250	248	4.710	145	6.010	103	4.851	121	5.630	127
1876-1880 (20-24)	5.513	197	4.977	133	6.625	64	4.968	95	6.020	102
1871-1875 (25-29)	5.659	164	4.972	109	7.018	55	5.795	78	5.535	86
1886-1870 (30-34)	6.344	128	5.875	80	7.125	48	6.222	72	6.500	56
1861-1865 (35-39)	6.686	70	5.902	41	7.793	29	6.842	38	6.500	32
1856-1860 (40-44)	6.566	45	6.038	26	7.263	19	6.704	27	6.333	18
1851-1855 (45-49)	7.348	23	5.182	11	9.333	12	5.600	10	8.692	13
1850 and earlier (50+)	7.200	20	7.389	18	5.500	2	6.400	15	9.600	5

Source: Sample of enumerators' manuscripts.

[a] Lackawanna, Luzerne, Northumberland, Schuylkill, Susquehanna, Wayne, and Wyoming.
[b] Number of women.

census (U.S. Bureau of the Census, 1943a, b). For example, as may be seen in Table IV-15, white women aged 45–54 in 1900 had an average parity of 4.830 children ever born for the whole United States and 5.329 in the anthracite counties. The only area in which the United States exceeded the average for the anthracite region in this comparison was in the fertility of native white women. The United States averages were below those for the Pennsylvania counties for urban, rural, and foreign-born populations.

Parity data would have been more useful if the U.S. census had asked the question earlier in the nineteenth century. Unfortunately, the U.S. census first asked this question only in 1890. The data from this census were never adequately tabulated and neither were those from 1900. If more detailed information on fertility is desired, it is necessary to use own-children methods. The overall and standardized marital child–woman ratios presented in the last section pointed to fertility declines, at least after 1860, for the total population along several dimensions of the population, including occupation of husband, nativity of parents, literacy of parents, residence, labor-force status of wife, and, to a limited degree, wealth. These child–woman ratios do suffer, as has been noted, a number of deficiencies. Furthermore, as Tables IV-6 and IV-14 show, there were also declines in overall (as opposed to marital) fertility. It is of interest to evaluate the role of marriage in the decline of overall fertility.

In order to overcome some of the shortcomings of age-specific child–woman ratios the next step is to estimate age-specific fertility rates. These provide a basis for analysis of the age pattern of fertility decline which, in turn, is an important clue to the ability of couples to control fertility within marriage over time. In order to convert age-specific child–woman ratios to age-specific fertility rates, three types of correction factors are required.

TABLE IV-15 Average Parities for White Women Aged 45-54 in 1900. United States and Seven Pennsylvania Counties.[a] By Residence and Nativity

Women aged 45-54 in 1900	Total women	Rural	Urban	Native	Foreign
United States	4.830	4.724[b]	4.316	4.805	5.836
Anthracite counties	5.329	5.410	5.248	4.649	6.526

Source: U.S. Bureau of the Census, *U.S. Census of Population 1940*, "Differential Fertility, 1940 and 1910. Fertility for States and Large Cities," (Washington, D.C.: G.P.O., 1943). Sample of enumerators' schedules from the 1900 census.

[a] Lackawanna, Luzerne, Schuylkill, Northumberland, Susquehanna, Wayne and Wyoming.

[b] Rural nonfarm.

1. An adjustment for children not living with their mothers at the time of the census
2. An adjustment for the underenumeration of children relative to adult women in the childbearing ages
3. A correction for mortality of children and women over the previous 5 years (since children aged 0–4 are being used here).

The procedure used here closely follows the methods suggested by Grabill and Cho (Grabill and Cho, 1965; Cho, Grabill, and Bogue, 1970, Chap. 9).[34]

The first adjustment, the correction for children not living with their mothers at the time of the census, is relatively straightforward. It is simply the ratio of total children aged 0–4 in the census sample to total *own* children aged 0–4 tabulated from the same sample. This correction is applied to women of all ages because there is no information on which to base age-specific corrections. Although there is some evidence that the incidence of missing own-children may vary with age of mother (Cho, Grabill, and Bogue, 1970, pp. 318–321), the error introduced is not likely to be too great. The error will tend somewhat to understate fertility of younger women and overstate that of older women. Separate corrections were done for rural and urban populations, but not for native- and foreign-born, since most of the children of foreign-born women were actually native born and therefore it would be impossible to compute correct adjustment ratios. The overall upward adjustments of the child–woman ratios ranged from 8.4% in 1850 to 2.5% in 1900.

The second adjustment, for relative underenumeration of children, is considerably more difficult. What is required is a factor for underenumeration of all children aged 0–4 and a series of factors for women in the reproductive ages.[35] Fortunately, there are some relatively reliable estimates of underenumeration for the total United States by Coale and Zelnik (1963) going back to 1880. The Coale and Zelnik estimates for the total white population were compared to the census population at each date, and correction factors were calculated. This was done for 1880 and 1900. For 1860, an estimate was given for underenumeration of white females aged 0–4 (Coale and Zelnik, 1963, Table 5). All the 1880 underenumeration relationships were then scaled upward to the higher underenumeration of children in 1860, and this was taken as the underenumeration for 1860. For

[34] These methods might be termed standard or conventional own-children methods, since the adjustments for mortality, underenumeration, and children missing are made to grouped data after they are tabulated. An alternative, when data on children ever born and children surviving are available, is to construct fertility histories for individual women based on various probabilities of death and children missing, women missing, etc. This is considerably more complex initially, but once the fertility histories are reconstructed, the estimates may be produced simply by tabulation. For a discussion, see Avery (1976).

[35] Ideally, there should be a correction for children for all ages of women 15–49, but it would seem extremely unlikely that this sort of information could be acquired without special surveys.

1850 and 1870, a round number of 10% (similar to the 1860 magnitude) was assumed for underenumeration of children and the 1880 underenumeration of adult females was scaled proportionately. The results are presented, along with an explanation, in Table IV-16. The relative underenumeration of children was then derived by dividing the correction factor for children by the correction factor for the appropriate age group of women. It should be noted that a number of assumptions have been made. First, it is assumed that the level and age pattern of underenumeration in the anthracite counties was similar to that for the white population of the whole United States. Second, the patterns for 1850, 1860, and 1870 were assumed similar to that for 1880, and only the levels were assumed to be slightly different. Third, underenumeration was taken to be roughly constant between 1850 and 1870 and quite similar to that for 1880. All these assumptions may be questioned, but it can be stated, in defense of these procedures, that there is relatively little information on underenumeration. One other set of estimates of underenumeration, those of Grabill, Kiser, and Whelpton (1958, pp. 410–411), gave only factors for children aged 0–4 and used less reliable methods

TABLE IV-16 Assumed Correction Factors for Underenumeration of Young Children and White Females, 15-49

	1900[a]	1880[b]	1870[c]	1860[d]	1850[c]
Total children (White) 0-4	1.071	1.091	1.10	1.101	1.10
White females					
15-19	1.021	1.001	1.009	1.010	1.009
20-24	.991	.978	.986	.987	.986
25-29	1.058	1.067	1.075	1.077	1.075
30-34	1.101	1.161	1.170	1.172	1.170
35-39	1.101	1.153	1.162	1.164	1.162
40-44	1.170	1.170	1.189	1.181	1.180
45-49	1.164	1.164	1.174	1.175	1.174

Source: Ansley J. Coale and Melvin Zelnik, *New Estimates of Fertility and Population in the United States: A Study of Annual White Births From 1855 to 1960 and of Completeness of Enumeration in the Censuses From 1880 to 1960*, (Princeton, N.J.: Princeton University Press, 1963), Tables 5, 14-17.

[a] 1900. Taken directly from Coale and Zelnik.

[b] 1880. Taken from Coale and Zelnik up to age 25-29. For ages 30-34 and 35-39, the correction factors for these ages for 1890 were assumed. For ages 40-44 and 45-49, the correction factors for 1900 were assumed.

[c] 1870 and 1850. Assumed as 1.10 for children 0-4. Then the 1880 factors were scaled upward by the ratio 1.10/1.091 [i.e. (C_{0-4}) 1880/ (C_{0-4}) 1870].

[d] 1860. For ages 0-4, assumed the same as for white females in Coale and Zelnik (page 59). The 1880 factors were scaled upward by the ratio 1.101/1.091 .

than Coale and Zelnik.[36] Therefore the Coale and Zelnik figures, as adjusted, were assumed to be better than any set of more arbitrary assumptions about underenumeration.[37]

The third set of adjustments, corrections for mortality of young children and adult women, also posed problems. The state of knowledge concerning mortality in nineteenth-century America is far behind that for fertility. There is some disagreement as to trends and levels of nineteenth-century American mortality. Thompson and Whelpton, for instance, state that there was a decline in mortality throughout the nineteenth century with an acceleration after the 1880s (Thompson and Whelpton, 1933, p. 230). Taeuber and Taeuber thought there was little improvement before about 1850 but substantial and continuous mortality decline thereafter (Taeuber and Taeuber, 1958, p. 269). Vinovskis (1972), working with Massachusetts data, saw little change in mortality between 1800 and 1860, while Edward Meeker (1972) believes that changes in public health, nutrition, and levels of living were only able to lower death rates after 1880. They are supported in this by Higgs (1973), who has tried to estimate death rates for rural America after 1870. On the other hand, Coale and Zelnik (1963, pp. 7–9, 168–170) assumed a linear decline in mortality from 1850 to 1900, constructing a model life system and anchoring it on the Jacobson Massachusetts–Maryland life table of 1850 (Jacobson, 1957). The Jacobson table has, however, recently been called into question as having been based on rather defective data and also because Massachusetts suffered a severe cholera outbreak in the summer of 1849 (Vinovskis, 1976b).

Given the uncertainty regarding mortality in the later nineteenth century, another approach was adopted. Based on work with the 1900 census sample

[36] Grabill, Kiser, and Whelpton used forward survival of children 0–4 and compared them with children 10–14 in the next census. For native whites aged 0–4 they found the following correction factors:

1850	1.109
1860	1.087
1870	1.131
1880	1.066
1900	1.020

The results for 1860, 1880, and 1900 are considerably lower than those by Coale and Zelnik, whose methods were more sophisticated. Coale and Zelnik used a set of model life tables which they specified; Grabill, Kiser, and Whelpton did not specify their life tables and may have used contemporary tables of less certain reliability (Grabill, Kiser, and Whelpton, 1958, Appendix A). Also Coale and Zelnik used data already adjusted for age misstatement and averaged several sets of backward survival estimates. The only improvement suggested by the findings of Grabill, Kiser, and Whelpton might have been to assume a higher correction factor for 1870, a census of less reliability than those of 1860 or 1880. But much of the heavy undercounting took place in the South, and Pennsylvania was probably about as well enumerated in 1870 as it was in 1850 or 1860.

[37] The population of the anthracite region was almost entirely white so that there is virtually no bias introduced by the fact that the Coale and Zelnik estimates only applied to the white population of the United States.

and a 5% sample of the 1865 New York State census for seven counties, child mortality was estimated for total, rural–urban, and native–foreign-born populations[38] (Haines, 1977c). Roughly, the technique used was to "survive" the age structure of own children backward until they just equaled the number of children ever born. Only the children of younger women (aged 20–34) were chosen in order to minimize the number of older children who would have left the home. The vector of survival probabilities can be chosen from some one parameter family of model life tables. The Coale and Demeny West model tables were used in this instance (Coale and Demeny, 1966). The model table allowed the child mortality estimates to be extended to adult mortality. In this way, direct estimates of mortality were derived for the Pennsylvania anthracite region for the period just prior to the census of 1900.

These own-children mortality estimates were then compared to death rates calculated from census questions on deaths in the year previous to the census. The conclusion was that death rates from census mortality data for the ages 5–9, 10–14, and 15–19 were close to the estimates derived from the own-children methods. Therefore, death rates for these ages were calculated for Pennsylvania for the census years[39] 1850, 1860, 1870, 1880, 1890, and 1900 for males, females, and both sexes together. West model life tables were fitted to each death rate for each sex (and both sexes together) at each date. The tables for each sex at each date were then averaged to obtain a single mortality estimate at each date. Annual mortality data for Massachusetts were examined to determine if any of the census years had abnormally high mortality relative to the preceding several years, and, as it turned out, none did with the exception of 1850. (See, for example, U.S. Bureau of the Census, 1975, Series B-193.) (This is only a very crude check, however, since the correlation of annual mortality fluctuations between Massachusetts and Pennsylvania was certainly not perfect.) The main point was to determine if any of the years were exceptional. They were not and so, with the exception of the census year 1850, the results give a good idea of the trend in mortality in Pennsylvania from 1860. Even for the census year 1850, however, it might be argued for the purposes of making own-children fertility estimates that the high mortality of the year prior to the census is the most important one, even if it is not typical. The slight rise in child–woman ratios between 1850 and 1860 (see Table IV-6) might indeed have been due to the effects of the 1849 cholera epidemic. Thus, using census year mortality data is appropriate for making fertility estimates.

These Pennsylvania mortality estimates were probably a good approximation of mortality in the anthracite counties. Bearing in mind that the West

[38] For foreign-born populations, child mortality was related to the nativity of the mother, not of the child.

[39] The census year was essentially June 1 of the previous year to May 31 of the year in which the census took place.

TABLE IV-17 Expectation of Life at Birth Fitted from Census Mortality Data and Data on Own Children to West Model Life Tables.[a] Pennsylvania Anthracite Region, 1850-1900. By Sex, Residence, and Nativity

$\mathring{e}_0$	Total	Rural	Urban	Native	Foreign
Total					
1850	44.87	45.46	41.71	45.84	41.30
1860	47.15	47.69	43.75	48.33	43.54
1870	43.91	44.87	41.43	45.38	40.16
1880	44.34	45.39	42.18	45.80	39.48
1900	46.49	47.96	45.11	50.14	41.42
Male					
1850	41.88	42.42	38.92	42.91	38.66
1860	45.12	45.62	41.85	46.32	41.73
1870	41.87	42.79	39.51	43.27	38.30
1880	42.73	43.74	40.65	44.24	38.13
1900	45.02	46.52	43.68	48.74	40.05
Female					
1850	47.82	48.47	44.47	48.69	43.86
1860	49.02	49.60	45.50	50.17	45.20
1870	45.97	46.98	43.38	47.51	42.04
1880	45.99	47.08	43.75	47.47	40.92
1900	48.02	49.47	46.62	51.61	42.86

Source: U.S. Bureau of the Census, *U.S. Census of Population for 1850...1860...1870...1880...1900.* Sample of enumerators' manuscripts for the Pennsylvania anthracite counties (Lackawanna, Luzerne, Schuylkill, Northumberland, Susquehanna, Wayne, and Wyoming) for 1900 and for seven New York counties (Allegheny, Dutchess, Montgomery, Rensselaer, Steuben, Tompkins, and Warren) from the New York State census of 1865.

[a] For 1900, data on the age distribution of surviving own children and data on children ever born and children surviving were used to fit West model life tables. [See Ansley J. Coale and Paul Demeny, *Regional Model Life Tables and Stable Populations* (Princeton, N.J.: Princeton University Press, 1966)].

For 1850-1880, census death rates were calculated for Pennsylvania for males, females, and both sexes together for the ages 5-9, 10-14, and 15-19. West model life tables were fitted to these rates and the tables averaged. The rural/urban and native/foreign-born differentials were estimated on the basis of differentials calculated directly in 1900 and on differentials also calculated directly from a census sample for seven New York counties in 1865. Relative differentials were interpolated between these two points and applied to the overall mortality level at each date.

model life table values for the anthracite counties fitted from child survivorship and the age distribution of own children to women 20–34 actually applied not to the census year 1900 but to the period roughly 1885–1900 and comparing these values (an $\mathring{e}_0$ for males of 45.02 years and for females of 48.02 years) to these for the census years 1890 and 1900 for Pennsylvania ($\mathring{e}_0$ values of 45.54 and 45.02 for males in 1890 and 1900, respectively, and of 50.87 and 49.23 for females), it was decided that mortality levels were sufficiently close to assume that the levels for 1850 through 1880 were the same in the anthracite counties as in Pennsylvania as a whole. This avoided further arbitrary assumptions about mortality differentials between the anthracite counties and the state, and seems plausible, since the anthracite egion was not greatly different from the rest of the state in terms of general haracteristics during the period 1850–1880. The results are presented in Table IV-17.

With respect to mortality differentials for rural–urban and native–oreign-born populations, no direct evidence on differentials was available rom deaths in the census year. The census sample from 1900 for the nthracite counties did, however, yield mortality estimates for these sub-groups, and the estimates for that date in Table IV-13 are taken directly rom those estimations. Additional information was also provided by the 1865 New York State census sample mentioned above.[40] The relative ural–urban and native–foreign-born differentials in the anthracite counties n 1850 and 1860 were assumed to be the same as those in the New York sample for 1865. The differentials were linearly interpolated between 1860 and 1900 to gain values for 1870 and 1880. The relative differentials were then combined with the shares of the population which were rural and urban or native and foreign in order to derive estimates whose weighted average would be the overall average expectation of life at birth.[41]

The mortality levels, as given by expectations of life at birth in Table IV-17, indicate some fluctuations in mortality over time and no real trend

[40] See Haines (1977c) for additional information on the samples and procedures.

[41] The relative differentials were defined as [$(\mathring{e}_0)$ rural/$(\mathring{e}_0)$ urban] and [$(\mathring{e}_0)$ native/$(\mathring{e}_0)$ foreign] and they had assumed values of:

Year	Rural/ urban (r_1)	Native/ foreign (r_2)
1850	1.090	1.110
1860	1.090	1.110
1870	1.083	1.130
1880	1.076	1.160
1900	1.063	1.211

The same values were assumed to hold for males, females, and the total population. The means of calculation for 1850–1880 were

$$(\mathring{e}_0)\text{ rural} = \frac{(\mathring{e}_0)\text{ total}}{w_1 + (w_2/r_1)},$$

$$(\mathring{e}_0)\text{ urban} = \frac{(\mathring{e}_0)\text{ total}}{w_1 r_1 + w_2},$$

$$(\mathring{e}_0)\text{ native} = \frac{(\mathring{e}_0)\text{ total}}{w_3 + (w_4/r_2)},$$

$$(\mathring{e}_0)\text{ foreign} = \frac{(\mathring{e}_0)\text{ total}}{w_3 r_2 + w_4},$$

where w_1 is the share of population which was rural, w_2 is the share of population which was urban, w_3 is the share of population which was native, w_4 is the share of population which was foreign, and where r_1 and r_2 are given as above.

before 1900. If, however, the 1860 census-year death rates might be regarded as unusually low then a pattern can be seen of no mortality trend prior to 1880 with some improvement thereafter. The 1860 census-year mortality was not especially low, however, when compared to some recent estimates for Massachusetts (Vinovskis, 1972) of 46.4 years for males and 47.3 years for females and for seven New York counties for the approximate period 1850-1865 (Haines, 1977c) of 45.8 years for males and 48.9 years for females. If then, the 1860 data were more typical and 1850 data were affected by a worse than average year for disease, then the pattern appears to have been one of deteriorating conditions after 1860 followed by some improvement after 1880.[42] This would have been true, if the assumptions that have been made are reasonable, of the rural and native-born populations as well. Thus the effects of increasing urbanization and higher mortality among the foreign born were not solely to blame for the trend. One conclusion can be drawn from these census mortality data, however. There were still considerable year to year fluctuations in mortality prior to 1880. To the extent that reduction in annual variation in mortality is an important step in human control of mortality, then it appears that progress was not too great up to 1880.

Some caveats must be kept in mind vis-à-vis these mortality figures. First, they are based on a large series of assumptions, although every effort has been made to stay as close to the data as possible. Second, they are only based on single years of experience in an era when mortality had significant annual fluctuations. More relevant for constructing own-children fertility estimates, the results do not cover the full 5-year period prior to the census. They do, however, cover the most recent and, from the viewpoint of child mortality, most important year. Third, the extension to adult mortality is less certain and, in fact, rests on the appropriateness of the choice of West model tables. Previous work with the Pennsylvania and New York data indicates that the West model gives adequate results (Haines, 1977c). On the other hand, mining populations do suffer peculiar mortality patterns, particularly among adult males as a result of occupationally related respiratory problems (see Chapter I.) Also, the pattern of mortality change over time within the West model system seems to be somewhat different than that which occurred in the United States in the late nineteenth century (Haines, 1977d.) This did not prove to be a great problem, however, and so the West model table estimates were kept.[43]

[42] The mortality level for the census year 1850 was not remarkably high, however, relative to mortality for 1870 and 1880. This was especially true for females.

[43] As the level of mortality improved over the late nineteenth century in the United States, infant and child mortality improved relative to adult mortality. This conclusion was based on an analysis of existing United States life tables from the late nineteenth century and some specifically constructed for the analysis. Using a Brass two-parameter model life table system using logits of life table ℓ_x values (see Carrier and Hobcraft, 1971, pp. 7–13, Appendix I; Brass,

To return to the original discussion of fertility, the correction factors for own children not with their mothers, for relative underenumeration, and for mortality of children and adult women were applied to age-specific child–woman ratios for the total, rural, urban, native-, and foreign-born population. The resulting total fertility rates (TFRs), gross reproduction rates (GRRs), and net reproduction rates (NRRs) are presented in Table IV-18. The estimated age-specific fertility rates, derived by interpolating the corrected age specific child–woman ratios to the required 5-year age categories, are presented in Table IV-19.[44] Relative declines in the age-specific rates, TFRs, and NRRs (with 1846–1850 = 100) are given in Table IV-20, and a comparison of the levels and decline of the TFR in the anthracite region with TFRs for the white population of the United States may be seen in Table IV-21.

Several points are worthy of note. One is that there was indeed a continuous and substantial decline in TFRs, NRRs, and age-specific fertility in the anthracite region between the late 1840s and the late 1890s. In this respect the results from the marital child–woman ratios are confirmed. Declines in overall fertility exceeded declines in the marital child–woman ratios, however. Between 1846–1850 and 1896–1900, for example, the overall marital child–woman ratio declined 20.5% while the TFR declined 32.6% and the NRR declined 28.4%. These declines were also not the result of fertility reductions only among the urban and native-born population, since rural and the foreign-born populations also experienced declines in TFRs and NRRs. The declines were not the same for all groups, however, as the urban population showed a slower relative decline than the rural (i.e., 21.0% for urban NRR versus 25.6% for rural NRR from 1846–1850 to 1896–1900). Since rural fertility was higher than urban fertility, some convergence of the relative differentials is implied by this, and Table IV-22 shows that this was

1975, Chapters XII–XIV, XVIII), life tables from the late nineteenth-century United States were compared for level and shape, with the 1900–1902 U.S. registration state table (Glover, 1921) as the standard table. The same was done for Coale and Demeny West model tables for Levels 9 through 15, which was the range of levels comparable to the actual tables. The result was that, as the level of mortality improved over the late nineteenth century in the United States, infant and child mortality improved relative to adult mortality. In the West model tables, up to about Level 13, precisely the opposite occurs. Adult mortality improves relative to child mortality. Some sensitivity analysis indicates that the differences introduced using the West model versus a Brass model were not very large. The West model tables performed quite well. For further details see Haines (1977d).

[44] The interpolation procedure, using Sprague osculatory multipliers as suggested by Grabill and Cho (1965, pp. 58–69), does introduce a certain amount of error, but mostly at the extreme ages (i.e., 15–19 and 45–49). The TFR (call it TFR_1) derived from the interpolated data (in Table IV-19) was never more than 1 or 2% away from the TFR derived directly from the corrected but uninterpolated child–woman ratios (call it TFR_2). Rather than apply the same overall adjustment to the interpolated age-specific birth rates at all ages, based on the ratio (TFR_2/TFR_1), it was decided to leave the age-specific rates as is, since the rates 20–24 to 40–44 are likely to be quite accurate.

TABLE IV-18 Total Fertility Rates, Gross and Net Reproduction Rates for the Pennsylvania Anthracite Region,[a] 1846/1850 - 1896/1900. By Residence and Nativity

Total fertility rate	Total	Rural	Urban	Native-born	Foreign-born
1846/1850	6.4196	6.6037	5.8025	6.2049	7.0350
1856/1860	6.3100	6.5086	5.3357	5.7841	7.0578
1866/1870	5.6958	6.0732	5.5594	5.3263	6.8278
1876/1880	5.4106	5.7226	5.2044	4.5137	7.1263
1896/1900	4.3281	4.5648	4.1438	3.5807	6.0636
Gross reproduction rate					
1846/1850	3.1315	3.2213	2.8305	3.0268	3.4317
1856/1860	3.0780	3.1749	2.6028	2.8215	3.4428
1866/1870	2.7784	2.9625	2.7119	2.5982	3.3306
1876/1880	2.6393	2.7915	2.5387	2.2018	3.4762
1896/1900	2.1113	2.2267	2.0214	1.7467	2.9578
Net reproduction rate					
1846/1850	2.0263	2.1111	1.7127	1.9842	2.0579
1856/1860	2.0504	2.1465	1.6090	1.9206	2.1475
1866/1870	1.8494	1.9142	1.6958	1.7105	1.9719
1876/1880	1.6700	1.7325	1.5438	1.4318	1.9908
1896/1900	1.4506	1.5706	1.3526	1.2750	1.8481

Source: Data are from a sample of enumerators' manuscripts. Rates were computed from data on own children corrected for mortality, children not with their mothers, and relative underenumeration of children.

[a] Lackawanna/Luzerne, Schuylkill, and Northumberland counties for 1850-1880. For 1900, Susquehanna, Wayne, and Wyoming counties were also included.

indeed precisely the case. Convergence of the differentials in TFR had mostly taken place by 1866–1870, however, and the differential for NRR even widened between 1876–1880 and 1896–1900. The situation for native- and foreign-born populations was quite different. There was a decline in foreign-born fertility, to be sure, but the declines in TFR and NRR were far less than those for the native born. Since foreign-born fertility exceeded that for native-born women throughout the period considered, a divergence of the relative differentials is implied and is what is found in Table IV-22. The NRR for foreign-born women was a mere 3.7% in excess of that for the native born in 1846–1850, while the differential had risen to almost 45% by 1896–1900. A portion of the explanation for this must lie in the fact that the composition of the foreign-born population was gradually shifting from groups with lower fertility in their area of origin (like the English, Scots, Welsh) to groups with progressively higher fertility in their homelands (e.g., the Irish and later the Slavic populations of Central and Eastern Europe). (See Table IV-3, page 92.) This contrasts with Spengler's findings for Massachusetts, for example, which found, over the period 1856–1860 through 1896–1900, that native- and foreign-born fertility declined about equally (Spengler, 1930, p. 33). Compensating for the greater proportion of younger married women among the foreign born, Spengler actually found that marital fertility among native-born women held relatively constant after

TABLE IV-19 Age-Specific Birth Rates for the Pennsylvania Anthracite Region,[a] 1846/1850 - 1896/1900. By Residence and Nativity of Mother. (per 1000 Women)

	Ages of women						
	15-19	20-24	25-29	30-34	35-39	40-44	45-49
Total							
1846/1850	74.5	256.8	308.3	268.0	222.8	129.4	39.7
1856/1860	80.0	260.4	309.7	258.1	206.5	132.2	30.3
1866/1870	66.6	226.9	291.1	268.2	192.0	89.4	16.6
1876/1880	69.8	226.3	276.6	233.6	179.2	97.1	8.7
1896/1900	59.4	180.9	225.8	215.3	138.5	44.4	8.1
Rural							
1846/1850	77.2	264.8	313.3	274.5	229.2	134.1	45.0
1856/1860	83.7	265.1	319.6	273.1	211.1	131.0	33.0
1866/1870	59.7	266.0	342.3	254.0	189.9	95.2	19.4
1876/1880	71.3	237.6	306.3	247.0	180.1	107.9	2.8
1896/1900	72.2	197.4	232.3	230.6	139.4	45.0	5.5
Urban							
1846/1850	66.8	233.1	294.2	243.5	199.0	114.6	18.3
1856/1860	63.0	236.6	269.6	280.0	176.6	137.8	10.6
1866/1870	67.2	219.6	275.1	275.2	203.8	71.2	9.2
1876/1880	68.0	190.2	265.9	274.8	157.0	74.0	22.1
1896/1900	49.1	167.7	221.4	203.1	137.2	44.1	10.8
Native-born							
1846/1850	69.6	252.2	304.2	260.4	208.0	121.0	42.9
1856/1860	75.3	244.5	289.4	223.4	178.2	134.1	26.8
1866/1870	56.0	224.6	289.1	242.2	170.5	71.7	22.0
1876/1880	64.5	207.0	234.4	197.3	138.5	58.2	13.0
1896/1900	48.8	152.9	185.8	162.9	115.9	48.4	6.7
Foreign-born							
1846/1850	94.1	267.9	316.3	284.7	254.0	159.5	41.4
1856/1860	95.3	293.6	339.4	292.4	234.3	136.0	35.9
1866/1870	79.6	305.3	368.4	284.2	220.8	109.4	11.3
1876/1880	102.0	307.6	375.4	295.1	217.2	129.9	6.4
1896/1900	94.7	270.5	316.8	310.1	184.4	35.4	11.0

Source: Data are from a sample of enumerators' manuscripts. Rates were computed from age-specific child-woman ratios corrected for mortality, children not with their mothers, and relative under-enumeration of children.

[a] Lackawanna/Luzerne, Schuylkill, and Northumberland counties for 1850-1880. For 1900, Susquehanna, Wayne, and Wyoming counties were also included.

about 1875 while that of foreign-born women declined. This, as we shall see (Tables IV-23 and IV-24), was decidedly not the case for either the native-born nor the foreign-born population of the anthracite region.

The fertility declines in the anthracite region from the late 1840s through at least the late 1880s took place without significant improvement in mortality. There may indeed have been some deterioration in mortality over the period to 1880 (see Table IV-17, page 122). If such was the case, the experience in this region would contrast sharply to the conventional view of the demographic transition in which mortality decline (particularly infant- and child-mortality decline) is supposed to precede, or at least accompany, the fertility transition. (For a statement of this see Taylor, Newman, and

TABLE IV-20 Relative Declines in Total Fertility Rates, Net Reproduction Rates, and Age-Specific Fertility Rates. Pennsylvania Anthracite Region,[a] 1846/1850-1896/1900. By Residence and Nativity of Mother (1846/1850 = 100)

	Age of women								
	15-19	20-24	25-29	30-34	35-39	40-44	45-49	TFR	NRR
Total									
1846/1850	100	100	100	100	100	100	100	100	100
1856/1860	107	101	100	96	93	102	76	98	101
1866/1870	89	88	94	100	86	69	42	89	91
1876/1880	94	88	90	87	80	75	22	84	82
1896/1900	80	70	73	80	62	34	20	67	72
Rural									
1846/1850	100	100	100	100	100	100	100	100	100
1856/1860	108	100	102	100	92	98	73	98	102
1866/1870	77	100	109	92	83	71	43	92	91
1876/1880	92	90	98	90	79	80	6	86	82
1896/1900	94	74	74	84	61	34	12	69	74
Urban									
1846/1850	100	100	100	100	100	100	100	100	100
1856/1860	94	101	92	115	89	120	56	93	94
1866/1870	100	94	93	113	102	62	49	96	99
1876/1880	102	82	90	113	79	64	117	90	90
1896/1900	73	72	75	84	69	38	57	71	79
Native-born									
1846/1850	100	100	100	100	100	100	100	100	100
1856/1860	108	97	95	86	86	111	62	93	97
1866/1870	80	89	95	93	82	59	51	86	86
1876/1880	93	82	77	76	67	48	30	72	72
1896/1900	70	61	61	63	56	40	15	57	64
Foreign-born									
1846/1850	100	100	100	100	100	100	100	100	100
1856/1860	101	110	107	103	92	85	87	101	104
1866/1870	85	114	116	100	87	69	27	97	96
1876/1880	108	115	119	104	85	81	15	101	97
1896/1900	101	101	100	109	73	22	27	86	90

Source: See Table IV-19.

[a] Lackawanna/Luzerne, Schuylkill, and Northumberland counties for 1850-1880. For 1900, Susquehanna, Wayne, and Wyoming counties were also included.

Kelly, 1976; T. P. Schultz, 1976b. See also Notestein, 1953.) This supports the notion that the fertility decline in the anthracite region was voluntary and not biological, unless the deteriorating mortality conditions were also accompanied by increased fecundity impairment.

Comparison of trends in TFR for the anthracite region with those for the white population of the United States as a whole shows that the anthracite counties had overall fertility substantially in excess of that for the United States (see Table IV-21). The relatively high proportion of foreign born plus an above-average representation of high-fertility occupational groups (farmers, in the early part of the period, as well as miners and laborers throughout) contributed to this. In addition, prior to 1880 the relative gap widened, since relative rates of decline were higher for whites in the United States

TABLE IV-21 Total Fertility Rates for the Pennsylvania Anthracite Region[a] and for the White Population of the United States, 1846/1850 - 1896/1900

Period	Pennsylvania anthracite counties			United States white population			
	TFR	Relative decline	Average annual decline in preceding decade (% p.a.)	TFR	Relative decline	Average annual decline in preceding decade (% p.a.)	Ratio of TFR in the anthracite counties to TFR for the United States
1846/1850	6.4196	100	NA[b]	5.42[c]	100	NA[b]	1.18
1856/1860	6.3100	98	-0.17	5.26	97	-0.40	1.20
1866/1870	5.6958	89	-1.02	4.54	84	-1.47	1.25
1876/1880	5.4106	84	-0.51	4.31	80	-0.52	1.26
1896/1900	4.3281	67	-1.12	3.63	67	-0.86	1.19

Source: (a) Pennsylvania anthracite counties, see Table IV-18. (b) United States, white population: Ansley J. Coale and Melvin Zelnik, *New Estimates of Fertility and Population in the United States* (Princeton, N.J.: Princeton University Press, 1963), Table 2. For 1856/1860 and later, the TFR's were taken as arithmetic averages of the single year TFR's.

[a] Lackawanna/Luzerne, Schuylkill, and Northumberland counties for 1850-1880. For 1900, Susquehanna, Wayne, and Wyoming counties were also added.

[b] NA = Not available.

[c] 1848/1852.

TABLE IV-22 Relative Fertility Differentials by Residence and Nativity. Pennsylvania Anthracite Region,[a] 1846/1850 - 1896/1900

Period	Total fertility rate		Net reproduction rate	
	Rural/urban	Foreign-born/native	Rural/urban	Foreign-born/native
1846/1850	1.138	1.134	1.233	1.037
1856/1860	1.220	1.220	1.334	1.118
1866/1870	1.092	1.282	1.129	1.153
1876/1880	1.100	1.579	1.122	1.390
1896/1900	1.100	1.693	1.161	1.449

Source: See Table IV-18.

[a] Lackawanna/Luzerne, Schuylkill, and Northumberland counties for 1850-1880. For 1900, Susquehanna, Wayne, and Wyoming counties were also included.

than for the population of the anthracite counties. After 1880, the gap began to narrow; but it should be added that this was mostly due to accelerated decline among the native-born population (−1.26% per annum of the period 1876–1880 to 1896–1900 for native-born TFR versus −0.81 for the foreign-born TFR).

With respect to the age pattern of the fertility decline, it is apparent in Table IV-20 that decreases in age-specific birth rates took place at all ages of women (except among younger foreign-born women). The declines were relatively greatest among older women (i.e., women aged 35–39 and 40–44), which is a strong indication of voluntary family limitation. A pattern in which older women begin to increase spacing and terminate childbearing at an early age has been characteristic of several developing areas which have experienced fertility declines, such as Taiwan and Hong Kong, and was apparently the case in eastern Pennsylvania in the late nineteenth century as well.

One of the difficulties in discussing fertility decline from the perspective of overall fertility is, of course, that the effects of changes in marital fertility and proportions married are confounded. In order to assess the importance of changes in marital fertility, age-specific marital fertility rates were calculated and are presented in Table IV-23. These rates might be slightly too high, since no correction for illegitimate births was made; but, it must be added, ascertaining illegitimacy from these census manuscripts is very difficult. In the sample, virtually no children were recorded as illegitimate or as the children of never-married women. So, for all practical purposes, all fertility was recorded as within marriage and is taken here as such. Table IV-24 gives the proportions married among women of various ages at each

TABLE IV-23 Age-Specific Marital Fertility Rates for the Pennsylvania Anthracite Region,[a] 1846/1850 - 1896/1900. By Residence and Nativity of Mother. (per 1000 Married Women)

	Ages of women						
	15-19	20-24	25-29	30-34	35-39	40-44	45-49
Total							
1846/1850	661.3	469.5	370.5	306.9	243.1	148.1	46.9
1856/1860	866.7	450.4	359.6	280.7	237.6	150.6	34.7
1866/1870	781.7	407.6	336.4	301.6	214.7	103.4	20.5
1876/1880	879.5	421.4	360.0	260.5	200.9	115.4	10.2
1896/1900	663.7	382.6	317.5	256.2	166.4	52.5	9.5
Rural							
1846/1850	701.2	471.3	371.1	309.0	252.1	152.7	51.7
1856/1860	899.8	450.4	365.4	298.9	241.1	148.0	37.9
1866/1870	649.5	463.0	392.2	285.8	213.2	109.8	22.6
1876/1880	820.0	436.2	386.1	277.7	205.3	127.0	3.3
1896/1900	845.8	372.9	311.3	271.2	163.8	51.1	6.3
Urban							
1846/1850	554.0	466.2	371.6	297.6	210.1	133.3	24.8
1856/1860	708.8	447.6	339.7	302.9	210.2	165.4	12.0
1866/1870	1169.3	428.0	324.2	309.1	225.2	83.1	13.6
1876/1880	1062.5	365.1	373.2	300.0	170.0	90.1	25.7
1896/1900	526.4	392.2	323.4	243.9	168.2	54.2	12.9
Native-born							
1846/1850	719.2	472.7	375.2	300.6	231.2	142.0	51.2
1856/1860	1026.6	429.4	342.6	252.3	216.9	158.0	29.8
1866/1870	709.3	433.6	354.6	278.9	199.2	86.9	28.5
1876/1880	1121.6	386.2	316.9	224.8	160.7	74.2	15.8
1896/1900	684.7	364.5	282.0	208.0	148.2	59.4	7.8
Foreign-born							
1846/1850	479.1	459.3	357.7	321.3	260.6	173.0	46.9
1856/1860	587.7	489.3	384.2	307.6	256.6	149.2	43.4
1866/1870	656.7	471.8	396.3	311.5	237.5	130.4	13.3
1876/1880	552.5	567.1	441.3	317.8	234.9	147.3	7.2
1896/1900	432.9	420.0	364.8	329.3	198.8	38.2	12.8

Source: Age-specific total fertility rates from Table IV-19 were multiplied by the ratio of total to married women at each census. Married women of each age were estimated for 1850, 1860, and 1870. Data on total and married women by age were obtained from samples of enumerators' manuscripts. No correction for illegitimate births was made.

[a] Lackawanna/Luzerne, Schuylkill, and Northumberland counties for 1850-1880. For 1900, Susquehanna, Wayne, and Wyoming counties were also included.

date. These were used in calculating the age-specific marital fertility rates (Table IV-23).[45] For the years 1850, 1860, and 1870, when marital status was not given directly in the census, the number of married women was estimated by adjusting the number of spouses in families upward by the ratio of married women to spouses at various ages in 1880 and 1900.

A comparison of the relative roles of marital fertility versus proportions married in determining age-specific overall fertility may be seen in Table IV-25. In this table, which takes 1846–1850 as the base year, the declines in

[45] The total age-specific fertility rates in Table IV-19 were multiplied by the inverse of the proportion married to obtain the age-specific marital fertility rates.

TABLE IV-24 Proportion of Women Married at Ages 15-19 through 45-49. By Residence and Nativity. Pennsylvania Anthracite Region, 1846/1850 - 1896/1900[a]

	Total proportion married	Rural proportion married	Urban proportion married	Native proportion married	Foreign-born proportion married
Women 15-19					
1846/1850	.1126	.1101	.1206	.0968	.1964
1856/1860	.0923	.0930	.0889	.0733	.1622
1866/1870	.0852	.0919	.0575	.0789	.1212
1876/1880	.0794	.0870	.0640	.0575	.1846
1896/1900	.0895	.0854	.0933	.0713	.2188
Women 20-24					
1846/1850	.5469	.5618	.5000	.5335	.5833
1856/1860	.5782	.5886	.5286	.5694	.6000
1866/1870	.5567	.5745	.5130	.5180	.6471
1876/1880	.5370	.5447	.5210	.5359	.5424
1896/1900	.4728	.5294	.4275	.4195	.6441
Women 25-29					
1846/1850	.8321	.8842	.7917	.8108	.8843
1856/1860	.8612	.8746	.7937	.8447	.8834
1866/1870	.8654	.8728	.8485	.8162	.9296
1876/1880	.7683	.7933	.7125	.7396	.8507
1896/1900	.7112	.7462	.6846	.6589	.8684
Women 30-34					
1846/1850	.8732	.8885	.8182	.8664	.8862
1856/1660	.9195	.9173	.9286	.8855	.9505
1866/1870	.8893	.8889	.8902	.8684	.9124
1876/1880	.8969	.8896	.9167	.8777	.9286
1896/1900	.8404	.8503	.8326	.7831	.9416
Women 35-39					
1846/1850	.9167	.9091	.9474	.8947	.9747
1856/1860	.8689	.8756	.8400	.8217	.9130
1866/1870	.8943	.8907	.9048	.8559	.9297
1876/1880	.8919	.8774	.9254	.8621	.9245
1896/1900	.8324	.8512	.8158	.7821	.9274
Women 40-44					
1846/1850	.8738	.8782	.8600	.8521	.9219
1856/1860	.8778	.8848	.8333	.8487	.9118
1866/1870	.8649	.8671	.8571	.8913	.8387
1876/1880	.8413	.8496	.8214	.7848	.8818
1896/1900	.8453	.8810	.8129	.8087	.9268
Women 45-49					
1846/1850	.8471	.8710	.7576	.8374	.8824
1856/1860	.8723	.8710	.8824	.8989	.8269
1866/1870	.8104	.8584	.6750	.7722	.8514
1876/1880	.8571	.8559	.8605	.8243	.8875
1896/1900	.8545	.8716	.8378	.8533	.8571

Source: Samples of census enumerators' manuscripts. For 1850, 1860, and 1870, proportions married were estimated from married women in families adjusted upward on the basis of the ratio of total married women to married women in families in 1880 and 1900.

[a] Lackawanna/Luzerne, Schuylkill, and Northumberland counties for 1850-1880. For 1900, Susquehanna, Wayne, and Wyoming counties were also included.

	Total[b]			Rural			Urban			Native			Foreign-born		
	(a)	(b)	(c)	(a)	(b)	(c)	(a)	(b)	(c)	(a)	(b)	(c)	(a)	(b)	(c)
Women 20-24															
1846/1850	100	100	100	100	100	100	100	100	100	100	100	100	100	100	100
1856/1860	101	96	106	100	96	105	101	96	106	97	91	107	110	107	103
1866/1870	88	87	102	100	98	102	94	92	103	89	92	97	114	103	111
1876/1880	88	90	98	90	93	97	82	78	104	82	82	100	115	123	93
1896/1900	70	81	86	74	79	94	72	84	86	61	77	79	101	91	110
Women 25-29															
1846/1850	100	100	100	100	100	100	100	100	100	100	100	100	100	100	100
1856/1860	100	97	103	102	98	104	92	91	100	95	91	105	107	107	100
1866/1870	94	91	104	109	106	103	93	87	107	95	94	101	116	111	105
1876/1880	90	97	92	98	104	94	90	100	90	77	84	91	119	123	96
1896/1900	73	86	85	74	84	88	75	87	86	61	75	81	100	102	98
Women 30-34															
1846/1850	100	100	100	100	100	100	100	100	100	100	100	100	100	100	100
1856/1860	96	91	105	100	97	103	115	102	113	86	84	102	103	96	107
1866/1870	100	98	102	92	92	100	113	104	109	93	93	100	100	97	103
1876/1880	87	85	103	90	90	100	113	101	112	76	75	101	104	99	105
1896/1900	80	83	96	84	88	96	84	82	102	63	69	90	109	102	106
Women 35-39															
1846/1850	100	100	100	100	100	100	100	100	100	100	100	100	100	100	100
1856/1860	93	98	95	92	96	96	89	100	89	86	94	92	92	98	94
1866/1870	86	88	98	83	85	98	102	107	96	82	86	96	87	91	95
1876/1880	80	83	97	79	81	96	79	81	98	67	70	96	85	90	95
1896/1900	62	68	91	61	65	94	69	80	86	56	64	87	73	76	95
Women 40-44															
1846/1850	100	100	100	100	100	100	100	100	100	100	100	100	100	100	100
1856/1860	102	102	100	98	97	101	120	124	97	111	111	100	85	86	99
1866/1870	69	70	99	71	72	99	62	62	100	59	61	105	69	75	91
1876/1800	75	78	96	80	83	97	64	68	96	48	52	92	81	85	96
1896/1900	34	35	97	34	33	100	38	41	95	40	42	95	22	22	100
Women 45-49															
1846/1850	100	100	100	100	100	100	100	100	100	100	100	100	100	100	100
1856/1860	76	74	103	73	73	100	56	48	116	62	58	107	87	92	94
1866/1870	42	44	96	43	44	99	49	55	89	51	56	92	27	28	96
1876/1880	22	22	101	6	6	98	117	104	114	30	31	98	15	15	101
1896/1900	20	20	101	12	12	100	57	52	110	15	15	102	27	27	97

Source: See Tables IV-19, 23, 24.

[a]Lackawanna/Luzerne, Schuylkill, and Northumberland counties for 1850-1880. For 1900, Susquehanna, Wayne, and Wyoming counties were also included

[b](a) = Births per woman (1850=100). (b) = Births per married woman (1850=100).
(c) = Married women as a proportion of total women (1850=100). (a) = (b) · (c).

overall fertility rates from 1846–1850 are found in the columns labeled (a) and may be compared to the relative declines in marital fertility in the columns headed (b) and the relative changes in proportions married in the columns headed (c).[46] As may be seen from these results, the reductions in overall fertility between 1846–1850 and 1896–1900, particularly among older women, originated largely in reductions in marital fertility. At the end of the period (1896–1900), there was some tendency among younger women (i.e., ages 20–24 and 25–29), to experience declines in proportions married as well as reductions in marital fertility. Nevertheless, the general impression is of substantial downward adjustment of marital fertility. Among the foreign born this was concentrated at ages above 35, but among the native born, and also to a certain degree among the rural and urban populations, this took place at all ages.

The importance of relative decreases in marital fertility among older women is illustrated in Table IV-26, which gives marital fertility at all ages above 20–24 as a percentage of the rate at age 20–24. This points to a decline of marital fertility among older women relative to peak marital fertility (which occurs, with but one exception, at age 20–24).[47] Thus, it appears quite clear that fertility control within marriage was occurring, most probably assisted by contraception, over the latter half of the nineteenth century. This control, while most vigorously exercised by older women, was also increasingly resorted to by younger, married, native-born women. One indicator of control among older women is the trend in the age of the mother at the birth of the last child. An approximation of this, measured by the difference in the mother's age and the age of the youngest child present, is set forth in Table IV-27 for women aged 40–44 and 45–49. The trend was generally downward for total women and for the rural–urban and native–foreign-born subgroups, indicating progressively earlier termination of childbearing among older women. After 1860 and 1870 foreign-born women generally completed childbearing later than native-born women, but there was little difference between the rural and urban women.

In an attempt to assess the magnitude of fertility control within marriage, a series of "m" values, based on the model fertility schedules of Coale and Trussell were calculated (Coale and Trussell, 1974). These "m" values try to measure the departure of an actual fertility schedule from a hypothetical, average natural marital-fertility schedule.[48] A value of zero for "m" indicates

[46] Fertility rates among women aged 15–19 are excluded from this table because of the high degree of unreliability of marital fertility rates of these ages.

[47] The age group 15–19 is excluded.

[48] The expression used for the model fertility rates is

$$r(a)/n(a) = Me^{m \cdot v(a)},$$

where $r(a)$ is the marital fertility at age(s) a in the population studied, $n(a)$ is the average natural fertility at age(s) a, M is a scale factor, and $v(a)$ is the "model" coefficient of departure from

TABLE IV-26 Relation of Age-Sepcific Marital Fertility Rates to the Rate at Age 20-24. Pennsylvania Anthracite Region, 1846/1850 - 1896/1900[a]

	Age					
	20-24	25-29	30-34	35-39	40-44	45-49
Total						
1846/1850	100	79	65	52	32	10
1856/1860	100	80	62	53	33	8
1866/1870	100	83	74	53	25	5
1876/1880	100	85	62	48	27	2
1896/1900	100	83	67	43	14	2
Rural						
1846/1850	100	79	66	53	32	11
1856/1860	100	81	66	54	33	8
1866/1870	100	85	62	46	24	5
1876/1880	100	89	64	47	29	1
1896/1900	100	83	73	44	14	2
Urban						
1846/1850	100	80	64	45	29	5
1856/1860	100	76	68	47	37	3
1866/1870	100	76	72	53	19	3
1876/1880	100	102	82	47	25	7
1896/1900	100	82	62	43	14	3
Native-born						
1846/1850	100	79	64	49	30	11
1856/1860	100	80	59	50	37	7
1866/1870	100	82	64	46	20	7
1876/1880	100	82	58	42	19	4
1896/1900	100	77	57	41	16	2
Foreign-born						
1846/1850	100	78	70	57	38	10
1856/1860	100	79	63	52	30	9
1866/1870	100	84	66	50	28	3
1876/1880	100	78	56	41	26	1
1896/1900	100	87	78	47	9	3

Source: Table IV-23.

[a]Lackawanna/Luzerne, Schuylkill, and Northumberland counties for 1850/1880. For 1900, Susquehanna, Wayne, and Wyoming counties were also included.

no deviation from average natural marital fertility, while a positive value indicates some reduction in marital fertility below a natural level. A negative value represents a marital fertility rate in excess of average natural fertility. For populations with fertility close to replacement (i.e., net reproduction rate equal to 1), "m" values may range up to 2.0 or more (Coale and Trussell, 1974, p. 189). Ideally, when "m" values are calculated for all the age-specific fertility rates for a particular group in a population at a particular date, they will come out roughly equal. When they were calculated individually in this way, the "m" values were found to vary a great deal and even become negative, especially at older ages of women. Therefore, another procedure, that suggested more recently by Coale and Trussell

natural fertility at age(s) a, and where $v(a) < 0$. The value "m," which varies between 0 and about 2.4, should give the degree of departure from natural fertility. Natural fertility is defined as fertility not subject to deliberate and intentional limitation.

TABLE IV-27 Estimated Mean Age at Last Birth. Married Women with Children and with Husband Present. By Residence and Nativity.[a] Pennsylvania Anthracite Region, 1850-1900[b]

	Total	Rural	Urban	Native	Foreign
Women 40-44					
1850	37.1	37.2	36.7	37.4	36.4
1860	36.7	36.8	35.7	37.3	36.0
1870	36.2	36.2	36.4	35.3	37.2
1880	36.0	36.3	35.1	34.7	36.7
1890	34.1	33.7	34.5	33.9	34.5
Women 45-49					
1850	40.6	40.9	39.3	40.7	40.1
1860	39.4	39.7	37.3	39.4	39.4
1870	38.1	38.5	36.8	37.7	38.6
1880	37.5	37.1	38.3	37.3	37.6
1900	35.8	36.8	34.9	35.1	37.5

Source: Sample of census enumerators' manuscripts.

[a]Estimated as the difference between the age of the mother and the age of the youngest child.

[b]Lackawanna/Luzerne, Schuylkill, and Northumberland counties for 1850-1880. For 1900, Susquehanna, Wayne, and Wyoming counties were also included.

(1978) has been applied.[49] It estimates average values of "m" and the scale factor M.

The results, presented in Table IV-28, indicate that there was a rather low average degree of intramarital fertility control in the 1840s and 1850s, but that this began to increase in the late 1860s and had substantially increased by the late 1890s. This is shown by the rising level of "m." The native-born population demonstrated the most regular pattern of departure from natural fertility, while that for the foreign born was much less regular and, in 1850, even had average fertility at ages 25–29 through 40–44 which was greater than that expected by the average natural fertility level. (This is implied by the negative "m" value.) By 1900, the anthracite region had achieved values of "m" somewhat above those for developing nations today (which range from near zero to .5 or so) but well below those for developed countries (Coale and Trussell, 1974, p. 189). The M value represents the ratio of age-specific marital fertility at ages 20–24 to average natural fertility at that same level. As may be seen in Table IV-28, the population of the Pennsyl-

[49] The procedure may simply be explained as follows: The expression for the model fertility schedules $r(a)/n(a) = Me^{m \cdot v(a)}$ is converted to natural logarithms $\ln\ [r(a)/n(a)\ ] = \ln M + m \cdot v(a)$. Since $n(a)$ and $v(a)$ are given by Coale and Trussell and since $r(a)$ is known for the population studied, it is possible to estimate "m" and $\ln M$ by ordinary least squares regression. The fit is generally improved by using only the age groups 20–24 through 40–44, since errors are generally more prevalent in the original data for the extreme age groups.

TABLE IV-28 Deviation of Age-Specific Marital Fertility from Natural Fertility as Measured by Coale-Trussel "m" Values. Pennsylvania Anthracite Region, 1846/1850 - 1896/1900 [a]

	M	"m"	Mean Square Error
Total			
1846/1850	0.921	0.110	.0084
1856/1860	0.870	0.075	.0130
1866/1870	0.870	0.243	.0007
1876/1880	0.867	0.237	.0070
1896/1900	0.898	0.645	.0104
Rural			
1846/1850	0.920	0.085	.0085
1856/1860	0.890	0.086	.0082
1866/1870	0.974	0.326	.0028
1876/1880	0.905	0.217	.0098
1896/1900	0.892	0.645	.0156
Urban			
1846/1850	0.930	0.207	.0103
1856/1860	0.844	0.035	.0243
1866/1870	0.922	0.367	.0077
1876/1880	0.873	0.360	.0092
1896/1900	0.903	0.643	.0069
Native-born			
1846/1850	0.933	0.155	.0092
1856/1860	0.805	0.032	.0259
1866/1870	0.935	0.419	.0001
1876/1880	0.823	0.463	.0011
1896/1900	0.779	0.544	.0006
Foreign-born			
1846/1850	0.880	-0.020	.0115
1856/1860	0.957	0.124	.0083
1866/1870	0.975	0.212	.0033
1876/1880	0.109	0.207	.0145
1896/1900	0.913	0.424	——

SOURCE: Calculated from data in Table IV-23 using the methods developed by Coale and Trussell (1974, 1978).

[a]Lackawanna/Luzerne, Schuylkill, and Northumberland counties for 1850-1880. For 1900, Susquehanna, Wayne, and Wyoming counties were also included.

vania anthracite region, especially the rural and foreign-born groups, had fertility at ages 20–24 quite close to natural fertility. For the foreign born for 1876–1880 it was even above natural fertility levels. The mean square error in Table IV-28 is an indication of the goodness of fit of the relationship which estimated "m" and M. According to Coale and Trussell (1978, p. 204), a mean square error of .005 is a mediocre fit whereas that of .01 is rather poor. By these standards, a number of the "m" values estimated in Table IV-28 must be regarded rather tentatively. On the other hand, the anthracite mining region experienced rather late marriage (see below) and rather high fertility. In these circumstances, marital fertility might be quite high in the age group 20–24, because of bridal pregnancies. The decline relative to a natural fertility pattern between the age groups 20–24 and 25–29 is really quite steep and not at all typical of the model. This may account, in part, for the relatively poor fit. Overall, however, there is evidence of deliberate family limitation within marriage certainly occurring by the 1860s and much stronger by the late 1890s.

Earlier, proportions of females married at various ages were examined to ascertain the role of marriage in changes in overall age-specific fertility (Tables IV-24 and IV-25). Some additional inquiries were made into marriage using census data. In Table IV-25, it seemed that changes in proportions married accounted for relatively little of the decline in overall fertility. Table IV-29, which tabulates the mean age of marriage for various age cohorts of women from data on duration of marriage in the 1900 census, tends to bear this out. For the most recent age cohorts, a rising age at marriage is expected (since women in this cohort were still marrying). Although those data were for currently married women and some effort was made to identify those women who had remarried, it was inevitable that remarriages were included. Thus, the data do not fully reflect age at first marriage, although the lack of a strong upward trend for women born between 1851–1855 and 1866–1870 indicates some stability in first-marriage age over that period.

In terms of differential nuptiality, it seems that average age at marriage for current marriage (Table IV-29) was higher among cohorts of foreign-born females born after 1851–1855. Rural and urban average current-marriage ages were quite similar with perhaps a slightly younger age among rural wives. Occupational marriage differentials are also examined in Table IV-30, which gives average age at marriage for current marriages for males by occupation and for their wives. Earlier it was noted for England and Wales that miners and their spouses both married early and that mining regions had low first-marriage ages. (See Chapter II, this volume.) Table IV-30 shows, however, that the picture was not especially clear in the anthracite region, insofar as census data bear on the issue. On average, miners' wives probably married as early as any of the groups, although the differences were small. On the other hand, the miners themselves often had below-average marriage ages, but the differences were small and the ranking of the groups unstable. The only consistent pattern was the relatively late marriage among professional males. The lack of differentials in age of marriage among males in different occupational groups is substantiated by information on average age of marriage of persons married during the census year. This question was asked in the censuses of 1850 through 1880 and the results from 1850 and 1880 are tabulated in Table IV-31. Because of small cell sizes for 1880, tabulations by occupation were made only for 1850, but these results confirm those from the census of 1900. The data in Table IV-31 also suggest that the decline in overall fertility was affected by a rising age of marriage, that the relatively high marital fertility among the foreign born (and especially among the Irish) was amplified by earlier female age of

TABLE IV-29 Estimated Female Age of Marriage[a] from 1900 Census Data for Seven Pennsylvania Counties, by Age, Nativity, and Residence. Currently Married Women

Age (year of birth)	Total		Native-born		Foreign-born		Rural		Urban	
	Mean age at marriage	*N*[b]	Mean age at marriage	*N*	Mean age at marriage	*N*	Mean age at marriage	*N*	Mean age at marriage	*N*
15-19 (1881-1885)	16.8	45	16.9	31	16.4	14	16.8	20	16.7	25
20-24 (1876-1880)	19.1	231	19.4	157	18.5	74	18.8	115	19.5	116
25-29 (1871-1876)	20.2	318	20.4	221	19.6	97	19.9	146	20.4	172
30-34 (1866-1870)	21.4	344	21.6	207	21.1	137	21.1	154	21.6	190
35-39 (1861-1865)	21.8	283	22.1	174	21.3	109	22.3	134	21.3	149
40-44 (1856-1860)	22.2	209	22.3	139	22.0	70	22.2	105	22.2	104
45-49 (1851-1855)	22.3	182	22.6	124	21.8	58	22.0	92	22.7	90
50-54 (1846-1850)	23.8	141	23.5	89	24.3	52	23.2	73	24.5	68
55-59 (1841-1845)	24.4	87	24.2	54	24.8	33	23.7	44	25.3	43
60-64 (1836-1840)	23.8	44	23.8	25	23.9	19	25.1	25	22.2	19
65 and over (1835 and earlier)	27.1	74	25.7	45	29.3	29	27.1	43	27.1	31
Total	21.6	1958	21.7	1266	21.5	692	21.6	951	21.7	1007

Source: Sample of enumerators' manuscripts.

[a] Calculated as age minus number of years married.

[b] Number of cases.

TABLE IV-30 Estimated Average Male and Female Age of Marriage[a] from 1900 Census Data for Seven Pennsylvania Counties by Occupation of Husband. Currently Married Spouses Both Present

Age (year of birth)	Farmer and farm worker	Laborer	Miner and mine worker	Manufacturing, etc.	Mercantile, etc.	Professional and other	Total
	Estimated average ages of females at marriage[b]						
15-19 (1881-1885)	(16.8)	(17.4)	16.5	(16.3)	(18.0)	—	16.8
20-24 (1876-1880)	18.9	18.8	18.8	19.1	19.6	20.1	19.1
25-29 (1871-1875)	19.4	19.4	19.9	20.7	20.2	22.7	20.1
30-34 (1866-1870)	21.0	21.2	21.2	21.0	21.8	20.9	21.3
35-39 (1861-1865)	22.6	21.9	21.6	21.5	22.0	22.6	21.9
40-44 (1856-1860)	22.6	22.2	21.5	21.9	22.1	23.7	22.1
45-49 (1851-1855)	21.2	23.5	22.2	21.7	22.2	21.9	22.1
50-54 (1846-1850)	22.5	26.6	(24.9)	21.4	20.2	(23.9)	23.3
55-59 (1841-1845)	24.7	25.6	24.4	23.2	23.1	23.5	24.1
60 and over (1840 and earlier)	25.7	27.1	(23.5)	25.9	(26.3)	24.1	25.4
	Estimated average ages of males at marriage[b]						
15-19 (1881-1885)	—	(18.3)	(15.0)	—	—	—	(17.5)
20-23 (1876-1880)	(21.0)	20.2	21.1	20.9	20.4	(21.5)	20.8
25-29 (1871-1875)	23.1	22.9	23.1	23.1	22.4	24.3	23.0
30-34 (1866-1870)	24.1	24.0	25.0	24.0	24.5	25.5	24.5
35-39 (1861-1865)	25.0	23.4	24.9	23.7	26.5	27.0	25.0
40-44 (1856-1860)	27.0	27.1	24.9	25.5	26.5	27.0	26.0
45-49 (1851-1855)	23.8	27.5	25.0	26.9	26.3	24.8	25.7
50-54 (1846-1850)	29.3	28.5	28.3	24.6	25.3	29.1	27.3
55-59 (1841-1845)	26.5	28.0	28.1	29.0	26.6	29.2	27.7
60 and over (1840 and earlier)	29.8	32.4	28.7	30.7	29.0	31.4	30.6

Source: Sample of enumerators' manuscripts.

[a] Calculated as age minus number of years married.

[b] Numbers in parentheses are based on less than 10 cases.

TABLE IV-31 Mean Age at Marriage by Nativity and Occupation of Husband, Males and Females, Lackawanna/Luzerne, Schuylkill, and Northumberland Counties, Pennsylvania, 1850 and 1880.

	1850		1880[a]	
	Male	Female	Male	Female
1. *Mean age of marriage*	23.9	21.0	26.8	21.4
2. *By nativity*				
Native-born	23.6	21.0	26.6	21.6
Foreign-born	24.4	20.8	27.5	20.0
British	24.5	21.2	—	—
Irish	24.3	20.1	—	—
Other foreign	24.7	20.8	—	—
3. *By occupation of husband*				
Farmer	23.6	23.8	—	—
Laborer	24.0	20.1	—	—
Miners	24.1	20.3	—	—
Manufacturing, etc.	23.5	20.5	—	—
Other	26.0	21.8	—	—

Source: Sample of census enumerators' manuscripts.

[a]Numbers of observations were too small to give reliable information for detailed nativity and occupation in 1880.

marriage, that miners and laborers had relatively high fertility in 1850 partly because of younger wives but not younger husbands, and that farmers had high fertility despite a higher age of marriage for wives. Regretably, these types of census data have a number of defects and so the results must be treated with caution.[50] Nonetheless, they do suggest a role for marriage in explaining ethnic and occupational fertility differentials.

In order to gain additional insight into ages at first marriage, Hajnal's method was applied to data by age, sex, and marital status from the 1880 and 1900 censuses to calculate a singulate mean age of marriage (SMAM) (Hajnal, 1953). These results for both males and females, along with data on proportions of the population married at ages 20–24, are given in Table

[50] Among the defects are (*a*) the data reflect total marriages and not first marriages; (*b*) census questions on vital events have what is called "reference period error," which means only those events close in time to the census itself are generally reported. Other biases are also present. It is likely that the high proportion of laborers in the 1850 sample (44.1%) reflects the fact that young men just entering the labor force and just married were perhaps more likely to have been laborers before they had found a more regular occupation. This is a general problem when working with cross-sectional occupation data. There is obviously occupational mobility over the life cycle and looking at, for example, age and occupation may give a biased notion of the relation of occupations to various life-cycle variables such as family size and income. For a discussion, see Anderson (1972, pp. 59–62).

IV-32. This SMAM could not, unfortunately, be calculated for earlier censuses since data on marital status were lacking, and it was felt that estimates of proportions single, which are necessary to calculate SMAM, could not be estimated with as much reliability as proportions married (which were estimated and presented in Table IV-20). The results do confirm the impression that some changes in marriage were taking place toward the end of the period considered here. Female SMAM rose from 23.2 to 23.8 years between 1880 and 1900, and male from 26.1 to 28.1 years. More impressive was the increase in native-born female SMAM from 23.4 to 25.0 years while foreign-born female SMAM was actually declining. The more rapid decline in native-born fertility relative to foreign-born fertility was partially due to this, but, as was seen in Table IV-25, most of the explanation lay in changes in marital fertility. Other interesting features of Table IV-32 include the very high, and increasing, male age at marriage and the fact that differentials between male and female SMAM were far greater among the foreign born than among the native born. The existence of the large differentials by ethnicity is confirmed by investigation of marriage registers. For example, Roberts found for Schyulkill County in 1899 that average age at first marriage was 25.7 years for native-born males and 27.2 for the foreign born. Similarly, it was 23.1 years for native-born females and

TABLE IV-32 Singulate Mean Age at Marriage and Percentage Married at Age 20-24. Pennsylvania Anthracite Region, 1880 and 1900[a]

	Singulate mean age at marriage			
	1880		1900	
	Male	Female	Male	Female
Total	26.1	23.2	28.1	23.8
Rural	26.0	23.3	28.0	23.5
Urban	27.6	23.0	28.2	24.5
Native-born	25.8	23.4	28.5	25.0
Foreign-born	27.5	22.3	27.7	21.2
	Percent married at age 20-24			
Total	25.07	53.70	19.21	47.28
Rural	27.50	54.47	22.43	52.94
Urban	19.82	52.10	16.60	42.75
Native-born	24.56	53.59	18.95	41.95
Foreign-born	27.14	54.24	20.00	64.41

Source: Samples of enumerators' manuscripts from the censuses of 1880 and 1900. Singulate mean age at marriage computed according to Hajnal's method.

[a] Lackawanna, Luzerne, Schuylkill, and Northumberland counties for 1880. For 1900, Susquehanna, Wayne, and Wyoming counties were also included.

22.7 for foreign-born females. The overall average for Schuylkill County for 1899 was 26.2 for males and 23.9 for females (Roberts, 1904, p. 64). These figures are slightly below the SMAM for males and females in 1900. This may be partly attributable to the higher proportion of Southern and Eastern European migrants, who had lower marriage ages, in Roberts' sample. But Hajnal's method also produces some upward bias under conditions of heavy net in-migration of single persons. This raises SMAM but also probably did not much alter the change in SMAM between 1880 and 1900, since there was probably no major change in the migration rate and age–sex composition of migrants between 1880 and 1900.

The overall pattern of much higher than average foreign-born male age at marriage and much lower than average foreign-born female age of marriage was a reflection of migration patterns and the economic structure of the region. The selective and large net in-migration of young adult males, which was so characteristic of mining and heavy-industrial areas, produced a large surplus of single, young, foreign-born males relative to marriageable females. The marriage market for young, unattached foreign-born females was so favorable that their mean age at first marriage declined while that of native-born females was rising. This phenomenon is reflected in sex ratios for young adults, which show a surplus of younger males relative to younger females. Sex ratios (males per 100 females) for the age group 20–29 for the anthracite counties and for the white population of the United States are presented in Table IV-33. Sex ratios in these peak marriage ages were very favorable to females among the foreign born relative to the native born. Sex ratios like those for the foreign-born population in the anthracite region or, for that matter, for the foreign-born population of the whole United States during this period, would not be found in a stable closed population, as is indicated by the last column of Table IV-33. West model stable populations with mortality and fertility patterns similar to those in the anthracite region would only generate sex ratios of about 102–103 males per 100 females aged 20–29. The actual sex ratios among the foreign born were considerably higher. Interestingly, prior to 1880, this was also true for native-born males; but, later, young native-born men did not find it an attractive area of opportunity. Roberts noted this phenomenon late in the century:

> *Among the foreign born in the eight counties where anthracite coal is produced we have 33,623 more males than females. Of the Sclav immigrants into our country an average of 70 percent are males. It has been shown by the census returns that the majority of male immigrants from southern Europe are workingmen between 15 and 40 years of age. From 1891 to 1900, 74.8 percent of the immigrants was classified in the above age group. This accounts for the large number of bachelors of foreign birth in the coal fields.*
>
> *Among the native born in the eight counties above mentioned, the females outnumber the males by 3,694. This is due to the migration of male descendants of foreign born parents who, anxious to leave the mines, are forced out of the coal fields, where ambitious young men have very few openings* [Roberts, 1904, p. 57].

TABLE IV-33 Sex Ratios (Males Aged 20-29 per 100 Females Aged 20-29) for the Pennsylvania Anthracite Region, the United States, and Selected Stable Populations [a]

Year of census	Pennsylvania anthracite region			United States (white population)			Stable population [b]
	Total	Native	Foreign-born	Total	Native	Foreign-born	
1850	123.5	108.1	124.6	106.3	NA [c]	NA	102.2
1860	110.1	105.7	118.0	103.2	NA	NA	102.7
1870	111.3	104.5	123.4	97.4	94.4	108.7	102.1
1880	99.2	96.4	110.3	104.4	101.1	126.2	102.1
1900	105.9	95.0	140.1	101.3	100.1	107.7	102.2

Source: Sample of census enumerators' manuscripts. U.S. Bureau of the Census, *Historical Statistics of the United States, Colonial Times to 1970* (1975), Series A119-134. Ansley J. Coale and Paul Demeny, *Regional Model Life Tables and Stable Populations* (Princeton, N.J.: Princeton University Press, 1966).

[a] Lackawanna/Luzerne, Schuylkill, and Northumberland counties for 1850-1880. For 1900, Susquehanna, Wayne, and Wyoming were also included.

[b] The West model stable populations are taken as follows:

Year	e_0^0 females	GRR
1850	47.5	3.0
1860	50.0	3.0
1870	45.0	2.5
1880	45.0	2.5
1900	47.5	2.0

[c] NA = Not available.

The interaction between migration selectivity, sex ratios, and marriage was augmented by the relatively low degree of intermarriage across ethnic lines. “Between the Sclav bachelor and the Anglo-Saxon native born or foreign born spinster there is not fellowship [Roberts, 1904, p. 57].” In a study of marriage records in Lackawanna County for 1886, Berthoff found that about 80% of men born in Wales or of Welsh ancestry married women of the same ethnic background. Similar proportions were also found for the Irish (94%) and Germans (92%). The English were less opposed to exogamy: Only about 40% of marriages were between persons born in England or of English parents. The same things were apparently true in 1910 of immigrants from Poland, Russia, Hungary, Austria, and Italy (Berthoff, 1965, p. 270). In the 1900 sample from the anthracite counties, only 11.5% of the 702 foreign-born spouses in families with husbands present were married to native-born husbands. The percentage of foreign-born males married to native-born females was, as might be expected, somewhat higher (24.4%) given the relative shortage of foreign-born males. Table IV-34 gives some notion of the amount of endogamy by place of birth. Native-born women were most likely to marry a person from outside their place of birth whereas foreign-born women were often least likely. On the other hand, native-born men were highly likely to seek a native-born wife. In 1850, less than 1% of

TABLE IV-34 Percent of Family Heads and Wives with Spouses Born in the Same Geographic Area, Pennsylvania Anthracite Region, 1850, 1880, 1900[a]

Year	Pennsylvania	Total native-born	Britain[b]	Ireland	Germany	Italy	Slavic[c]	Other	Total
Percentage of family heads born in the area with spouses born in the same area									
1850	95.9	99.1	78.1	90.4	76.5	NI[d]	NI	(33.3)[e]	87.9
1880	89.2	93.7	80.9	82.0	56.9	NI	NI	60.4	79.8
1900	88.4	93.3	58.1	59.6	53.8	97.2	93.3	52.6	78.0
Percentage of wives born in the area with family heads born in the same area									
1850	86.1	92.9	92.6	97.7	94.8	NI	NI	(25.0)	87.9
1880	79.7	85.5	80.4	91.4	86.6	NI	NI	69.0	79.8
1900	78.4	84.4	70.6	74.3	72.7	100.0	99.3	62.5	78.0

Source: Sample of census enumerators' manuscripts.

[a]Lackawanna/Luzerne, Schuylkill, and Northumberland counties. In 1900 Susquehanna, Wayne, and Wyoming counties were also included.

[b]England, Wales, Scotland.

[c]Austria-Hungary, Poland, Czechoslovakia, Russia.

[d]NI = Not included.

[e]Figures in parentheses are based on less than 10 cases.

native-born husbands had foreign-born wives. By 1900 things had loosened up a bit but the pattern remained.

It thus seems clear that young, single, foreign-born women were especially desirable as spouses for young foreign-born men but not for native-born men. They were in sufficiently short supply, however, that a large proportion were married at an early age. As Table IV-32 (lower panel) shows, in 1900, 64.4% of foreign-born females aged 20–24 were already married whereas only 42.0% of native-born females had experienced matrimony. Foreign-born males experienced difficulty finding brides, and, perhaps, in reaching a position of sufficient economic security to enable them to marry early. Therefore, despite the fact that foreign-born males had slightly higher proportions married than native-born males at ages 20–24 (Table IV-32), the foreign born had higher singulate mean ages at first marriage in both 1880 and 1900.[51] Overall, it seems clear that migration played a vital role in determining marriage patterns and hence fertility.

It is of some interest to note in passing that the extent of endogamy weakened over time for virtually all the groups categorized in Table IV-34. This is to a good indicator of the gradual, slow assimilation process which was taking place. For example, the Irish and Germans began, in 1850, with very restricted intermarriage for females, but this gradually eased over the next half century. On the other hand, newer groups, the Italian and Slavic migrants of the late nineteenth century, began with the same patterns of restricted exogamy in 1900 that had characterized the Irish 50 years before. The same drama was being reenacted with a new cast of players.

Finally, with respect to marriage age, it is important to see whether marriage was early in the anthracite region relative to other areas. It was suggested in Chapter I that mining regions had low marriage ages. For the anthracite region, the SMAM was 26.1 for males and 23.2 for females in 1880 and 28.1 for males and 23.8 for females in 1900. As may be seen in Table IV-35, the anthracite region had relatively low SMAMs and proportions single at ages 20–24 for both sexes in 1880 and for females in 1900. This is in relation to the United States in 1890 and 1900, England and Wales in 1881 and 1901, and Prussia in 1880 and 1900. Within England and Wales and Prussia, two mining and metallurgical areas each were selected for comparison. *Regierungsbezirke* Oppeln (Upper Silesia) and Arnsberg (Ruhr) both showed lower ages at marriage and lower proportions single at ages 20–24 for both sexes than for Prussia as a whole. This was especially true for Arnsberg, with its very low proportion of agricultural population (see Table I-10, page 26). The same was true for the counties of Durham in England and Glamorganshire in South Wales for females, though not particularly for

[51] It must be remembered, however, that the singulate mean age at first marriage can be upward biased by net in-migration of single persons. Thus foreign-born SMAM in Table IV-32 might be a bit too high, but sensitivity analysis on this measure indicates that the bias is not large. (See Agarwala, 1962.)

TABLE IV-35 Singulate Mean Age of First Marriage and Proportions Single at Ages 20-24. Anthracite Region of Pennsylvania, United States, Prussia, Areas of Prussia, England, and Wales, and Areas of England and Wales, 1880-1881, 1900-1901 [a]

	Singulate mean age at marriage		Percent single at 20-24	
	Male	Female	Male	Female
1. *Anthracite region*				
1880	26.1	23.2	74.9	45.8
1900	28.1	23.8	80.0	52.3
2. *United States*				
1890	27.6	23.6	80.7	51.8
1900	27.4	23.7	77.6	51.6
3. *Prussia*				
1880	28.2	25.6	92.1	73.8
1900	27.6	25.4	90.3	70.2
a. R.B. Arnsberg -- 1880	27.9	23.8	90.9	62.7
1900	27.4	23.9	90.3	70.2
b. R.B. Oppeln -- 1880	27.5	25.4	91.1	71.3
1900	27.0	25.0	87.8	64.3
4. *England and Wales*				
1881	26.6	25.3	77.7	66.5
1901	27.3	26.2	82.6	72.6
a. County Durham -- 1881	26.6	23.4	77.0	52.1
1900	26.9	24.9	79.6	60.8
b. County Glamorganshire -- 1881	26.8	24.3	77.9	57.9
1900	27.3	25.0	81.6	62.6

Source: a. Anthracite region: sample of enumerators' manuscripts, b. United States: U.S. Censuses of 1890 and 1900. c. Prussia: *Preussische Statistik*. d. England and Wales: Censuses of England and Wales, 1881 and 1901.

[a] Lackawanna, Luzerne, Schuylkill, and Northumberland counties. In 1900, Susquehanna, Wayne, and Wyoming counties were also included.

males. Both counties contained large mining and smelting centers, and areas within them will be discussed in the next chapter. Comparing marriage ages in the Pennsylvania anthracite region with these selected mining areas in Prussia and England and Wales, it appears that, for females, the anthracite region was even more extreme in its pattern of early marriage than the other mining areas. This was not the case for males in 1900, although it was in 1880. It is probable that the very extreme migration selectivity for young, single males in the eastern Pennsylvania coalfields played a role in this.

Differential Mortality, 1900

Since vital statistics were of unreliable coverage and accuracy in late nineteenth-century Pennsylvania, it is difficult to discuss mortality levels, trends, or differentials. This problem has already been encountered in the course of estimating age specific birth rates using own-children methods. In that case, some results from the census of 1900 were used to establish levels of differentials for that point in time. The method, as explained above, was to survive the age structure of surviving own children backward until they just equaled the number of children ever born. This was done for younger women only (i.e., women aged 20–34) to reduce the incidence of children missing from the home for reasons other than mortality. West model tables (Coale and Demeny, 1966) were used to obtain the necessary survival probabilities. The methods are explaïned in more detail elsewhere (Haines, 1977c; Preston, 1976; Hill and Trussell, 1977). Also, the fit provided by the appropriate West model table to the 1900 United States life table for the registration area was quite good, lending some support to the choice of the West model (Coale and Zelnik, 1963, pp. 168–169; Haines, 1977d).

The results of these estimations yield childhood mortality probabilities, which are presented in Table IV-36. So, for example, ${}_2q_0$ is the probability of a child (both sexes combined) of dying between birth and age 2. Similarly, ${}_{10}q_0$ is the probability of dying between birth and age 10. An extension of these results to adult mortality is much more conjectural and so Table IV-36 gives expectations of life at birth ($\mathring{e}_0$) for males and females, separately, which are *implied* in the West model system by that particular level of childhood mortality. This is included to provide a notion of differentials in overall mortality levels. One particular advantage of these own-children mortality estimates is that they give childhood mortality by the characteristic of the mother and/or father. For example, the children of foreign-born parents are likely to be native born themselves. Registered deaths usually do not classify deaths by nativity of parents, and so it is usually only possible to examine mortality differences only among the foreign born, not among their children. Those methods circumvent that problem. In many ways it is preferable to have mortality estimates for children because this was such an impor-

TABLE IV-36 Differential Infant and Child Mortality by Residence, Nativity, and Literacy of Spouse, and Occupation of Family Head. Seven Pennsylvania Counties, 1900 (Families with Husband and Wife Present)[a]

	$_2q_0$	$_3q_0$	$_5q_0$	$_{10}q_0$	Implied e_0^0 Male[b]	Implied e_0^0 Female[b]
I. *Total*	.17642	.19223	.21023	.22860	45.02	48.02
II. *Residence*						
Rural	.16533	.17995	.19661	.21395	46.52	49.47
Urban	.18708	.20388	.22304	.24232	43.68	46.62
III. *Nativity of spouse*						
Native	.14871	.16144	.17593	.19172	48.74	51.61
Foreign-born	.21730	.23686	.25913	.29910	40.05	42.86
IV. *Literacy of spouse*						
Illiterate	.26882	.29271	.31991	.34514	34.47	37.06
Literate	.17915	.19587	.21423	.23289	44.60	47.58
V. *Occupation of family head*						
Farmer and farm worker	.10710	.11647	.12952	.14139	54.03	57.38
Laborer	.20615	.22471	.23584	.26669	41.36	44.21
Mine and mine worker	.24584	.26786	.29292	.31668	36.87	39.55
Manufacturing/crafts/construction	.14360	.15578	.16965	.18493	49.41	52.33
Mercantile/lodging/transport/servants	.13890	.15058	.16388	.17869	50.04	53.03
Professional and other	.12772	.13850	.15195	.16576	51.37	54.50

Source: Data from a sample of enumerators' manuscripts. Calculated using the age distribution of surviving children and the numbers of children ever born and children surviving. The method is explained in Haines (1977c), Preston (1976), and Hill and Trussell (1977).

[a] Lackawanna, Luzerne, Schuylkill, Northumberland, Susquehanna, Wayne, and Wyoming.

[b] The implied e_0^0 (expectation of life at birth) is calculated for males and females separately assuming a sex ratio at birth of 105. It is the extension to total mortality of the results from childhood mortality, using West model life tables.

tant part of total mortality in this period and because childhood mortality is a good indicator of general social wellbeing. One additional point of importance is that the mortality levels in Table IV-36 do not represent mortality in 1900 but rather a weighted average of mortality in the previous 10 to 15 years. Since most of the mortality occurs in the previous few years, however, the weights are heaviest for the years approximately 1895 through 1900.

The substantive results indicate that children of native-born mothers had distinctly more favorable mortality experience than the children of foreign-born women. The children of native-born mothers had approximately 32% lower probabilities of dying at young ages. Also, urban environments appeared somewhat less healthy than rural ones. Illiterate mothers were much more likely to have had children die at young ages than literate mothers. This differential was quite large. Finally, among the various occupational groups, it does appear here that childhood mortality among miners and mine workers was the highest among all the groups considered. Previous work on occupational mortality differentials has dealt with the mortality of adults. (See discussion in Chapter I, pages 29–36.) An analysis of United States data for the period 1890–1910 by Uselding (1976) did reveal substantially higher adult-male mortality in mining and in manufacturing than among other occupational groups. These results for the anthracite region indicate in addition, that miners had high mortality among their children, higher even than among even common laborers. Farmers and farm workers had very favorable childhood mortality, as did professionals, whereas the manufacturing– crafts– construction and mercantile– lodging– transport– servant groups were intermediate, although relatively favorably situated. There is, of course, the complicating factor that miners and mine workers and laborers were much more likely to be foreign born and thus experience higher mortality, while, at the other extreme, farmers and professionals were much more likely to be native born. There were too few cases in the sample, however, to standardize for this by finer cross-classification.

The higher mortality among the children of coal miners would be consistent with the hypothesis that the higher fertility among miners' families was partly a consequence of higher infant and child mortality. The mechanism could have been behavioral (i.e., more children were conceived in a conscious attempt to obtain a targeted surviving family size) or biological (e.g., interruption of lactation shortening birth intervals). If the differentials also extended to adults, the higher mortality among males, in particular, might have encouraged earlier marriage. It would also, however, have broken more marital unions and thus tended to lower fertility.

It is plausible that urban mortality levels might have been higher than rural, because of environmental conditions more favorable to disease in urban areas, for example. On the other hand, it is not at all clear why foreign-born children should have been at higher risk of dying than native-born children. The same is true of differentials by literacy and occupation of husband. The higher childhood mortality among miners' families is also puzzling in view of the reasonable levels of living which they enjoyed. The mortality differentials are probably at basis due to differences in socioeconomic wellbeing, which were, in turn, partly related to the ethnic composition of the population. Miners were more likely to have been foreign born and have less literate wives and were thus more subject to the disadvantages, socially and economically, consequent upon these states of being.[52] Again the importance of the particular environment and context of the differential demographic behavior is important.

SUMMARY AND CONCLUSIONS

This chapter has utilized one case study, the Pennsylvania anthracite region over the period 1850 through 1900, in order to examine some of the characteristics of mining populations and areas. Using samples of enumerators' manuscripts from the U.S. censuses of 1850–1880 and 1900, overall and age-specific marital child–woman ratios were calculated for the anthracite counties and for various dimensions of the population within the counties, including occupation of husband, literacy and nativity of husband and spouse, and rural–urban residence. It was shown that occupational fertility differentials existed in the Pennsylvania anthracite region from the mid- to late-nineteenth century. While theoretical reasons and empirical evidence from other areas in the nineteenth and twentieth centuries would indicate that coal-mining families would have the highest fertility, this was not the case in eastern Pennsylvania at mid-century. The relative lower marital fertility of miners' wives in 1850 (as measured by standardized ratios of children aged 0–4 to married women aged 15–49) was undoubtedly partly due to specific factors such as ethnic composition, residence, and education (as measured by literacy), but it was also due to the very high fertility of native-born farmers at that time. The situation had by 1900, however, changed to the more usual pattern of a longer settled region and was more similar to that of Europe. Between 1850 and 1900 there was a substantial decline in marital fertility for all occupational groups except miners' families, who actually experienced an *increase* in age-standardized child–woman ratios between 1850 and 1880. Regression (both ordinary least squares and multinomial logit) and multiple classification analysis were applied to try to control for the simultaneous influence of variables such as

[52] In the 1850 sample, 88.0% of all miners were foreign born, whereas 96.9% of all farmers were native born. Even among laborers, only 52.3% were foreign born. By 1900, only 63.5% of all miners or mine workers were foreign born, but this was still the highest proportion among all occupational groups.

residence, wealth, literacy, ethnic composition, and age, but the high fertility of miners' wives persisted. Marriage practices (age of marriage and proportions married at various ages) also apparently played a role and helped amplify the differentials in marital fertility, but differences in marital fertility appear most important in overall occupational fertility differentials.

A number of factors inducing high marital fertility and early marriage in mining areas were discussed, and it was shown that the anthracite region conformed to most expectations about these factors. Thus, the region urbanized only gradually, showed a low level of extrahousehold female labor-force participation, had high sex ratios in the young adult years, and offered differentially more favorable opportunities to young adult males in mining. Data availability precluded, however, a consistent microanalysis over time of the influence of female labor participation on fertility. The analysis of families in 1850 through 1900 did show, however, that residence (rural or urban), ethnic background, literacy, and, above all, husbands' occupation were influential variables in the fertility decision. The interaction of labor-force structure, age and sex selectivity of migration, sex ratios, marriage, and marital fertility was also examined and found to favor high fertility and earlier marriage in mining areas.

This chapter has also treated the issue of fertility decline. It has, in contrast to other work on nineteenth-century fertility (see Easterlin, 1977, pp. 140–146), concentrated on an area that became quite urban and industrial over the course of the nineteenth century. Since the forces and factors influencing fertility were increasingly associated with urbanization and industrial change, the decline in the United States birth rate after mid-century should be seen as much from this perspective and as from the viewpoint of rural, agricultural populations.

Child–woman ratios indicated a steady decline in fertility in the anthracite region from 1800 onward. Standardization of marital child–woman ratios to the age structure of all married women in 1880 somewhat reduced the magnitude of the declines in the total marital child–woman ratio, since the age structure of married women became, in fact, less favorable to fertility between 1850 and 1900. But the declines remained substantial. The same proved true for the various subgroups of the population considered. The differentials also remained after standardization, with the fertility of illiterate parents generally being greater than that of literate parents, of rural parents greater than urban parents, of foreign born greater than native born, and of miners and laborers greater than most other occupational groups. The differentials also changed between 1850 and 1900 with most (occupation of husband, literacy and nativity of parents) showing divergent patterns while only fertility differentials by rural–urban residence showed convergence.

A better view of fertility change is provided by knowledge of the change in age-specific fertility rates over time. These were estimated from age-specific child–woman ratios using own-children methods. In order to transform the child–woman ratios into fertility rates, estimates of mortality were necessary. These were obtained by applying other own-children techniques to the census of 1900 and by using death rates from census mortality data for persons 5–19 to fit West model life tables. Age-specific fertility was examined only along two dimensions: rural–urban residence and nativity of mother (native versus foreign born).

The findings on age-specific fertility showed a persistent decline in the total fertility rate and the net reproduction rate for the total, rural, urban and native populations. The foreign-born population exhibited a reduction in fertility, but it was slower and less regular. Most of the declines took place among older women (i.e., above age 35), especially for the foreign born. Between 1876–1880 and 1896–1900, however, some considerable declines took place among younger women (i.e., aged 20–34). Breaking down age-specific overall fertility rates into age-specific marital fertility and age-specific proportions married, the declines at older ages of women were seen to derive mostly from reductions in age-specific marital fertility and not from changes in proportions married. There were somewhat larger declines in proportions married among younger women, but age-specific marital fertility also declined for them, except among the foreign born. A further indication of the fertility adjustment among older women was the progressive decline in the estimated mean age at last birth.

Adjustments in marriage do not appear to have been notable in the anthracite region until after 1880. At that time there was some tendency toward increasing mean age at first marriage for both males and females, especially among the native born. Again the foreign born were exceptional, with female first-marriage age declining between 1880 and 1900. Part of the explanation for this latter fact lay in the very favorable marriage market for foreign-born females at the end of the century.

This analysis presented a case in which fertility continued a steady decline without any apparent reduction in mortality before about 1880. This would make the anthracite region (and possibly much of the rest of urban, industrial America) a most unusual type of demographic transition. Also, in terms of the relationship of differentials to the decline, the basic findings confirmed those of Okun that declines within each group were more important than the shifting weights of the different subgroups within the population. Nevertheless, the slow decline in foreign-born fertility did noticeably retard the decline in overall fertility. The decline between 1846–1850 and 1896–1900 in TFR would have been almost 30% greater if foreign-born fertility had declined at the same rate as native-born. Thus the changing fertility of subgroups was quite important to overall trends.

How do the findings here change or confirm our views on fertility in nineteenth-century America? The data definitely show that occupational and class fertility differences existed at mid-century and widened over time.

Education (as represented by adult-female literacy) seems to have had a negative effect on fertility, though not significant, and probably deserves more treatment as an independent variable (Vinovskis, 1976, pp. 392–393). Urbanization and ethnic composition also appear to have become increasingly important over time, although their role may be limited, as suggested by Okun (1958, pp. 98–101). When standardized to the age structure of married women in 1880, there was a decline in fertility for both rural and urban areas, although that for rural areas was more pronounced. Native-born fertility declined dramatically; that of foreign-born parents showed little decline. When taken in conjunction with the overall decline in fertility, rapid urbanization and industrialization, and changes in ethnic and occupational composition characteristic of post civil-war America, it would appear that the study of fertility for the second half of the nineteenth century should place more emphasis on urban and nonagrarian populations.

It should be further noted that the study of fertility, marriage, and occupation can be usefully viewed at two levels of analysis. First, the specific setting of each occupation has a series of general or expected characteristics which influence fertility and nuptiality behavior. In the case of coal mining these included a relatively lower level of extrahousehold female labor-force participation than in other nonagricultural populations, a considerable lower level of urbanization than that surrounding most other industrial populations, relatively high sex ratios in the young adult years because of differential male net-in-migration, very favorable male income-earning opportunities, and possibly higher mortality and debility levels. Second, however, there are characteristics that vary with the specific context of the region at each date which will affect the relationship of fertility and occupation. These include ethnic composition, level of literacy, and similar personal characteristics. While it has not always been possible to analyze all suggested variables at all dates considered, both levels of analysis have been pursued, and it appears that both sets of factors acted to influence marital fertility and marriage in the Pennsylvania anthracite region 1850–1900.

In concluding the chapter, data from the sample of the 1900 census were used to construct estimates of differential mortality. Miners' and mineworkers' families were shown to have had higher childhood mortality than the other occupational groups considered, suggesting further reason for higher marital fertility. Complicating this was, however, the fact that foreign-born and illiterate mothers, both overrepresented in the mining population, also had above-average mortality among their children.

The next chapter will deal with two more case studies: Durham and Easington in northern England and Merthyr Tydfil in South Wales for the period 1851–1871. The data do not permit as detailed an analysis as for the Pennsylvania anthracite region, but the contrast of the same economic structures in differing social, cultural, and geographic settings will be instructive.

V

Durham and Easington, England, and Merthyr Tydfil, South Wales, 1851–1871

INTRODUCTION AND BACKGROUND

The importance of coal mining and metallurgy in the industrial revolution in nineteenth-century Britain is beyond question (Chambers, 1968, pp. 28–35; Deane and Cole, 1969, pp. 214–229; Mathias, 1969, pp. 267–271). By 1851, roughly 2.7% of all adult males in England and Wales (aged 20 and over) were engaged in coal mining and a further 1.3% were employed in ferrous metallurgy. The absolute numbers were 128,086 and 63,355, respectively. The fertility and nuptiality patterns among the mining and industrial populations and regions in England and Wales in the nineteenth and twentieth centuries have already been examined in Chapters I and III. In this chapter, two case studies, one from England and one from Wales, will be studied.

The English case study consists of the Durham and Easington registration districts in the large northeastern coalfield, which was producing about 24% of all of Britain's coal in 1854 (Mitchell and Deane, 1971, p. 115). The geographically adjacent registration districts of Durham and Easington were located within this coalfield at the northern end of County Durham. The ancient city and bishop's seat of Durham is found on the Wear River, south of the Tyne River, and southwest of the cities of Newcastle-upon-Tyne (County Northumberland) and Sunderland (County Durham). The surrounding northeastern coalfield was "one of the earliest to be developed and has always been an important supplier of coal to the coastwise and export trades [House, 1954, p. 35]." The London coal trade from Newcastle was flourishing by the sixteenth century (Nef, 1932). To the east of the Durham district was the registration district of Easington, which bordered the North Sea coast at Seaham Harbor. Although these registration districts ceased to exist after 1910, they are a convenient means of organizing census and vital statistics for this period. For the purposes of analysis, the Durham and Easington districts will be combined.

These two districts were heavily engaged in the mining trade. As Table V-1 indicates, almost 43% of adult males were employed in mining and metallurgy in 1851. Of these, almost all were in coal mining. These districts were relatively late in developing. As may be seen in Table V-2, population growth there was below the average for England and Wales up to the 1830s, when growth suddenly spurted to almost 7%. The districts then continued to enjoy above-average population growth for the remainder of the century. During the 1840s, 1850s, and 1860s, they had positive rates of net in-migration (Table V-1). The districts shared in the mid-century surge in demand for coal which characterized the northeastern field, where output increased at an annual rate of 3.46% between 1854 and 1873, and mining employment increased at 2.45% per year from 1851 to 1871 (calculated from Mitchell and Deane, 1971, p. 115; House, 1954, Table 6). This growth induced a strong demand for labor which, in turn, drew workers from throughout the British Isles (House, 1954, pp. 38–39). In 1871, for example, among male heads of families in the Durham and Easington districts, less than half (48.4%) were born in Durham. Over 22% came from the adjacent counties of Northumberland, Cumberland, and Yorkshire, and 13.4% originated in Ireland. As was the case in the Pennsylvania anthracite region, the in-migration was heavily sex and age selective. The large preponderance of young adult males was reflected in sex ratios (males per 100 females) well above 100 in the adult years. This may be seen in Tables V-1 and V-3. The contrast to the sex ratios for England and Wales as a whole, which was a net loser of population over the mid and late nineteenth century, was dramatic. The ratios were well below 100 among adults, especially younger adults (Tables V-1 and V-3).

In terms of the selected characteristics presented in Table V-1, the Durham and Easington districts conformed closely to the pattern expected of mining areas. By 1851 almost 43% of the adult male population was engaged in mining and metallurgy, and less than 15% was still in primary employment (agriculture, forestry, fishing). This was in contrast to over 30% still in primary employment for England and Wales as a whole. As mentioned earlier, Durham and Easington were net in-migration areas (unlike the nation overall) and the migration favored adult males. Female labor-force participation was only about 14% of the total adult female population, less than half the proportion for England and Wales, indicating a paucity of

1861, and 1871

	1851			1861			1871		
	Durham and Easington	Merthyr Tydfil	England and Wales	Durham and Easington	Merthyr Tydfil	England and Wales	Durham and Easington	Merthyr Tydfil	England and Wales
1. Percentage of Males aged 20 and over in primary employment (excluding mining)	14.05	5.22	30.43	10.50	4.46	23.46	7.00	2.80	18.48
2. Percentage of males aged 20 and over in mining and metallurgy	42.76	52.32	4.05	42.78	53.16	5.38	54.99	60.25	10.14
3. Percentage of population in urban areas[a]	16.96	82.13	50.15	17.09	78.31	54.62	28.33	84.48	61.82
4. Density (persons per acre)	0.57	0.68	0.48	0.71	0.95	0.54	0.84	1.49	0.61
5. Infant mortality rate[b]	159.40	174.00	152.60	143.60	156.40	147.50	179.10	155.10	155.70
6. Net migration in the previous decade (per 1000 population per annum)	14.72	23.20	-0.16	2.69	16.99	-0.97	3.68	-4.94	-0.83
7. Percent of females aged 20 and over employed outside the home	14.39	16.21	29.59	13.87	15.79	29.49	14.06	20.85	33.63
8. e_0^0 for females (years)	38.21[c]	31.21[d]		41.79[e]	34.85[e]	43.03[f]	42.16[g]	38.97[g]	42.43[h]
9. Sex ratio (males per 100 females aged 20-29)	120.70	137.60	91.0	113.20	121.20	88.40	123.60	129.80	90.20
10. Total population (000's)	77.70	76.80	17,927.6	97.60	107.10	20,066.2	125.7	104.2	22,712.3

Source: Birth and death statistics are from the Annual Reports of the Registrar General. Population data were obtained from the censuses of 1841, 1851, 1861, and 1871. Expectations of life at birth for Durham and Easington and for Merthyr Tydfil were calculated from census and vital data. For England and Wales for 1861 and 1871, the e_0^0 was taken from Nathan Keyfitz and Wilhelm Flieger, *World Population (1968)*, pp. 522-525.

[a] Classified by official definition of principal town, municipal borough, or town.

[b] 1850/1852, 1860/1862, and 1870/1872.

[c] Durham only for 1847/1850.

[d] 1846/1850.

[e] 1851/1860.

[f] 1861.

[g] 1861/1870.

[h] 1871.

TABLE V-2 Average Annual Rates of Population Growth by Decade. Durham and Easington Registration Districts, Merthyr Tydfil Registration District, and England and Wales, 1801-1911

Decade	Percent per annum		
	Durham and Easington[a]	Merthyr Tydfil[b]	England and Wales
1801/1811	0.46	3.75	1.34
1811/1821	1.63	2.97	1.66
1821/1831	1.15	2.46	1.47
1831/1841	6.98	4.36	1.36
1841/1851	3.54	3.74	1.19
1851/1861	2.27	3.32	1.13
1861/1871	2.53	1.14	1.24
1871/1881	2.62	-0.27	1.34
1881/1891	1.08	1.44	1.10
1891/1901	1.37	1.45	1.15
1901/1911	2.41	2.51	1.03

SOURCE: Computed from the Censuses of England and Wales, 1851-1911, assuming exponential growth.

[a] After 1871, includes Lanchester Registration District which was separated from Durham in 1875.

[b] Adjusted for a loss of area in 1863 which went to Pontypridd.

female employment opportunities. The degree of urbanization, measured as the proportion of the population living in principal towns, was only 17% in 1851 and 28% in 1871.[1] This was considerably less than those for England and Wales (50 and 62%, respectively). Durham and Easington were, however, somewhat more densely populated than the national average, reflecting their rural but nonagrarian character. Durham and Easington had female mortality (as measured by expectation of life at birth) slightly *below* the national average in 1861 and very close to it in 1871. Infant mortality was, however, above the national average in 1851 and 1871 but below in 1861. The relatively favorable mortality picture, despite being mining areas, may have reflected the low degree of urbanization in Durham and Easington.

Finally, these two districts were characterized by high fertility and relatively early and more extensive marriage. As may be seen in Table V-4, the crude birth rate (CBR) was considerably above the national rate. The decade CBRs in Durham and Easington averaged 24.4% higher than those for England and Wales for the period 1841–1850 through 1901–1910. In addition, given that the crude death rate (CDR) for Durham and Easington

[1] Urban areas were defined as Durham City in Durham Registration District for all three census dates, 1851, 1861, and 1871, and Seaham Harbor (Dawdon Parish) in Easington Registration District for 1861 and 1871.

TABLE V-3 Sex Ratios by Age. Durham and Easington R.D.'s, Merthyr Tydfil R.D., and England and Wales; 1851, 1861, 1871

Age	Sex ratios, 1851			Sex ratios, 1861			Sex ratios, 1871		
	Durham and Easington	Merthyr Tydfil	England and Wales	Durham and Easington	Merthyr Tydfil	England and Wales	Durham and Easington	Merthyr Tydfil	England and Wales
0-4	105.9	100.7	100.5	102.9	99.4	100.7	103.1	99.9	100.1
5-9	104.4	98.4	100.8	104.1	99.5	100.2	100.3	101.5	99.6
10-14	111.3	106.1	101.5	109.1	111.9	101.4	107.3	107.7	101.4
15-19	113.2	120.0	98.8	118.3	117.8	98.3	116.4	126.2	99.0
20-24	124.2	137.5	91.3	112.0	122.5	88.7	122.1	134.6	90.4
25-29	116.9	137.8	90.7	114.7	119.7	88.0	125.3	124.3	90.0
30-34	113.4	133.7	93.9	111.8	116.2	91.2	117.5	114.0	91.7
35-39	113.9	127.8	95.8	113.6	120.4	93.1	112.5	111.4	91.5
40-44	108.2	134.0	95.9	115.0	121.7	94.5	118.6	109.9	92.2
45-49	112.1	133.6	96.7	107.1	114.3	94.9	117.1	114.9	92.8
50-54	107.7	117.1	95.4	106.0	118.9	94.6	113.4	119.1	93.2
55-59	101.2	102.3	93.9	109.9	118.5	94.9	116.0	109.8	92.9
60-64	103.7	97.9	89.4	100.3	99.9	91.3	104.3	103.6	89.8
65-69	91.3	89.2	86.2	96.9	89.1	87.3	100.0	104.6	87.1
70+	80.8	78.6	80.6	81.7	76.5	80.4	89.3	71.2	81.8
Total	110.4	117.1	96.0	108.6	111.1	95.0	110.9	111.7	94.9

Source: Census of England and Wales, 1851, 1861, 1871.

TABLE V-4 Components of Population Change: Durham and Easington R.D.'s, Merthyr Tydfil R.D., and England and Wales, 1841/1850 - 1901/1910[a]

	Per 1000 population per annum						
	1841/ 1850	1851/ 1860	1861/ 1870	1871/ 1880	1881/ 1890	1890/ 1900	1901/ 1910
A. Durham and Easington R.D.'s							
1. CBR	42.92	42.66	42.46	46.70	37.68	36.40	35.11
2. CDR	22.75	22.18	21.63	24.38	18.79	19.12	16.76
3. RNI	20.17	20.48	20.83	22.32	18.89	17.28	18.35
4. RNM	14.72	2.69	3.68	4.64	-8.07	-3.61	5.72
5. RTI	34.89	23.17	24.51	26.96	10.82	13.67	24.07
B. Merthyr Tydfil R.D.							
1. CBR	42.94	45.28	42.39	39.63	34.21	37.63	35.90
2. CDR	28.78	29.01	26.05	24.23	22.36	23.01	18.82
3. RNI	14.16	16.27	16.34	15.40	11.85	14.62	17.08
4. RNM	23.20	16.99	-4.94	-18.12	2.59	-0.09	7.98
5. RTI	37.36	33.26	11.40	-2.72	14.44	14.53	25.06
C. England and Wales							
1. CBR	34.25	34.78	35.48	35.15	32.13	29.56	26.94
2. CDR	22.17	22.54	22.26	21.11	18.95	18.00	15.21
3. RNI	12.08	12.24	13.22	14.04	13.18	11.56	11.73
4. RNM	-0.16	-0.97	-0.83	-0.62	-2.15	-0.09	-1.39
5. RTI	11.92	11.27	12.39	13.42	11.03	11.47	10.34

Source: *Annual Reports of the Registrar General* and *Census of England and Wales, 1851 ... 1861 ... 1871 ... 1881 ... 1891 ... 1901 ... 1911.*

[a]CBR = crude birth rate
CDR = crude death rate
RNI = rate of natural increase
RNM = rate of net migration
RTI = rate of total increase

was quite close to that for the nation, the rate of natural increase was also considerably above the national average (57% above). Table V-5 presents Coale's indices of overall fertility (I_f), marital fertility (I_g), proportions married (I_m), and illegitimate fertility (I_h). There it is also clear that fertility was considerably higher in the Durham and Easington districts. For the average of the periods 1850–1852 through 1900–1902, the I_f for Durham and Easington was 37.8% above the national average. For the period 1850–1852 through 1890–1892, I_g was 12% higher; I_m, 12% higher; and I_h almost 66% higher. The high fertility and early marriage in these districts, in addition to their representative character for mining areas, were important factors in their selection as a case study.

The other case study was that of Merthyr Tydfil in Glamorganshire in southeastern Wales. Although the proportion of adult males employed in mining and metallurgy was also quite high, ranging from 52.3% in 1851 to 60.2% in 1871 (Table V-1), it was a rather different area. It was much more involved with iron manufacture than were Durham and Easington. In 1851, 29.0% of the adult male population was in iron manufacture as opposed to 23.3% in coal mining. In the 1840s, the famous Dowlais iron works of Sir John Guest near Merthyr Tydfil employed nearly 6000 workers, produced annually over 25,000 tons of pig iron per year, and had a capital of over

TABLE V-5 Indices of Overall Fertility (I_f), Marital Fertility (I_g), Illegitimate Fertility (I_h), and Proportions Married (I_m) for Durham and Easington R.D.'s, Merthyr Tydfil R.D., and England and Wales, 1850/1852 - 1900/1902

Date	Durham and Easington R.D.'s[a]				Merthyr Tydfil R.D.				England and Wales			
	I_f	I_g	I_m	I_h	I_f	I_g	I_m	I_h	I_f	I_g	I_m	I_h
1850/1852	.465	.755	.572	.077	.451	.722	.595	.053	.355	.686	.483	.046
1860/1862	.485	.756	.601	.077	.441	.668	.630	.054	.359	.671	.502	.044
1870/1872	.519	.784	.632	.064	.463	.719	.613	.058	.369	.685	.509	.041
1880/1882	.485	.718	.648	.056	.407	.670	.580	.044	.352	.663	.506	.033
1890/1892	.431	.713	.582	.038	.428	.723	.574	.030	.308	.613	.482	.024
1900/1902	.391	--	--	--	.412	--	--	--	.272	.549	.476	.020

Source: Birth statistics are from the Annual Reports of the Registrar General. Births are adjusted for underregistration on the basis of factors for counties and for the nation estimated by Michael S. Teitelbaum, "Birth Underregistration in the Constituent Counties of England and Wales, 1841 - 1910," *Population Studies*, Vol. 28, No. 2 (July, 1974), pp. 329-343.

Population data were obtained from the Censuses of England and Wales for 1851, 1861, 1871, 1881, and 1900. Some interpolation was necessary to obtain population by marital status in 5 year age groups.

For an explanation and definition of I_f, I_g, I_m, and I_h, see Ansley J. Coale, "Factors Associated with the Development of Low Fertility: An Historic Summary," United Nations, *World Population Conference: 1965*, Vol. II (New York: U.N., 1967), pp. 205-209.

[a]Includes Lanchester R.D. after 1870/1872.

£1 million. The iron works in South Wales were generally the largest i Britain at that time (Mathias, 1969, p. 269). In 1847, the South Wales iro industry produced over one-third (35.3%) of the total British production c 1,999,608 tons of pig iron (Mitchell and Deane, 1971, p. 131; Thomas, 1930 p. 276); South Wales was then the largest single pig iron producing regio in the British Isles (although it soon lost its supremacy to Scotland). The iro industry was of long standing, the Dowlais works having been founded i 1759 (Minchinton, 1969, p. xii). The growth of the industry there was rapid especially after the development of puddling and rolling in 1784. A majo problem for Merthyr Tydfil was transportation. This was partially solved i the 1790s when the Glamorganshire Canal from Merthyr to Cardiff wa opened. Later, of course, railways were built. The Taff Vale line fron Cardiff to Merthyr Tydfil was completed in 1841 and ushered in a new era o industrial development. In 1823, Dowlais had 8 blast furnaces, and by 1830 i was operating 12, all of which were new, larger, and more efficient. By th 1850s, Dowlais was called the "greatest ironworks in the world," had 18 blas furnaces, and employed almost 7000 workers in all capacities. Dowlais ha been able to quadruple its production between 1817 and 1850 to over 25,00 tons per year (Minchinton, 1969, pp. xiv, xxi).

The town of Merthyr Tydfil showed the most spectacular populatio growth in Wales over the century from 1750 to 1850. From a small hamlet i 1750, it grew to a town of 7705 in 1801. It was larger than Swansea (6831) Cardiff (1870), and Newport (1087). By 1851 the town of Merthyr Tydfil itsel (which was only a part of the registration district) was, with 63,080 persons the largest town in Wales. As Table V-2 makes clear, the growth rate of th registration district of Merthyr Tydfil was extremely rapid over the first hal of the nineteenth century, averaging 3.45% per annum over the 1801–185 period. Since (as Table V-4 shows for the end of the period) natural increas was very unlikely to have accounted for even as much as half of this growth the progress in population was due very much to heavy net in-migration The net in-migration of the 1840s and the 1850s was considerably greater i Merthyr Tydfil than in Durham and Easington for the same period (Tabl V-4). In 1851, of the 35,093 persons aged 20 and above enumerated in tha year, only 9120 (26.0%) were born within the town of Merthyr Tydfil an only an additional 4146 (11.8%) within Glamorganshire but outside th town. Of the remaining 21,827 persons (62.2%) who were born outside th county, 14,189 (40.4%) came from the neighboring four Welsh counties o Carmarthan, Brecknock, Pembroke, and Cardigan. Over 2330 Irish (6.6% had already made their way to Merthyr by 1851. There was also a tremen dous turnover of population, as was also the case in many urban areas in th United States (for the United States, see Thernstrom and Knights, 1971). I 1849, for example, the town of Merthyr Tydfil was estimated as having 10,000–11,000 person turnover annually. This was slightly over 16% of th

›pulation (*Westminster Review*, 1849, cited in John, 1950, p. 72). This ›ntributed to "the turbulence and unrest which characterized the coal field this time [John, 1950, p. 72]." There was also considerable seasonal .igration to the iron works (John, 1950, p. 66), although this tended to minish over time. Many left agriculture in Wales, and complaints were eard that "agricultural laborers are less numerous than they formerly were ving to their being drained off to Merthyr and the manufacturing districts Royal Commission on Education, 1847, xxvii, p. 309 quoted in John, 1950, p. 64–65]." Many workers came long distances to work in Merthyr Tydfil ermanently; the Irish have already been mentioned. In 1851, about 11% of Merthyr's adult population had been born in England. But, in the main, the igrants were Welsh. The migrants, especially those in mining, "were ainly drawn from the counties bordering upon the coal field . . . and from mong the agricultural workers of the mining district [Evans, 1961, p. 6]."

After approximately 1850, however, the character of the region began to hange from one with an emphasis on iron manufacture to one in which oal mining showed the most rapid growth. Between 1851 and 1861, for xample, the number of adult males in coal mining increased from 5579 to 887, or roughly 77%. During the same period, the number of males in iron anufacture (excluding iron mining) increased from only 3741 to 4766, or nly about 27%. The main growth was in demand for the "steam coals"— xcellent fuel for ships, railway locomotives, and stationary steam engines. Much of the growth here took place in the southern part of the Merthyr Tydfil district, outside the town of Merthyr Tydfil in the subdistrict of Gelligaer near the Rhondda valleys. Further rail connections were necesary to tap these coal seams, and they were completed in the 1850s (Minhinton, 1969, p. xix). Evidence of this development is furnished by the nore rapid growth of the nonurban than the urban portions of Merthyr Tydfil registration district which led to a decline in the proportion urban etween 1851 and 1861. Most of the rapid growth in the steam coal industry lid not, however, take place within Merthyr Tydfil, but rather in the Rhondda valleys and areas to the south and west (E. D. Lewis, 1959, Chaps. IV and V). A portion of the southern edge of the Merthyr Tydfil registration listrict was, in fact, removed in 1863 and placed in the newly created district of Pontypridd. Thus, having lost most of the area of rapid development, the growth of Merthyr (adjusted for boundary changes) slowed from 3.32% per year in the 1850s to 1.14% in the 1860s. Depressed times struck the iron ndustry after the boom of 1872–1874. Iron ore deposits were being depleted, and it was expensive to ship it to places far inland like Merthyr. As a result, when the iron industry rationalized and converted to Bessemer and openhearth steel production, it also relocated near the coast, where iron ore could be cheaply imported. The Dowlais Company finally moved some of its operations to Cardiff when it opened a new plant there in 1891.

The characteristics of the Merthyr Tydfil registration district, therefo make it an appropriate case study and an interesting contrast to the Durha and Easington districts. As the previous discussion made clear and as may seen in Table V-1, Merthyr had a very high proportion of its adult ma population in mining and metallurgy (up to 60% by 1871). By 1851, it alrea had a very small proportion of its population (5.2%) in agriculture. It w thus considerably less agricultural than Durham and Easington. Merth was also a very urban area, unlike many other mining regions. It was 82 urban by 1851 and 84.5% by 1871.[2] This reflected its orientation toward ir manufacture. This extensive urbanization created a high density, whi exceeded the averages both for the nation as a whole and for Durham a Easington. The rapid growth prior to the 1860s and 1870s was, as mention previously, due largely to heavy net in-migration. Net in-migration h become net out-migration by the 1860s, and the whole district showed negative total increase during the economically depressed decade of t 1870s (Table V-4). The earlier large net in-migration was concentrat among younger adults, as the sex ratios in Table V-3 demonstrate. The s ratios in Merthyr were even higher than those in Durham and Easingt and were clearly in contrast to the low ratios in England and Wales as whole.

As far as mortality was concerned, the crude death rate (CDR) in Merth Tydfil was considerably higher than either in Durham and Easington or England and Wales as a whole for the entire period 1841–1850 throu 1901–1910 (Table V-4). This is also demonstrated by the considerably low female expectation of life in Merthyr in 1846–1850, 1851–1860, and 186 1870, than in Durham and Easington or in England and Wales. The infa mortality rate was also somewhat higher in Merthyr Tydfil until 1870–187 This higher mortality, combined with fertility levels generally comparable those in Durham and Easington (with the exception of the 1870s), led to a ra of natural increase below that of Durham and Easington but still above th for England and Wales. The average rate of natural increase over the peri 1851–1860 through 1901–1910 was 20% above the national average (opposed to 57% for Durham and Easington). Fertility, although not quite high in Merthyr Tydfil as in the Durham and Easington districts, was st quite high in relation to the nation as a whole. The index of overall fertili in Table V-5 (I_f) was an average of 29% above the national I_f for the perio 1850–1852 through 1900–1902. The index of marital fertility was, howeve only 5.5% above the average for England and Wales for 1850–1852

[2] Urban areas were defined as the town of Merthyr Tydfil, which included the registrati subdistrict of Aberdare, most of the registration subdistricts of Upper and Lower Merth Tydfil, and part of the parish of Vainor from Brecknockshire. The decline in proportion urb between 1851 and 1861 was due to a more rapid growth of the nonurban areas in the southe part of the district. Much of this area was removed from Merthyr in 1863.

90–1892. (Durham and Easington had an I_g 12.2% above the national ·el.) Marriage, as measured by the index of proportions married, was as rly and extensive as in Durham and Easington. The level of I_m for erthyr Tydfil was, in fact, above that for Durham and Easington in 50–1852 and 1860–1862 and averaged 20.5% above the national average er the period 1850–1852 through 1890–1892. Finally, illegitimate fertility s measured by I_h) was below that for the Durham and Easington area t still well above (27%) the national level.

Merthyr Tydfil was clearly not the same type of area as Durham and isington. It was more urban and more concentrated in heavy industry ıetallurgy) in addition to coal and iron mining. Merthyr was also in a very fferent ethnic setting than the English case study. It was, indeed, chosen rtly for its contrasts to Durham and Easington. In addition to these fferences, Merthyr had considerably higher mortality and a development ttern which slacked off in the 1860s. It was geographically rather more mote. But Merthyr Tydfil also had high fertility, early and extensive arriage, and an in-migration pattern that favored young adult males. hese were features which it held in common with Durham and Easington ıd with many other mining and heavy-industrial areas. Both are therefore ›tentially fruitful areas to analyze and compare.

For both case studies, it is clear from Table V-5 that the analysis, which is ›nfined to the censuses of 1851, 1861, and 1871, covers a period preceding e decline in marital fertility or any major adjustments in marriage pat- rns. Earlier censuses were not used because they lacked full information ı each individual. No censuses after 1871 have yet been released by the ritish government for public use. It is unfortunate that the fertility decline ınnot be analyzed as it was for the Pennsylvania anthracite region, but the udy of differential fertility can be conducted in much the same way as it as in Chapter IV. The census data are, in many ways, very similar to those r the United States in the same time period, except that the British ensuses of 1851, 1861, and 1871 all asked questions on marital status and on lationship to head of household. For this reason, the British own-children rtility estimates may be regarded as somewhat more reliable than those for ıe United States for 1850, 1860, and 1870, since the attribution of children › their mothers in the British samples was only infrequently a matter of ıference. In addition, the published mortality data for England and Wales llow more dependable estimates of survivorship to be used in the own- hildren estimating techniques. On the other hand, there is no information n literacy, duration of marriage, children ever born or children surviving in ny of these British censuses.[3] So more can be done in some areas, such as ıortality analysis, but less in others, such as secular fertility change.

[3] The first British census to inquire about marital duration, parity, and child survivorship as the special census of marriage and fertility of 1911.

THE SAMPLE

Systematic samples of approximately 10% were taken from the origin enumerators' manuscripts for the registration districts of Durhar Easington, and Merthyr Tydfil for the censuses of 1851, 1861, and 187 These censuses were enumerated individually into "census families" defined in the instructions to enumerators.[5] The sample was taken as eve tenth household (as defined by the census) with a random starting poin Most information in the manuscripts was recorded for each individual. Th included exact age (at last birthday), sex, marital status, relationship to hea of household, occupation, place of birth (county and parish in the Unit Kingdom or simply the country if born outside the United Kingdom), plac of residence, and labor-force status (i.e., apprentice, employer). For th head of household, name and address were coded and, for 1851 and 18 (when such information was given), number of men employed and/or acr of farm land owned were recorded. Institutional populations were inte tionally omitted from the sample, but the resulting bias was not great.

During coding, a household and family structure (or, alternatively, family and a subfamily structure) was imposed on the data. They were th same procedures used with the U.S. censuses of 1880 and 1900. The hous hold (basically a coresiding unit) was taken as defined in the census. The were seldom any ambiguities here, although they occasionally occur Then, using name, age, sex, marital status, and relationship to househol head, a family structure within the household was created. A family wa defined as two or more persons who constituted a conjugal unit or th remains of a conjugal unit. One exception was boarders and lodgers, wh were part of a household but considered separate families (even if singl individuals). Domestic or farm servants were considered part of the primar family in the household unless they were part of a conjugal unit themselve and other members of the unit were present.

The household and family structure was used to create household an family files, which, in turn, contained all the individual information on th head and spouse of head of household or family, as well as summar information on other members. Some other variables were created, such a number of children aged 0–4, 5–9, 10–14, and 15 and over; number o boarders; age of mother at last surviving birth; number of children in scho at various ages; and number of other relatives present. The family was th unit used for fertility analysis, and age-specific child–woman ratios wer

[4] The manuscripts have been microfilmed and are available through the Public Reco Office in London. All the "piece numbers" for the geographic units within these registratio districts were used.

[5] For some of the problems in defining families and households for census purposes se Tillott (1972, pp. 90–105).

[6] Some examples are given in Tillott (1972, pp. 90–116).

created using the number of own children aged 0–4 present from the family file.

In order to verify the representativeness of the sample, published distributions by age and sex were compared to sample distributions. Other dimensions such as marital status, occupation, and place of birth were also examined. The sample distributions were all quite close to the published ones, and chi-square tests generally showed statistically insignificant differences between the distributions.

The result was a series of samples ranging in size from 7391 individuals and 1370 households in Merthyr Tydfil in 1851 to 12,527 individuals and 2499 households in Durham and Easington in 1871.[7] The sample sizes are comparable to those for the Pennsylvania anthracite region 1850–1900 and are quite adequate to perform the analysis.

DEMOGRAPHIC DIFFERENTIALS AND CHANGE, 1851–1871

Differential Fertility

The analysis of fertility in these British census samples will begin with a study of overall and age-standardized marital child–woman ratios. The overall child–woman ratios (children 0–4 per 1000 women aged 15–49) are presented for the censuses of 1851, 1861, and 1871 for Durham and Easington in Table V-6 and for Merthyr Tydfil in Table V-7. The standardized ratios are given in Table V-8 for Durham and Easington and Table V-9 for Merthyr Tydfil. These are, as before, direct standardizations, using the actual age-specific child–woman ratios and applying them to a standard age structure. Three standardizations were done: first, to the age structure of total married women in each area at each date (Standardization A); second, to the age structure of total married women in England and Wales at each date (Standardization B); and, third, to the age structure of

[7] The sample sizes and sampling fractions were as follows:

	1851	1861	1871
Durham and Easington			
Individuals	7,684	9,555	12,527
Households	1,503	1,818	2,499
Families	1,896	2,480	3,338
Sampling percentage	9.93%	9.79%	10.05%
Merthyr Tydfil			
Individuals	7,391	11,119	10,595
Households	1,370	2,167	2,005
Families	2,381	3,475	3,192
Sampling percentage	9.62%	10.38%	10.16%

TABLE V-6 Overall and Marital Child-Woman Ratios (Children 0-4 per 1000 Women Aged 15-49). Durham and Easington R.D.'s, England, 1851, 1861, 1871 (per 1000 women)[a]

	1851	*N*	1861	*N*	1871	*N*
I. *Total population*						
A. Total	663.	1794	715.	2178	715.	2797
B. Rural	715.	1416	769.	1575	737.	2036
Urban	466.	378	576.	603	656.	761
II. *Married women with husband present*						
A. Total	1030.	993	1099.	1227	1054.	1730
B. Rural	1059.	832	1153.	919	1063.	1302
Urban	882.	161	938.	308	1026.	428
C. Occupation of husband						
1. Farmer, farm laborer	1071.	98	1174	69	973.	74
2. Laborer	1043	70	1101	69	981.	106
3. Miner, mine worker	1080.	424	1125.	544	1093.	835
4. Manufacturing, crafts, construction	953.	235	1065.	306	1066.	456
5. Mercantile, food, lodging, transport, servant	982.	109	1113.	133	951.	164
6. Professional and clerical	1114.	35	871.	62	1033.	61
7. Other	(773.)	22	1181.	44	871.	31
D. Social class (1911 categories)						
1. Higher business and professional	1303.	33	1000.	50	854.	48
2. Lower business and professional	1061.	99	1085.	117	1071.	155
3. Skilled manual workers	911.	158	1027.	187	1071.	254
4. Semiskilled workers	1039.	127	1154.	136	1064.	124
5. Unskilled workers	969.	130	1104.	163	1044.	249
6. Textile workers	(818.)	11	(667.)	9	(733.)	15
7. Miners	1085.	412	1130.	532	1091.	816
8. Agricultural laborers	—	—	—	—	611.	36
E. Social class (1951 categories)						
1. Higher business and professional	(1368.)	19	(1000.)	24	(917.)	12
2. Lower business and professional	1092.	98	1093.	107	1086.	152
3. Skilled manual workers	1035.	630	1100.	781	1079.	1170
4. Semiskilled manual workers	984.	126	1126.	174	1019.	207
5. Unskilled manual workers	1000.	99	1085.	106	930.	156
F. Place of birth of spouse						
1. Durham	1037.	599	1113.	666	1048.	939
2. Northumberland	1039.	154	1173.	173	1043.	235
3. Other England	1022.	137	1025.	162	1058.	311
4. Scotland, Wales, Ireland	957.	93	1061.	212	1099.	233
5. Other	(1300.)	10	(1000.)	14	(750.)	12
G. Does spouse work?						
1. Not working	1030.	969	1109.	1171	1057.	1686
2. Working	(1042.)	24	893.	56	932.	44

Source: Sample of enumerators' manuscripts.

[a]Numbers in parentheses are based on fewer than 30 cases.

TABLE V-7 Overall and Marital Child-Woman Ratios. (Children 0-4 per 1000 Women Aged 15-49). Merthyr Tydfil R.D., Wales, 1851, 1861, 1871 (per 1000 Women)[a]

	1851	*N*	1861	*N*	1871	*N*
I. *Total population*						
A. Total	634.	1725	636.	2639	627.	2421
B. Rural	572.	668	685.	590	778.	198
Urban	673.	1057	622.	2049	614.	2223
II. *Married women with husband present*						
A. Total	943.	1001	935.	1633	963.	1395
B. Rural	899.	365	943.	389	1129.	124
Urban	969.	636	932.	1244	946.	1271
C. Occupation of husband						
1. Farmer, farm laborer	(1000.)[a]	21	1000.	37	(538.)	13
2. Laborer	842.	82	788.	113	745.	102
3. Miner, mine worker	974.	463	969.	778	986.	652
4. Manufacturing, crafts, construction	997.	311	923.	532	936.	441
4a. Iron worker	903.	144	928.	251	977.	218
5. Mercantile, food, lodging, transport, servant	716.	88	912.	114	1073.	124
6. Professional and clerical	(929.)	28	933.	45	1164.	55
7. Other	(571.)	7	(714.)	14	(875.)	8
D. Social class (1911 categories)						
1. Higher business and professional	867.	45	836.	61	1185.	54
2. Lower business and professional	824.	68	989.	93	1010.	95
3. Skilled manual workers	1000.	150	935.	230	852.	189
4. Semiskilled manual workers	986.	71	852.	122	1068.	103
5. Unskilled manual workers	925.	266	918.	441	923.	337
6. Textile workers	(667.)	3	(1000.)	2	(833.)	6
7. Miners	966.	386	973.	659	978.	600
8. Agricultural laborers	(800.)	5	(857.)	14	(625.)	8
E. Social class (1951 categories)						
1. Higher business and professional	(1100.)	10	(692.)	13	(1118.)	17
2. Lower business and professional	817.	93	945.	109	1010.	95
3. Skilled manual workers	973.	655	987.	1062	992.	931
4. Semiskilled manual workers	973.	110	853.	265	884.	206
5. Unskilled manual workers	853.	116	785.	172	837.	141
F. Place of birth of spouse						
1. Glamorganshire	948.	408	963.	590	988.	560
2. Other Wales	954.	418	941.	659	899.	527
3. England	882.	110	892.	212	1026.	193
4. Ireland	948.	58	873.	157	980.	100
5. Other	(800.)	5	(800.)	10	(1375.)	8
G. Does spouse work?						
1. Not working	947.	974	944.	1543	963.	1368
2. Working	(815.)	27	789.	90	(963.)	27

Source: Sample of enumerators' manuscripts.

[a]Numbers in parentheses are based on fewer than 30 cases.

TABLE V-8 Standardized Overall and Marital Child-Woman Ratios. Durham and Easington R.D.'s, England, 1851, 1861, 1871 (per 1000 Women)[a]

	Standardization A[b]			Standardization B[c]			Standardization C[d]		
	1851	1861	1871	1851	1861	1871	1851	1861	1871
I. *Total population*									
A. Total	853.	902.	894.	848.	884.	890.	812.	855.	865.
B. Rural	918.	966.	916.	916.	948.	912.	876.	917.	886.
Urban	616.	755.	835.	593.	720.	830.	579.	696.	809.
II. *Married women with husbands present*									
A. Total	1027.	1098.	1053.	1014.	1060.	1035.	1006.	1059.	1037.
B. Rural	1056.	1140.	1060.	1046.	1106.	1042.	1036.	1102.	1043.
Urban	896.	978.	1032.	874.	937.	1014.	871.	940.	1019.
C. Occupation of husband									
1. Farmer, farm laborer	1032.	1263.	1065.	1025.	1213.	1061.	981.	1222.	1027.
2. Laborer	960.	1112.	993.	949.	1101.	980.	933.	1084.	969.
3. Miner, mine worker	1076.	1115.	1070.	1062.	1077.	1046.	1062.	1076.	1057.
4. Manufacturing, crafts, construction	961.	1047.	1049.	951.	1006.	1041.	935.	1004.	1029.
5. Mercantile, food, lodging, transport, servant	935.	1087.	994.	916.	1038.	978.	917.	1044.	975.
6. Professional and clerical	1115.	968.	1043.	1096.	953.	1046.	1056.	929.	1001.
7. Other	(961.)	1213.	892.	(969.)	1183.	855.	(928.)	1176.	932.
D. Social class (1911 categories)									
1. Higher business and professional	1256.	1055.	826.	1241.	1040.	836.	1187.	1011.	813.
2. Lower business and professional	986.	1091.	1131.	971.	1038.	1118.	955.	1069.	1101.
3. Skilled manual workers	917.	1015.	1064.	905.	977.	1055.	897.	971.	1045.
4. Semiskilled manual workers	1032.	1163.	1122.	1028.	1116.	1107.	1003.	1116.	1107.
5. Unskilled manual workers	918.	1138.	1012.	907.	1118.	1001.	893.	1095.	984.
6. Textile workers	(615.)	(652.)	(716.)	(647.)	(552.)	(710.)	(624.)	(650.)	(690.)
7. Miners	1085.	1121.	1064.	1071.	1084.	1040.	1071.	1083.	1052.
8. Agricultural laborers	--	--	711.	--	--	711.	--	--	685.
E. Social class (1951 categories)									
1. Higher business and professional	(1481.)	(1128.)	(640.)	(1443.)	(1096.)	(634.)	(1406.)	(1081.)	(635.)
2. Lower business and professional	1010.	1120.	1137.	1002.	1059.	1121.	974.	1080.	1115.
3. Skilled manual workers	1037.	1079.	1070.	1023.	1039.	1050.	1027.	1043.	1056.
4. Semiskilled manual workers	981.	1177.	1041.	971.	1152.	1032.	925.	1119.	1013.
5. Unskilled manual workers	959.	1112.	907.	949.	1088.	898.	940.	1075.	881.
F. Place of birth of spouse									
1. Durham	1051.	1117.	1045.	1037.	1084.	1028.	1029.	1078.	1029.
2. Northumberland	1016.	1225.	1040.	1007.	1177.	1018.	996.	1181.	1029.
3. Other England	973.	1016.	1103.	966.	974.	1083.	934.	979.	1090.
4. Scotland, Wales, Ireland	901.	1037.	1037.	885.	1010.	1025.	886.	1007.	1012.
5. Other	(1284.)	(700.)	(386.)	(1302.)	(642.)	(392.)	(1184.)	(625.)	(351.)
G. Does spouse work?									
1. Not working	1025.	1108.	1057.	1012.	1070.	1039.	1004.	1070.	1040.
2. Working	(791.)	912.	818.	(771.)	896.	813.	(768.)	866.	795.

Source: Sample of enumerators' manuscripts.

[a]Numbers in parentheses are based on fewer than 30 cases.

[b]Standardization A = standardized to the age structure of married women at each date.

[c]Standardization B = standardized to the age structure of married women in England and Wales at each date.

[d]Standardization C = standardized to the age structure of married women in the Pennsylvania anthracite region in 1880.

TABLE V-9 Standardized and Marital Child-Woman Ratios. Merthyr Tydfil R.D., Wales, 1851, 1861, 1871 (per 1000 Women)[a]

	Standardization A[b]			Standardization B[c]			Standardization C[d]		
	1851	1861	1871	1851	1861	1871	1851	1861	1871
I. *Total population*									
A. Total	790.	786.	800.	772.	763.	809.	734.	738.	780.
B. Rural	768.	827.	934.	749.	807.	947.	716.	781.	924.
Urban	802.	777.	788.	786.	754.	797.	745.	729.	767.
II. *Married women with husbands present*									
A. Total	946.	936.	960.	910.	897.	956.	895.	898.	953.
B. Rural	908.	946.	1116.	872.	906.	1111.	858.	922.	1122.
Urban	964.	938.	945.	929.	899.	941.	914.	897.	937.
C. Occupation of husband									
1. Farmer, farm laborer	(948.)	919.	(473.)	(902.)	892.	(503.)	(857.)	828.	(468.)
2. Laborer	825.	817.	745.	804.	773.	743.	775.	784.	763.
3. Mine, mine worker	986.	959.	978.	953.	921.	974.	930.	923.	967.
4. Manufacturing, crafts, construction	994.	905.	950.	958.	870.	946.	945.	858.	942.
4a. Iron workers	891.	910.	978.	873.	884.	980.	859.	868.	970.
5. Mercantile, food, lodging, transport, servant	732.	952.	1072.	701.	896.	1060.	700.	930.	1065.
6. Professional and clerical	(982.)	943.	1052.	(892.)	923.	1037.	(958.)	883.	1044.
7. Other	(500.)	(628.)	(423.)	(422.)	(587.)	(429.)	(530.)	(614.)	(388.)
D. Social class (1911 categories)									
1. Higher business and professional	962.	865.	1184.	924.	833.	1175.	896.	829.	1165.
2. Lower business and professional	801.	1100.	1012.	768.	1041.	990.	747.	1058.	1013.
3. Skilled manual workers	1000.	937.	889.	948.	899.	883.	942.	884.	880.
4. Semiskilled manual workers	1048.	866.	1044.	1010.	817.	1047.	993.	827.	1053.
5. Unskilled manual workers	916.	915.	928.	889.	880.	925.	881.	874.	923.
6. Textile workers	(358.)	(438.)	(447.)	(358.)	(396.)	(453.)	(322.)	(358.)	(432.)
7. Miners	975.	959.	971.	943.	921.	968.	923.	924.	958.
8. Agricultural laborers	(872.)	(716.)	(461.)	(798.)	(683.)	(485.)	(716.)	(640.)	(452.)
E. Social class (1951 categories)									
1. Higher business and professional	(1418.)	(515.)	(919.)	(1317.)	(506.)	(920.)	(1329.)	(474.)	(960.)
2. Lower business and professional	834.	982.	981.	811.	938.	978.	764.	956.	959.
3. Skilled manual workers	977.	969.	993.	944.	930.	988.	926.	929.	985.
4. Semiskilled manual workers	958.	879.	880.	914.	849.	877.	901.	834.	863.
5. Unskilled manual workers	832.	829.	832.	795.	783.	828.	793.	802.	846.
F. Place of birth of spouse									
1. Glamorganshire	977.	960.	987.	944.	927.	984.	923.	925.	976.
2. Other Wales	942.	964.	914.	904.	922.	912.	880.	930.	905.
3. England	887.	896.	1028.	856.	853.	1016.	867.	841.	1022.
4. Ireland	863.	822.	967.	802.	770.	952.	797.	798.	990.
5. Other	(728.)	(672.)	(1100.)	(660.)	(630.)	(1140.)	(625.)	(579.)	(1060.)
G. Does spouse work?									
1. Not working	951.	947.	958.	916.	906.	954.	900.	908.	951.
2. Working	(770.)	755.	(1030.)	(711.)	739.	(1021.)	(693.)	721.	(1014.)

Source: Sample of enumerators' manuscripts.

[a] Numbers in parentheses are based on fewer than 30 cases.

[b] Standardization A = standardized to the age structure of married women at each date.

[c] Standardization B = standardized tc the age structure of married women in England and Wales at each date.

[d] Standardization C = standardized to the age structure of married women in the Pennsylvania anthracite region in 1880.

total married women in the Pennsylvania anthracite region in 1880 (Standardization C). Overall and standardized ratios were calculated for the total population of females aged 15–49, and for the rural and urban subgroups of these women separately. The same overall and standardized ratios were also calculated separately for married women aged 15–49 with husband present. For this group, ratios were calculated for the total group as well as for a number of subgroups categorized by rural–urban residence, occupation of husband, social class of husband (using the 1911 and 1951 Registrar General's categories),[8] and place of birth and labor-force participation of spouse.

Dealing with the total population of women first, it is quite apparent that Durham and Easington had higher total fertility than Merthyr Tydfil at all three census dates. Durham and Easington had overall ratios which averaged 10.3% higher over the period. In terms of rural–urban differences, urban fertility in Durham and Easington was consistently less than rural, although the differential was converging as urban fertility rose over time.[9] For Merthyr Tydfil, on the other hand, urban fertility was considerably above rural fertility in 1851 (17.7% above), but then rural fertility rose dramatically while urban fertility declined. This was partly a function of the growth of the urban area, the town of Merthyr Tydfil gradually growing until only the high fertility subdistrict of Gelligaer remained as rural. There was virtually no trend in overall fertility in either Durham and Easington or in Merthyr Tydfil over the period. Notable was the rise in fertility in Durham and Easington between 1851 and 1861, the rapid rise of urban fertility throughout in the Durham and Easington districts, and finally the contrasting decline in urban fertility in Merthyr.

Standardization of the ratios for the total population notably affected the levels of fertility, since the age distribution of married women (as opposed to total women) assigns much larger relative weight to the ages with the highest child–woman ratios. The age distributions of married women within each region (Standardization A) were generally more conducive to higher fertility than those for England and Wales as a whole (Standardization B) or for the Pennsylvania anthracite region in 1880 (Standardization C). Notably, the age distribution of married women in England and Wales was much more weighted toward women in their late 30s and 40s where age-specific fertility was relatively lower. The still lower ratios using the age structure of married women in the Pennsylvania anthracite region was not the result of an older age structure for married women but rather a much younger age structure that assigned more weight to the age-specific ratios for ages 15–19 and 20–24

[8] For a discussion of these social stratification schemes, see Armstrong (1972, pp. 198–211).

[9] This convergence was partially due to the changing composition of the designated urban areas. Between 1851 and 1861, Seaham Harbor (Easington) was added to Durham City in the urban category.

rather than the peak age groups 25–29 and 20–34. Standardization C has the effect of holding age structure constant over time, and the result of this was to confirm a small *upward* trend in fertility in both the Durham and Easington districts and Merthyr Tydfil. As the population of total women aged because of reductions in mortality and because of a reduced impact of in-migration on younger cohorts, the age structure became somewhat less favorable to high overall fertility over time. Standardization C has corrected for that.

Considering the marital child–woman ratios in Tables V-6 to V-9, the first impression is of the expectedly higher level of the marital child–woman ratios relative to the total ratios.[10] For both case studies there was no real trend over time, with 1861 being a high year in Durham and Easington and a low year in Merthyr Tydfil. The relative positions of rural and urban fertility were the same as for the total population but the differentials had narrowed somewhat. In Durham and Easington the average excess of rural over urban was only 15% for married women as opposed to 33% for total women. The reason was the later age of marriage among women in the urban areas for 1851 and 1861 (see Table V-15, page 192). The same pattern of a reversal in the rankings of rural and urban fertility for Merthyr Tydfil between 1851 and 1861 appears for the marital ratios as well as those for total women. The standardizations do little to change these patterns, indicating that variations in the age patterns of married women had much less effect on the fertility of spouses from the family sample than on fertility in the total female population.

The classification of marital child–woman ratios by the occupation of the husband makes it clear that miners and mine workers had high fertility relative to other occupational groups in both regions and at all three dates. An extra subcategory, Iron Workers, was added to the Merthyr Tydfil tables in order to examine the fertility behavior of that large subgroup of the Manufacturing–Crafts–Construction category. The iron workers had fertility below the coal miners in Merthyr Tydfil for 1851 and 1861, but were quite close (for the standardized ratios) and somewhat above (for the overall ratios) for 1871. The relative rankings of the occupations were not particularly stable, however, as Table V-10 shows. The rankings are given for both the overall ratio and Standardization A (i.e., the age structure of all married women at each date in each region). Farmers and farm laborers had relatively high fertility in Durham and Easington in 1851 and 1861 and also for 1871 when standardized for the age structure of all wives. For Merthyr

[10] One point that must be borne in mind, however, is that the child–woman ratios for the total female population were adjusted for children not included in the own children tabulations. Thus each ratio was adjusted by the factor Total Children 0–4/Own Children 0–4. This was not done for the marital child–woman ratios, and it may be that some children were missing from their mothers for reasons other than mortality.

TABLE V-10 Rankings of Occupational Groups by Level of Overall and Standardized Marital Child-Woman Ratios[a]

Durham and Easington

Overall			Standardization A		
1851	1861	1871	1851	1861	1871
Professional/ Clerical	Other	Miners, etc.	Professional/ Clerical	Farmers, etc.	Miners, etc.
Miners, etc.	Farmers, etc.	Manufacturing, etc.	Miners, etc.	Other	Farmers, etc.
Farmers, etc.	Miners, etc.	Professional/ Clerical	Farmers, etc.	Miners, etc.	Manufacturing, etc.
Laborers	Mercantile, etc.	Laborers	Manufacturing, etc.	Laborers	Professional/ Clerical
Mercantile, etc.	Laborers	Farmers, etc.	(Other)	Mercantile, etc.	Mercantile, etc.
Manufacturing, etc.	Manufacturing, etc.	Mercantile, etc.	Laborers	Manufacturing, etc.	Laborers
(Other)	Professional/ Clerical	Other	Mercantile, etc.	Professional/ Clerical	Other

Merthyr Tydfil

Overall			Standardization A		
1851	1861	1871	1851	1861	1871
(Farmers, etc.)	Farmers, etc.	Professional/ Clerical	Manufacturing, etc.	Miners, etc.	Mercantile, etc.
Manufacturing, etc.	Miners, etc.	Mercantile, etc.	Miners, etc.	Mercantile, etc.	Professional/ Clerical
Miners, etc.	Professional/ Clerical	Miners, etc.	(Professional/ Clerical)	Professional/ Clerical	Miners, etc.
(Professional/ Clerical)	[Iron workers]	[Iron workers]	(Farmers, etc.)	Farmers, etc.	[Iron workers]
[Iron workers]	Manufacturing, etc.	Manufacturing, etc.	[Iron workers]	[Iron workers]	Manufacturing, etc.
Laborers	Mercantile, etc.	(Other)	Laborers	Manufacturing, etc.	Laborers
Mercantile, etc.	Laborers	Laborers	Mercantile, etc.	Laborer	(Farmers, etc.)
(Other)	(Other)	(Farmers, etc.)	(Other)	(Other)	(Other)

Source: Tables V-6 through V-9.

[a] Groups in parentheses are based on less than 30 cases. Iron workers are placed in brackets to indicate that they are a subset of the group "Manufacturing, etc."

Tydfil, the numbers of farmers and farm laborers in the sample were quite small and the estimates are much less reliable, but their fertility, once standardized for age structure, was quite a bit lower. Laborers demonstrated consistently low fertility relative to the average, especially in Merthyr. This was in marked contrast to the Pennsylvania anthracite area.[11] For the other groups, the rankings were quite changeable from one census to the next. Manufacturing–Crafts–Construction was generally near the middle or top, but Professional–Clerical fluctuated a great deal in Durham and Easington and Mercantile–Food–Lodging–Transport–Servants did the same in Merthyr Tydfil. In Durham and Easington, however, the Mercantile, etc., group generally experienced below-average fertility, while in Merthyr Tydfil the Professional–Clerical group had above-average marital child–woman ratios. The latter is most puzzling since it is usually the higher socioeconomic strata which have the lowest fertility and earliest decline. (See, for example, Innes, 1938.) This could mean that occupational fertility differentials were not well established at this time, but could also reflect defects in the categorization scheme and large sampling errors surrounding some of the smaller groups (such as Farmers–Farm Laborers and Professional–Clerical). Nonetheless, the consistently high fertility of miners and mine workers and the comparatively high fertility of iron workers (in Merthyr Tydfil) does substantiate the fact that the high fertility which had been observed among these groups in 1911 (see Chapter I) was indeed true at mid-century in these two areas. Finally, it might also be observed that some of the same factors that influenced high fertility among miners and iron workers, such as lack of employment opportunities for women, relatively high wages, and above-average infant and child mortality, might also have influenced other occupational groups to have had above-average fertility. Wages and incomes might have been higher among the other groups because high wages for miners and iron workers[12] would have tended to bring the wages and incomes for other groups up as well. Marital and overall fertility for both the Durham–Easington and the Merthyr Tydfil districts was well above the national level, as Table V-5 shows.

As an alternative to categorization by industrial–occupational groups, two schemes of social-class stratification that were used by the Registrar General in the 1911 and the 1951 censuses of England and Wales are presented. While the former has been characterized as a "wholesale assignment of occupations to social classes in a rough and ready way [Armstrong, 1972, p. 203]," it does have the virtue of being comparable to the findings of the 1911

[11] The more specific designation of occupation in the British censuses from 1851 onward may have had something to do with this, since workers simply classified as laborers in the U.S. censuses may, in fact, have been more than common laborers. This misidentification was less common in the British censuses.

[12] See Evans (1961) and Minchinton (1969) on the very high wages paid to the iron and coal workers in Merthyr Tydfil.

census on completed fertility (see Table I-1, pages 6–7). The 1951 scheme was rather more rational in its assignment pattern, and its wider use in historical research has been suggested by Armstrong (1972, pp. 209–211). Neither scheme gives the results that were found later; that is, that there was a smooth inverse gradation in completed fertility from the lowest to the highest social classes. The census of marriage and fertility of 1911 found these clear, monotonic class differentials (Innes, 1938, Chap. 2), as did the subsequent censuses of 1951 and 1961. This was not the case for Durham and Easington or for Merthyr Tydfil for 1851, 1861, and 1871, however. The most common pattern was somewhat of a U-shaped pattern, with skilled workers having the highest fertility and with professionals, semiskilled, and unskilled workers having somewhat lower levels. Standardization did little to change these basic patterns.

It may be that the social-class differentials observed for the late nineteenth and for the twentieth centuries were not well established by the mid-nineteenth century. In this connection it should be pointed out that Anderson, working with the textile factory town of Preston in 1851, rejected the use of the Registrar General's schemes of stratification on the grounds that they represented more modern notions of stratification not appropriate to the mid-nineteenth century (Anderson, 1971, pp. 25–29 and Chap. 4, note 23). Katz has also suggested that, for historical work on small, local areas or even specific cities, occupational groupings should really reflect the questions asked and the nature of the local economy rather than some a priori scheme (Katz, 1972, 1975, p. 343). Specialized local economies, such as Durham and Easington (concentrated in coal mining), Merthyr Tydfil (specializing in coal mining and iron manufacture), and Preston (dominated by cotton textiles), may not provide adequately diversified social–occupational groupings. Also, fertility is measured here in terms of current fertility and not completed parity, as in the 1911 census. Differences can appear, especially if the various groups experienced different patterns of timing of births and fertility decline. Nonetheless, the basic patterns of differentials should still appear. Perhaps the best solution to the problem is, indeed, to construct classification schemes most appropriate to the specific context.[13]

Classification of fertility by place of birth of spouse (one alternative among the possible uses of the nativity data from the census) reveals for the Durham and Easington districts that those women born in County Durham or in neighboring County Northumberland were most likely to have had the

[13] As an alternative, and very empirical, approach to the problem, Theodore Hershberg, Michael Katz, Stuart Blumin, Lawrence Glasco, and Clyde Griffin compared their subjective social-status rankings of occupations for the five cities each had been studying for the mid-nineteenth century (Philadelphia; Hamilton, Ontario; Kingston, New York; Buffalo, New York; and Poughkeepsie, New York). The rankings proved to be quite similar, although the economic structures of the cities were quite different in some cases. See Hershberg *et al.* (1974).

largest families in 1851 and 1861, but that migrants from elsewhere in England (mostly from Yorkshire and Cumberland) had the highest standardized fertility by 1871. Spouses born in Scotland, Wales, or Ireland showed marital fertility that increased over time. They had the highest overall fertility in 1871 but, when standardized, they dropped to second rank. Most of these spouses were born in Ireland (67% in 1851 and 72% in 1871). It is possible that the lower child–woman ratios in 1851 might have reflected considerably higher differential infant and child mortality of the late 1840s, particularly among the Irish fleeing the famine and its aftermath. The differential mortality may have alleviated somewhat by the late 1850s and 1860s and resulted in the rise in relative rankings. There also might have been an improvement in family stability. The situation in 1851 and 1861 in which the nonmigrant or short-distance migrant population had high fertility relative to the longer-distance migrants resembles that in the Pennsylvania coal fields in 1850 and contrasts with the American experience later in the century.

In Merthyr Tydfil it was the spouses born locally, in Glamorganshire, who showed generally high fertility. For the age-standardized ratios, spouses born in Glamorganshire had the highest fertility in 1851 and were close to the highest in 1861. By 1871, although they had experienced an increase in marital child–woman ratios, the first rank had been taken by migrants from England. This is somewhat the same pattern as found in Durham and Easington. Migrants from elsewhere in Wales (largely from the adjacent counties of Carmarthenshire, Brecknockshire, Pembrokeshire, and Cardiganshire) had fertility close to that of spouses born in Glamorganshire in 1851 and 1861, but they experienced a decline in marital child–woman ratios between 1861 and 1871. The Irish spouses in Merthyr Tydfil had low fertility initially (as in Durham and Easington) but their fertility rose after 1861 to higher levels, although not as high as in Durham and Easington. Again the persistently high fertility of the local residents as well as the rising marital child–woman ratios of the English and Irish in-migrant wives is notable.

The final tabulation in Tables V-6 through V-9 contrasts the fertility experience of working versus nonworking wives. The proportion of spouses in the age group 15–49 who were enumerated as employed was very small, ranging from 2.4 to 5.5%.[14] As a result, several of the samples of working

[14] The percentage of spouses who were listed as employed was

	1851	1861	1871
Spouses 15–49			
Durham and Easington	2.42	4.56	2.54
Merthyr Tydfil	2.70	5.51	1.94
All spouses			
Durham and Easington	1.48	2.70	1.68
Merthyr Tydfil	1.36	2.88	1.25

wives had fewer than 30 cases. This low proportion certainly accords with expectations about the low level of labor-force participation among women, and especially among married women, in mining and heavy-industrial areas. The effect on fertility was clear, however. When adjusted for age composition, working wives had fewer younger children present in both Durham and Easington and in Merthyr. The one exception was Merthyr Tydfil in 1871, but the number of cases of wives working was rather small in that instance and the difference was statistically insignificant.

In sum, the overall and age-standardized marital child–woman ratios do support the contentions that miners and metallurgical workers did have relatively high marital fertility and that fertility among working wives, the few that there were in these areas, was lower than that for nonworking wives. There were fewer predictable patterns of occupational fertility differentials among the other groups: Farmers' wives had above-average fertility in 1851 and 1861; wives of men in Manufacturing–Crafts–Construction groups were close to the average throughout; and laborers' wives had generally below-average child–woman ratios. Attempts to use occupation to observe class differentials did not reveal the patterns which were common later in the nineteenth or the twentieth centuries. Fertility patterns by nativity demonstrated mixed results, with increases in fertility among Irish-born spouses and a relative constancy among the locally born, who often had the highest current fertility.

In order to assess the simultaneous effects of several of these dimensions on current fertility, regression equations were estimated for all three dates for each of the two areas. The units of observation were married women aged 15–49 with husband present. The dependent variable was the number of young own children present. The independent variables included age of wife, age of wife squared (to account for the curvilinear relationship between fertility and woman's age), residence (whether rural or urban), and two series of dummy variables, one for occupation of husband and one for place of birth of spouse. For the latter two variables, one category had to be omitted in order to permit estimation. The variable on wife working was also omitted because of the small number of working wives in the samples. The method of estimation was ordinary least squares. In view of the encouraging results in Chapter IV, it was felt that OLS was sufficiently robust and that estimation of multinomial logit was unnecessary.

The results are presented in Table V-11, with three equations for each of the two case studies. The equations explained between 7.8 and 17.7% of total variation in the dependent variable, and each equation was jointly significant at a 1% level (as measured by the F-ratio). The β-coefficients show that age of wife and age of wife squared were the most influential variables in explaining variation in the number of young own-children present, as was the case for the Pennsylvania data. Many of the other coefficients were neither very large nor significant. The other β-coefficients showed that the dummy variables for occupation of husband, place of birth of spouse, and rural–urban residence were not too influential.

For Durham and Easington, urban residence moved from having a significant negative effect on current fertility in 1851 and 1861 to a small and insignificant negative impact by 1871. The reverse was true for Merthyr Tydfil, where urban residence had a small but insignificant positive effect on current marital fertility in 1851 and 1861, but this had become negative and significant by 1871. Both these sets of results were suggested by the overall and age-standardized marital child–woman ratios.

The categories of dummy variables for occupation of husband were almost uniformly insignificant for both Durham–Easington and Merthyr Tydfil. (The omitted dummy variable category was "Professional and Clerical" group.) This result suggests that differentiation of fertility behavior by occupational grouping within these mining and industrial regions during the mid-nineteenth century was much less the case than indicated for the late nineteenth century (Innes, 1938, Chap. 2; see also Chap. I, this volume). The results from Chapter III indicate also that, for mid-century, differential fertility might have been larger *between* regions with differing economic structures rather than within regions having a particular type of economic structure. The lack of success of the 1911 and 1951 Registrar General's social-stratification schemes when applied to Durham–Easington and Merthyr Tydfil in 1851–1871 might well be attributable to this smaller degree of differentiation with respect to reproductive behavior for occupational groups within mining and industrial areas. In looking at the occupational dummy variables, a few points do emerge. In both regions, wives of farmers and farm laborers had generally high current marital fertility. The fact that a woman's husband was a miner or a mine worker generally had a larger upward effect on fertility than if the husband had been a member of some other occupational group. This was true also in Merthyr Tydfil for the group Manufacturing–Crafts–Construction (with its large representation of iron workers) in 1851 and 1861. Place of birth of spouse also did not furnish results that were easy to interpret. In general for 1861 and 1871, birth locally had an upward effect on fertility, but again, the dummy variable coefficients were mostly insignificant. No really clear patterns emerged.

The results of applying regression analysis to these case studies were not particularly striking nor surprising. Most could have been anticipated by the results from the child–woman ratios in Tables V-6 through V-9. The strength of the curvilinear pattern with respect to age was confirmed as were the changing rural–urban differentials. For occupation of husband, wives of miners and mine workers had usually high fertility but not the highest. The results on place of birth were not clear, as they were for the United States in the later nineteenth century. Indeed one is struck more by the lack of really

TABLE V-11 Regression Equations with Number of Children Aged 0-4 as the Dependent Variable. Durham and Easington R.D.'s, England; Merthyr Tydfil R.D., Wales; 1851, 1861, 1871. (Families with Both Husband and Wife Present. Wife Aged 15-49)

	1851			1861			1871		
	Coefficient	Significance	β-Coefficient	Coefficient	Significance	β-Coefficient	Coefficient	Significance	β-Coefficient
I. *Dependent variable*									
Children 0-4					*Durham and Easington*				
II. *Independent variables*									
1. Constant	-2.7819	NC[a]	NC	-2.575	NC	NC	-2.7293	NC	NC
2. Age of spouse	.2573	***	2.2607	.2540	***	2.1527	.2732	***	2.4205
3. Age of spouse squared	-.0041	***	-2.5079	-.0042	***	-2.3819	-.0045	***	-2.7110
4. Occupation of husband									
a. Farmer, etc.	-.0994	n.s.[b]	-.0326	.1674	n.s.	.0418	.0354	n.s.	.0078
b. Laborer	-.0820	n.s.	-.0232	.0836	n.s.	.0206	-.0742	n.s.	-.0193
c. Miner, etc.	-.1035	n.s.	-.0564	.0468	n.s.	.0250	.0388	n.s.	.0210
d. Manufacturing, etc.	-.1832	n.s.	-.0857	.0368	n.s.	.0172	.0190	n.s.	.0091
e. Mercantile, etc.	-.1900	n.s.	-.0656	.0605	n.s.	.0202	-.0236	n.s.	-.0075
f. Other	-.1892	n.s.	-.0279	.1606	n.s.	.0309	-.1596	n.s.	-.0233
5. Place of birth of spouse									
a. This county	.2819	**	.1514	.0769	n.s.	.0413	-.0360	n.s.	-.0194
b. Adjacent counties	.1981	*	.0940	.1041	n.s.	.0464	-.0338	n.s.	-.0151
c. Rest of Britain	.3287	**	.0960	-.1189	n.s.	-.0373	-.0504	n.s.	-.0185
d. Other	.4970	*	.0549	-.0903	n.s.	-.0104	-.2033	n.s.	-.0183
6. Residence	-.1593	**	.0645	-.1508	***	-.0704	-.0181	n.s.	-.0084
Number of cases		983			1211			1722	
Adjusted R^2		.135			.129			.177	
F-Ratio		12.826 ***			14.748 ***			29.418 ***	

	Merthyr Tydfil								
III. *Independent variables*									
1. Constant	-2.1212	NC	NC	-2.2759	NC	NC	-1.9195	NC	NC
2. Age of spouse	.2067	***	1.8426	.2257	***	2.1164	.2287	***	2.0745
3. Age of spouse squared	-.0033	***	-2.0038	-.0037	***	-2.3863	-.0037	***	-2.3136
4. Occupation of husband									
a. Farmer, etc.	.1500	n.s.	.0252	.0474	n.s.	.0084	-.4953	*	-.0527
b. Laborer	-.0501	n.s.	-.0160	-.1244	n.s.	-.0374	-.3602	**	-.1038
c. Miner, etc.	.0908	n.s.	.0529	-.0184	n.s.	-.0109	-.1071	n.s.	-.0591
d. Manufacturing, etc.	.0993	n.s.	.0538	-.0620	n.s.	-.0345	-.1323	n.s.	-.0681
e. Mercantile, etc.	-.1726	n.s.	-.0567	-.0392	n.s.	-.0118	-.0488	n.s.	-.1534
f. Other	-.5142	n.s.	-.0537	-.1585	n.s.	-.0154	.2202	n.s.	.0130
5. Place of birth of spouse									
a. This county	-.0366	n.s.	-.0210	.1027	n.s.	.0568	-.0371	n.s.	-.0201
b. Adjacent counties	-.0846	n.s.	-.0483	.0824	n.s.	.0479	-.0751	n.s.	-.0397
c. Rest of Britain	-.0728	n.s.	-.0293	.1069	n.s.	.0435	-.0451	n.s.	-.0185
d. Other	.2406	n.s.	.0218	.4321	*	.0401	-.1398	n.s.	-.0317
6. Residence	.0635	n.s.	.0357	.0116	n.s.	.0059	-.1996	**	-.0624
Number of cases		993			1626			1390	
Adjusted R^2		.078			.140			.128	
F-Ratio		7.488 ***			21.346 ***			16.667 ***	

Source: Sample of enumerators' manuscripts.

*$p < .1$.

**$p < .05$.

***$p < .01$.

[a] NC = Not calculated.

[b] n.s. = Not significant at least at a 10% level.

consistent differentials with respect to residence, nativity of spouse, and occupation of husband than with any patterns. Since the results and coefficients seemed relatively stable with respect to age of spouse and because no real patterns emerged with respect to the other variables, it was decided to estimate one equation with both regions for all three dates pooled together. The resulting equation (not presented) explained about 14% of total variation in number of own young children present to married couples and was jointly significant at a 1% level. The most important variables were, as before, age of wife and age of wife squared, which also had the expected signs. A dummy variable for location showed that residence in Merthyr Tydfil had a significant and negative effect on current fertility. In this equation, however, the occupational dummy variables showed some improvement, with wives of farmers and farm laborers having the highest expected fertility and wives of miners and mine workers having the next highest. Both coefficients were significant. The expected fertility for wives of laborers was significantly lower than for any other group. Thus a pattern of sorts could be discerned, and it was somewhat like that for the anthracite region of eastern Pennsylvania at mid-century (see Table IV-10, page 107) when farmers and miners had relatively higher current fertility while laborers experienced the lowest expected rates.

Fertility Change, Marriage, and Migration

From the census sample discussed previously, the age-specific child–woman ratios (for women aged 15–19 through 45–49) were used to calculate age-specific overall and marital fertility rates. The only differential aspect of fertility discussed in this section is that of rural–urban. For Durham and Easington, the urban area in 1851 consisted of Durham City. For 1861 and 1871, Seaham Harbor (in Easington) was also included as an urban area. For Merthyr Tydfil, it was the town of Merthyr Tydfil (which included most of the subdistricts of Aberdare and Upper and Lower Merthyr Tydfil). The procedures employed are those suggested by Cho and Grabill (Grabill and Cho, 1965; Cho, Grabill, and Bogue, 1970, Chap. 9) and are the same as those used in Chapter IV.

The original age-specific child–woman ratios were obtained by tabulating the number of young children by age group for women in families (either as the spouse or the head). To obtain the overall ratios, the numbers of these children for each age of mother were divided by the total number of women in the sample in each age category of women. These ratios were then adjusted for children not present with their mothers by multiplying by the ratio of total children aged 0–4 in the whole sample to total own children present aged 0–4 tabulated from families in the sample (to mothers of all ages).[15] The age-specific ratios were then "survived" backward to account for children who had died between birth and the census but who would have been aged 0–4 at the census and women who were a risk of having those births in the previous 5 years but who had died before the census. To accomplish this it was necessary to calculate life tables for the populations in question.

When using English census manuscripts for the censuses of 1851, 1861 and 1871, one is fortunate to have published mortality data by age and sex available. These, along with published data on infant deaths, births, and population by age and sex, are available for registration districts (from the Annual Reports of the Registrar General and the censuses) and form the materials from which life tables may be constructed. Life tables were constructed using straightforward methods of converting age-specific death rates to life table probabilities of dying (i.e., the q_x function).[16] It was felt that use of any more sophisticated techniques were unwarranted, given the quality of the data. With these q_x values, life tables can then easily be computed.[17]

The actual life tables were constructed for males and females separately and both sexes together for Durham Registration District and Merthyr Tydfil Registration District for 1846–1850, and for Durham–Easington and for Merthyr Tydfil for 1851–1860 and 1861–1870. Only Durham was used for 1846–1850 because the mortality data for Easington were combined with those for some other districts during part of that period. Although the death rates were somewhat higher in Durham at that time,[18] Durham constituted 72.0% of the total population of the two districts combined in 1851. Thus little error was introduced. The periods 1851–1860 and 1861–1870 were chosen for the other life tables partly for reasons of convenience, because the Registrar General published summary mortality volumes for both of those

[15] The ratios for the total population were:

	1851	1861	1871
Durham and Easington	1.0780	1.0591	1.0373
Merthyr Tydfil	1.0560	1.0294	1.0498

Separate corrections were not made for rural–urban populations because the ratios were so similar. Also separate corrections were not made for women of different ages because no estimation of this could be made.

[16] That is ${}_nq_x = 2n\,{}_nM_x/(2 + n\,{}_nM_x)$, where ${}_nq_x$ is the probability of dying between ages x and $x + n$, ${}_nM_x$ is the death rate for persons aged x to $x + n$, and n is the size of the interval in use. The infant mortality rate (infant deaths per live birth per annum) yields ${}_1q_0$.

[17] For the methodology of life table construction, see U.S. Bureau of the Census (1971, pp. 433–446).

[18] The crude death rate for 1841–1850 was 23.01 for Durham and 20.36 for Easington. The infant mortality rate for 1847–1850 was 166.7 for Durham and 127.2 for Easington.

decades. Again, not much error was introduced by using a life table for the decades 1851–1860 and 1861–1870 rather than for the relevant subperiods 1856–1860 and 1866–1870, since mortality was not substantially different later in the decade relative to the decade average. For example, the infant mortality rate, a good indicator of the effect of different mortality levels on birth-rate estimation was usually only a few percentages different between the whole decade and its second half.[19] Finally, tables were not estimated for the rural and urban populations separately because the data were not available. Rather than shift to a model life table system, it was deemed more appropriate to remain with the actual mortality experience. In calculating the life tables, no adjustment was made for underregistration of deaths, although several other minor adjustments had to be made.[20]

Finally, it was necessary to consider the issue of relative underenumeration of children. Information on this is scarce for England and Wales. Some recent authors have felt that the only serious general underenumeration occurred in 1801 and 1811 (Krause, 1958; Taylor, 1951). Contemporaries suspected that there was some underenumeration of young children in the 1861 census (Farr, 1865; Sargant, 1865), but there was disagreement as to the magnitude and whether it was truly underenumeration or really age misstatement. Nothing about relative underenumeration of young children was treated. There is some evidence from the United States in the late nineteenth century that children were less completely enumerated than women in the younger childbearing years (Coale and Zelnik, 1963, pp. 179–180), but this is only suggestive. Furthermore, the real problem may have been age misstatement rather than underenumeration, in which case the broad age group 0–4 would capture most of the effect. On the other hand, if there was a systematic tendency to misstate ages of young children as higher, then the age group 0–4 would be too small and some correction should be applied. In the absence of any firm information, 5% relative underenumeration was assumed.

[19] The ratios of the infant mortality rate in the second half of the decade to the whole decade are:

	1851/60	1861/70
Durham and Easington	.984	1.027
Merthyr Tydfil	.993	.971

[20] For the decades 1851–1860 and 1861–1870, deaths by age were given for 10-year age groups above age 25 (i.e., 25–34, 35–44) instead of the needed quinquennial groupings. Deaths were interpolated using the gradations between the 5-year death rates in the life tables for England and Wales for 1861 and 1871 calculated by Keyfitz and Flieger (1968, pp. 520–522). The mid-period population by age, used as the base at risk for the age-specific death rates, was calculated by an exponential interpolation between the census age groupings, making allowance for the dates of the censuses. Because no age structure for registration districts was given in the census of 1841, the 1851 age groupings were simply projected backward using the growth rate of the total population over that decade.

Using this information on children missing from their mothers, on child and adult mortality, and on relative underenumeration of children, the standard own-children techniques were applied to the age-specific child–woman ratios for the total female population. Total fertility rates (TFRs), gross reproduction rates (GRRs), and net reproduction rates (NRRs) were calculated for Durham and Easington and for Merthyr Tydfil for 1846–1851, 1856–1861, and 1866–1871. These are presented for the total, rural, and urban populations in Table V-12. Also included, for purposes of comparison, are GRRs for counties Durham and Glamorganshire for 1851, 1861, and 1871 and TFRs, GRRs, and NRRs for England and Wales for 1850–1852, 1860–1862, and 1870–1872, all calculated by Glass (1938) using a type of indirect standardization. This was necessary because, according to Glass (1938, p. 162), age-specific birth data did not exist for England and Wales in the nineteenth century. In addition, TFRs, GRRs, and NRRs were calculated from data provided by Keyfitz and Flieger (1968, pp. 520–522) for England and Wales for 1861 and 1871. In light of the comments by Glass and because the source of the age-specific birth data in Keyfitz and Flieger remains unclear, these rates must be viewed with some caution. All rates for counties Durham and Glamorganshire and for England and Wales were adjusted for birth underregistration, as indicated in Table V-12.

Overall, the rates in Table V-12 confirm the higher fertility in these mining and metallurgical areas relative to the national average, making due allowance for the slightly differing time periods for Durham and Easington and for Merthyr Tydfil versus England and Wales. Also, the large differentials between rural and urban fertility, suggested by the marital child–woman ratios, was also confirmed for Durham and Easington and, after 1851, for Merthyr Tydfil. In Durham and Easington, the differential declined over time, with rural fertility about 60% above urban in 1851 and only approximately 15% by 1871. In Merthyr Tydfil, in contrast, the rural TFR moved from being about 5% below urban fertility in 1851 to being about 25% above it in 1871. The GRRs for Durham and Easington were quite close to those estimated by Glass for County Durham in 1851, 1861, and 1871, but rural fertility was well above the county average. This was undoubtedly because these rural areas were more heavily populated with miners. For Merthyr Tydfil, the overall GRR was rather close to the county average, though generally above. For 1861 and 1871, rural fertility was, however, quite a bit above the GRR for County Glamorganshire. The urban GRR for Merthyr Tydfil remained virtually constant throughout the period.

The TFRs and GRRs for Durham and Easington were also substantially above the national average, which is what was expected for a mining region. For GRRs, the differential was 21% around 1851 and approximately 25% around 1861 and 1871. Interestingly enough, this was about the same excess of fertility in the Pennsylvania anthracite region over the national average during approximately the same time period. The differentials were some-

TABLE V-12 Total Fertility Rates (TFR), Gross Reproduction Rates (GRR), and Net Reproduction Rates (NRR). Durham and Easington R.D.'s, England; Merthyr Tydfil R.D., Wales; 1846/1851, 1856/1861, and 1866/1871; Durham County, 1861 and 1871; England and Wales, 1850/1852, 1860/1862, 1861, 1870/1872, 1871

	Durham and Easington R.D.'s			Durham County	Merthyr Tydfil R.D.			Glamorganshire	England and Wales	
	Total	Rural	Urban		Total	Rural	Urban			
	1846/1851			1851	1846/1851			1851	1850/1852	
TFR	5.733	6.253	3.820	-	5.296	5.115	5.415	-	4.663	
GRR	2.755	3.005	1.836	2.675	2.551	2.464	2.608	2.408	2.281	
NRR	1.518	1.655	1.014	-	1.170	1.131	1.195	-	1.377	
	1856/1861			1861	1856/1861			1861	1860/1862	1861
TFR	5.935	6.454	4.609	-	5.432	5.749	5.364	-	4.714	4.614
GRR	2.876	3.127	2.233	2.846	2.655	2.810	2.622	2.513	2.306	2.256
NRR	1.707	1.855	1.326	-	1.320	1.396	1.304	-	1.442	1.393
	1866/1871			1871	1866/1871			1871	1870/1872	1871
TFR	6.101	6.317	5.515	-	5.497	6.746	5.387	-	4.824	4.698
GRR	2.957	3.062	2.673	2.984	2.684	3.294	2.630	2.673	2.365	2.308
NRR	1.782	1.845	1.611	-	1.450	1.770	1.421	-	1.532	1.419

Sources: Total fertility rate (TFR), gross reproduction rate (GRR), and net reproduction rate (NRR) for Durham and Easington and for Merthyr Tydfil Registration districts were estimated from tabulations of age-specific child-woman ratios from samples of enumerators' manuscripts from the censuses of 1851, 1861, and 1871. The methods of Grabill and Cho were used (Grabill and Cho, 1965; Cho, Grabill, and Bogue, 1970, Chapter 9). Life-table data were calculated from published statistics. Relative underenumeration of children was assumed at 5%.

The measures for Durham County and Glamorganshire (1851, 1861, 1871) and for England and Wales for 1850/1852, 1860/1862, and 1870/1872 are from D.V. Glass, "Changes in Fertility in England and Wales, 1851-1931," in Lancelot Hogben, ed., *Political Arithmetic* (1938), pp. 173-191. The measures for England and Wales for 1861 and 1871 were calculated from data given in Nathan Keyfitz and Wilhelm Flieger, *World Population* (1968), pp. 520-523. All these rates were adjusted for birth underregistration on the basis of correction factors estimated by Michael Teitelbaum, "Birth Underregistration in the Constituent Counties of England and Wales: 1841-1910," *Population Studies*, Vol. 28, No. 2 (July, 1974), pp. 329-343.

what less for NRRs because of the slightly higher mortality in Durham and Easington than in England and Wales (see Table V-1). The quite high mortality in Merthyr Tydfil meant that NRRs there dropped below the national average NRRs. Thus, the high fertility in Merthyr did not compensate for its high mortality to the extent that this occurred nationally and certainly not to the extent in Durham and Easington.

Urban fertility was, in Durham and Easington, rather low in relation to the national average early in the period. For 1846–1851, fertility in Durham City was below the national rate, and, given the high level of mortality, the population was barely reproducing itself (in a period sense).[21] The GRR was quite close to that for London (1.762) in 1851 (Glass, 1938, p. 179). This was reminiscent of the situation of many premodern urban areas which did not reproduce themselves through natural increase. (Wrigley, 1969, pp. 97–98). The situation had greatly changed by 1856–1861 and 1866–1871, as both fertility rose and mortality declined.[22] The NRRs were all now well above one and had, by 1861, risen above the national average. The GRRs compared favorably to those for a number of other urban areas and county boroughs in England in 1871: London (2.022), Leeds (2.456), Leicester (2.280), Liverpool (2.063), Northampton (2.557). Still the urban areas were below other, more industrial urban areas (county boroughs) in County Durham in 1871: Gateshead (3.018), South Shields (2.982), West Hartlepool (3.063) (Glass, 1938, pp. 179, 182–183). The rural mining areas had, however, relatively high fertility. For urban areas in Merthyr Tydfil, the GRRs remained roughly constant at about 2.6 from the period just prior to 1851 to that just before 1871. This was well above the national average and compared well with other urban areas, including Swansea (with a GRR of 2.570 in 1871) in Glamorganshire. Again, however, it was the rural area, more heavily concentrated in coal mining, that had higher fertility and grew more rapidly after 1851.

The TFRs, GRRs, and NRRs for Durham and Easington and for Merthyr Tydfil were, unlike those computed by Glass, calculated directly from age-specific child–woman ratios.[23] The age-specific total and marital fertility rates, estimated using these same age-specific child–woman ratios, are presented in Table V-13 for the total, rural, and urban populations. Also given are some age-specific fertility rates for England and Wales for 1861 and 1871 computed with data from Keyfitz and Flieger (1968, pp. 520–522). The age-specific marital fertility rates were calculated by multiplying the age-

[21] If no relative underenumeration of children had been assumed, the NRR would have been less than one, implying that the population was not reproducing itself in a period sense.

[22] The inclusion of Seaham Harbor with Durham City in 1861 and 1871 makes changes between 1851 and 1861 not strictly comparable. But Durham City dominated the averages with 70% of the urban population in 1861 and 67% in 1871.

[23] The TFRs, GRRs, and NRRs in Table V-12 were calculated directly from the age-specific child–woman ratios without first estimating the individual age-specific fertility rates.

TABLE V-13 Age-Specific Total and Marital Fertility Rates for Durham and Easington R.D.'s, Merthyr Tydfil R.D., and England and Wales, 1846/1851, 1856/1861, 1866/1871 (per 1000 women)

	Overall fertility rates							
	Age							
	15-19	20-24	25-29	30-34	35-39	40-44	45-49	TFR
A. *Total*								
1. Durham and Easington								
1846/1851	36.9	181.8	280.9	301.3	222.3	92.9	45.0	5850.
1856/1861	53.3	214.6	291.7	272.6	229.7	117.5	18.3	5988.
1866/1871	59.6	237.2	308.3	288.6	234.3	91.9	10.4	6152.
2. Merthyr Tydfil								
1846/1851	39.2	176.0	254.1	223.4	220.1	146.9	7.6	5336.
1856/1861	47.8	198.7	290.7	265.9	184.4	90.2	19.2	5484.
1866/1871	43.3	199.6	277.4	245.8	213.5	112.2	17.0	5544.
3. England and Wales								
1861	27.3	154.5	224.3	217.0	181.5	100.2	—	4524.
1871	26.8	159.0	231.2	224.9	188.1	103.9	—	4670.
B. *Rural*								
1. Durham and Easington								
1846/1851	42.9	194.9	298.1	330.2	250.3	105.3	44.0	6328.
1856/1861	60.3	232.4	317.1	290.9	239.9	138.7	24.6	6519.
1866/1871	59.8	245.8	321.0	298.9	242.7	93.9	11.7	6369.
2. Merthyr Tydfil								
1846/1851	48.7	167.2	227.7	221.6	226.0	152.4	0.0	5218.
1856/1861	49.4	201.4	295.5	295.9	212.5	77.3	26.8	5794.
1866/1871	72.3	252.5	274.5	293.6	286.0	138.6	53.4	6854.
C. *Urban*								
1. Durham and Easington								
1846/1851	14.2	126.3	209.4	204.1	130.6	44.2	46.5	3876.
1856/1861	33.0	166.7	223.1	219.2	208.7	72.2	4.1	4635.
1866/1871	58.2	212.6	271.2	261.5	214.7	85.9	7.4	5558.
2. Merthyr Tydfil								
1846/1851	34.1	179.1	268.5	224.9	216.7	145.8	22.1	5456.
1856/1861	47.5	197.8	288.6	259.4	179.4	93.8	17.2	5418.
1866/1871	40.8	195.1	277.7	241.0	205.9	110.7	14.9	5430.

A. *Total*								
1. Durham and Easington								
1846/1851	1028.4	455.1	377.0	375.1	259.0	112.2	54.6	8165.
1856/1861	1000.6	437.4	390.7	338.4	267.1	138.4	24.9	7984.
1866/1871	843.3	467.7	389.9	344.8	267.3	104.8	12.9	7937.
2. Merthyr Tydfil								
1846/1851	1113.3	391.5	359.3	267.1	258.5	169.3	10.2	7280.
1856/1861	982.1	397.4	364.2	304.7	213.0	101.3	24.9	7028.
1866/1871	980.1	412.0	366.7	287.6	251.6	131.1	20.7	7348.
3. England and Wales								
1861	895.4	466.2	366.1	297.6	237.3	131.8	——	7495.
1871	849.4	463.3	370.6	305.8	245.6	137.0	——	7612.
B. *Rural*								
1. Durham and Easington								
1846/1851	1093.9	438.9	380.2	395.0	279.6	122.4	52.7	8344.
1856/1861	1071.2	444.4	410.5	345.0	277.5	163.7	33.0	8370.
1866/1871	854.3	466.3	397.5	352.1	268.5	104.6	14.1	8015.
2. Merthyr Tydfil								
1846/1851	1334.4	349.6	340.0	253.3	275.1	179.3	0.0	6986.
1856/1861	1514.9	406.3	373.8	310.1	220.7	83.2	31.3	7127.
1866/1871	1636.6	519.8	340.4	350.1	325.0	155.9	64.1	8776.
C. *Urban*								
1. Durham and Easington								
1846/1851	560.9	542.3	366.4	297.4	180.8	62.2	59.8	7544.
1856/1861	732.6	416.8	331.5	309.9	246.3	84.6	5.7	6974.
1866/1871	810.0	477.3	366.0	326.1	264.6	104.6	10.0	7743.
2. Merthyr Tydfil								
1846/1851	1002.5	415.9	369.2	275.0	249.2	166.2	27.4	7514.
1856/1861	900.0	394.6	360.5	307.2	211.3	107.0	23.0	7018.
1866/1871	942.5	402.8	369.2	281.5	243.5	129.8	18.2	7225.

Source: For Durham and Easington and for Merthyr Tydfil, birth rates were computed using data on own children by age of mother and data on the population of total and married women from a sample of census enumerators' manuscripts. Methodology is taken from Cho, Grabill, and Bogue (1970, Chapter 9); 5% relative underenumeration of children is assumed.

For England and Wales, 1861 and 1871 birth rates were calculated from data given in N. Keyfitz and W. Flieger, *World Population* (1968). Birth data were adjusted for underregistration on the basis of factors estimated by Michael Teitelbaum, "Birth Underregistration in the Constituent Counties of England and Wales: 1841-1910," *Population Studies*, Vol. 28, No. 2 (July, 1974), pp. 329-343.

specific total fertility rates by the inverse of the proportion married for each age group.[24]

Examining Table V-13 reveals that few changes took place in the age pattern of overall fertility over the 1846–1851 to 1866–1871 period. Although there was a change in the shape of the fertility schedules for Durham and Easington between 1846–1851 and 1856–1861 from a schedule peaking at ages 30–34 to one peaking at 25–29, there was little evidence of fertility change among older women and, hence, no sign of incipient fertility decline. All the other schedules for rural and urban, for Durham and Easington, for Merthyr Tydfil, or for England and Wales, showed peaks at the ages 25–29. For the marital fertility schedules there was also little evidence of any decline among older women.[25] Another point of note is that the lower level of overall fertility characteristic of the nation as a whole relative to Durham and Easington and to Merthyr Tydfil extended to all ages of women in 1861 and 1871. A glance at the marital fertility rates indicates that the differentials were far lower than for overall fertility. The levels of marital fertility in 1861 and 1871 were indeed higher at most ages in England and Wales than in Merthyr Tydfil. For Durham and Easington, however, marital fertility was higher at most ages. A summary measure of this was calculated and was called the Total Marital Fertility Rate (TMFR) and is given in Table V-13. It excludes the age group 15–19 where marital fertility rates are often unreliable because of small numbers of cases and very high because of large numbers of bridal pregnancies. For 1871, the TMFRs (per 1000 women) were 7937 for Durham and Easington, 7348 for Merthyr Tydfil, and 7612 for England and Wales. The source of the higher overall fertility in Merthyr Tydfil relative to the nation thus lay wholly in nuptiality patterns. For Durham and Easington, this was only partly the case. It is also apparent from the TMFRs that the origin of the rural–urban differentials in overall fertility was very much due to differences in marital fertility behavior.

The proportions of females married by age are given in Table V-14 for 1851, 1861, and 1871. The figures for Durham and Easington and for Merthyr Tydfil were calculated from the census samples. Some data from published census materials for 1861 and 1871 were included (for the whole population of each district) and indicate that the approximation by the samples was quite good. It is clear that women in the two mining/industrial areas were marrying earlier than the national average and also that far fewer remained unmarried in Durham and Easington and in Merthyr Tydfil. In addition, it also appears that at least some of the rural–urban fertility

[24] This is an alternative to the methods suggested by Cho, Grabill, and Bogue (1970, pp. 343–348) for calculating the rates directly from the age-specific marital child–woman ratios.

[25] The estimated rates for the age group 45–49 are relatively unreliable and should not be assigned much importance.

TABLE V-14 Proportions of Women Married at Ages 15-19 through 45-49. By Residence, Durham and Easington R.D.'s, England; Merthyr Tydfil, Wales; England and Wales; 1851, 1861, 1871

	Age						
	15-19	20-24	25-29	30-34	35-39	40-44	45-49
	Proportion married in Durham and Easington						
Total							
1851	.0358	.3994	.7451	.8033	.8584	.8276	.8247
1861	.0533	.4906	.7466	.8056	.8598	.8491	.7341
1871	.0707	.5072	.7907	.8369	.8764	.8766	.8034
Rural							
1851	.0392	.4441	.7840	.8360	.8953	.8603	.8346
1861	.0563	.5230	.7724	.8432	.8646	.8472	.7458
1871	.0700	.5272	.8076	.8489	.9040	.8978	.8303
Urban							
1851	.0253	.2329	.5714	.6863	.7222	.7105	.7778
1861	.0450	.4000	.6731	.7073	.8472	.8259	.7222
1871	.0719	.4454	.7411	.8019	.8113	.8214	.7391
Total from census[a]							
1861	.0650	.4749	.7854		.8429		.7973
1871	.0750	.5333	.8150		.8518		.7899
	Proportion married in Merthyr Tydfil						
Total							
1851	.0352	.4496	.7072	.8364	.8514	.8675	.7414
1861	.0487	.5000	.7982	.8726	.8656	.8901	.7696
1871	.0442	.4844	.7565	.8545	.8487	.8561	.8208
Rural							
1851	.0365	.4783	.6696	.8750	.8214	.8500	.6531
1861	.0326	.4957	.7905	.9541	.9454	.9286	.8571
1871	.0811	.4857	.8065	.8387	.8800	.8889	.8333
Urban							
1851	.0340	.4306	.7273	.8176	.8696	.8774	.8060
1861	.0528	.5013	.8006	.8444	.8491	.8768	.7486
1871	.0433	.4843	.7521	.8562	.8455	.8526	.8200
Total from census[a]							
1861	.0502	.4688	.8247		.8649		.7957
1871	.0491	.4800	.7969		.8520		.7938
	Proportion married in England and Wales						
Total							
1851	.0252	.3077	.5838	.7114	.7584	.7558	.7392
1861	.0305	.3314	.6127	.7292	.7648	.7605	.7436
1871	.0316	.3432	.6238	.7354	.7660	.7585	.7401

Source: Sample of enumerators' manuscripts and published census data, 1851, 1861, 1871.

[a]Age groups 15-19, 20-24, 25-34, 35-44, 45-54.

differences within Durham–Easington and Merthyr Tydfil were due to earlier and more extensive marriage in the rural areas (except for Merthyr in 1851 when the reverse was true).

In order to clarify this, some summary nuptiality measures were calculated and tabulated in Table V-15. The measures are presented for both sexes and include the singulate mean age at marriage (SMAM) calculated by Hajnal's method (Hajnal, 1953), Coale's index of proportions married (I_m), the proportion married at ages 20–24, and the proportion single at ages

TABLE V-15 Nuptiality Measures. Durham and Easington R.D.'s; Merthyr Tydfil R.D.; England and Wales; 1851, 1861, 1871

	Durham and Easington			Merthyr Tydfil			England and Wales
	Total	Rural	Urban	Total	Rural	Urban	Total
	Singulate mean age at marriage (SMAM)[a]						
Male							
1851	25.72	26.03	25.51	27.65	27.41	27.77	27.06
1861	26.77	26.74	26.85	26.71	28.30	26.10	26.47
1871	25.89	25.84	26.05	25.62	26.36	25.52	26.49
Female							
1851	24.02	23.48	26.59	23.55	23.80	23.46	25.83
1861	23.68	23.39	25.49	23.21	23.14	23.25	25.43
1871	22.74	23.15	22.10	23.80	22.80	23.88	25.17
	I_m						
1851	.572	.612	.434	.605	.577	.622	.483
1861	.606	.627	.527	.646	.679	.636	.502
1871	.630	.648	.582	.602	.643	.598	.509
	Proportions married at 20-24						
Male							
1851	.2097	.2182	.1887	.1861	.1869	.1856	.2004
1861	.2293	.2234	.2917	.2321	.2023	.2431	.2227
1871	.2197	.2235	.2083	.2367	.1930	.2416	.2303
Female							
1851	.3989	.4452	.2222	.4490	.4818	.4272	.3077
1861	.4749	.5224	.4000	.5000	.4957	.5013	.3314
1871	.5072	.5272	.4454	.4844	.4857	.4843	.3432
	Proportions single at 45-54						
Male							
1851	.1200	.1040	.1600	.1259	.1400	.1180	.1146
1861	.1097	.0987	.1368	.1075	.1217	.1028	.1050
1871	.1207	.1191	.1260	.1479	.1220	.1503	.0973
Female							
1851	.0827	.0663	.1379	.0762	.0805	.0735	.1225
1861	.0731	.0726	.0753	.0332	.0123	.0385	.1195
1871	.0600	.0311	.1250	.0261	.0435	.0250	.1205

Source: For Durham and Easington and for Merthyr Tydfil, data from census enumerators' manuscripts and published data were used. For England and Wales, published census data were used.

[a] SMAM was calculated using Hajnal's methods.

45–54. From these data it emerges that, while male marriage patterns in these two mining/industrial districts were rather similar to the national pattern (i.e., relatively late marriage and reasonably high proportions never marrying), female marriage in Durham and Easington and in Merthyr Tydfil was early and extensive. Female SMAM was about 23 years (as opposed to over 25 in England and Wales), and far fewer than 10% were never married (in contrast to about 12% in England and Wales as a whole). It is notable that this pattern of relatively early female marriage and late male marriage was also found in the Pennsylvania anthracite region later in the century. It was undoubtedly characteristic of such areas which experienced heavy net male in-migration and high sex ratios. As a result, the male population still retained the distinctive "European marriage pattern [Hajnal, 1965]" of later marriage and high proportions never marrying, while females changed to earlier marriage and less permanent celibacy. Such patterns tend to support the view of Wrigley (1961, Chap. V) that it was earlier female marriage rather than earlier male marriage that resulted from the employment and labor-force patterns of heavy-industrial areas of Europe. On the other hand, it appears that in Merthyr Tydfil, male SMAM was declining over the decades of the 1850s and the 1860s. This might have been partly a reflection of increased prosperity among workers.

Rural–urban differences in overall fertility are partly explicable in terms of female age of marriage. In the case of Durham and Easington, female SMAM was lower for rural than urban areas (except in 1871), I_m was consistently higher, and proportions married at ages 20–24 were always larger. For Merthyr Tydfil the pattern was less clear, but in 1861 and 1871, when rural total fertility was higher, SMAM was lower in rural areas and I_m was higher. The opposite was true in 1851.

It is important then to emphasize that marriage, rather than marital fertility, played a large role in determining changes in overall fertility between about 1850 and about 1870. This is consistent with the finding in Chapter III that the equations explaining I_m were much more significant than those explaining I_g for England and Wales in 1861 and 1871. It was only after 1870 that declines in marital fertility began to be important (see Table V-5). In order to assess, to some extent, the relative roles of marriage versus marital fertility in changes in overall fertility over time, Table V-16 was constructed. It shows changes in overall fertility (columns labeled a), marital fertility (columns labeled b), and proportions married (columns labeled c) for each age group of women 20–24 through 45–49. The base is 100 and indexed at 1851 for Durham–Easington and Merthyr Tydfil and 1861 for England and Wales. Rural and urban subgroups are not considered. The results indicate that, for the younger age groups, especially women 20–24, changes in proportions married were usually more important in raising overall fertility. At older ages, however, changes in marital fertility (both up and down) were larger. For Merthyr Tydfil, there was a tendency for the age-specific marital fertility schedule to peak a bit more, and for England and Wales marital fertility rose for women above age 30 while proportions married changed little.[26]

The changes in marital fertility which took place over this period were not great, however. One indication of this is the mean age of the mother at last birth. This was estimated in Table V-17 for older married women (who had completed or nearly completed parity) as the difference between the age of the mother and the age of the youngest surviving child. It is generally an underestimate because of child mortality, but it did give consistent results

[26] The pattern of change for England and Wales is, in fact, so regular that one is tempted to speculate that the overall births by age were estimated by some proportional transformation from a base set of age-specific rates, perhaps somewhere in the early twentieth century.

TABLE V-16 Relative Changes in Age-Specific Overall and Marital Fertility Rates and in Proportions Married for Women 20-24 to 45-49. Durham and Easington, R.D.'s, England; Merthyr Tydfil, Wales; England and Wales; 1846/1851 - 1866/1871

	Durham and Easington[a]			Merthyr Tydfil[a]			England and Wales[a,b]		
	(a)	(b)	(c)	(a)	(b)	(c)	(a)	(b)	(c)
Women 20-24									
1846/1851	100	100	100	100	100	100	---	---	---
1856/1861	118	96	123	113	102	111	100	100	100
1866/1871	130	103	127	113	105	108	103	99	104
Women 25-29									
1846/1851	100	100	100	100	100	100	---	---	---
1856/1861	104	104	100	114	101	113	100	100	100
1866/1871	110	103	106	109	102	107	103	101	102
Women 30-34									
1846/1851	100	100	100	100	100	100	---	---	---
1856/1861	90	90	100	119	114	104	100	100	100
1866/1871	96	92	104	110	108	102	104	103	101
Women 35-39									
1846/1851	100	100	100	100	100	100	---	---	---
1856/1861	103	103	100	84	82	102	100	100	100
1866/1871	105	103	102	97	97	100	104	104	100
Women 40-44									
1846/1851	100	100	100	100	100	100	---	---	---
1856/1861	126	123	102	61	60	102	100	100	100
1866/1871	99	93	106	76	77	99	104	104	100
Women 45-49									
1846/1851	100	100	100	100	100	100	---	---	---
1856/1861	41	46	89	252	244	104	---	---	---
1866/1871	23	24	97	224	203	111	---	---	---

Source: Tables V-13 and V-14.

[a](a) = Births per woman (1846/1851 = 100) = [(b)·(c)]/100 . For England and Wales, 1861 = 100.

(b) = Births per married woman (1846/1851 = 100).

(c) = Married women as a proportion of total women (1846/1851 = 100).

[b]For England and Wales, 1861 and 1871 only.

for the Pennsylvania anthracite region. As marital fertility declined there, so did the estimated mean age of mother at last birth. Such did not appear to be the case in Durham and Easington or in Merthyr Tydfil between 1851 and 1861. One possible exception might have been some decline among women aged 45–49 in Durham and Easington between 1861 and 1871. The lack of any trend was true for rural as well as urban areas.

Another indicator of change in marital fertility is found in Table V-18. Presented there are Coale–Trussell "m" values (Coale and Trussell, 1974, 1978).[27] These "m" and M values were fitted by the regression method explained in Chapter IV. Only the age groups 20–24 through 40–44 were

[27] An explanation of these measures can be found in Chapter IV, pages 134–138 and note 48.

TABLE V-17 Estimated Mean Age at Last Birth.[a] Married Women with Children and with Husband Present. By Residence: Durham and Easington R.D.'s, England, and Merthyr Tydfil, Wales, 1851, 1861, 1871

	Durham and Easington			Merthyr Tydfil		
	Total	Rural	Urban	Total	Rural	Urban
Women 40-44						
1851	36.7	36.8	36.0	37.7	38.1	37.5
1861	37.1	37.4	36.4	36.1	36.2	36.1
1871	37.1	37.0	37.4	37.2	37.5	37.2
Women 45-49						
1851	39.5	39.5	39.9	38.6	39.0	38.3
1861	39.5	40.0	38.1	38.4	38.3	38.4
1871	37.6	37.6	37.5	38.7	40.4	38.6

Source: Sample of census enumerators' manuscripts.

[a]Estimated as the difference between the age of the mother and the age of the youngest child.

used because it was either necessary (as in the case of England and Wales) or because this procedure gave a better fit. A mean-square error below .005 is considered good by Coale and Trussell and one above .01 as rather poor (Coale and Trussell, 1978, p. 204). With the caution in mind that not all the estimates were equally good, it does appear that marital fertility was not subject to a great deal of control. As Coale and Trussell state: "We believe that any value of 'm' of less than .2 can be taken as evidence of no control [Coale and Trussell, 1978, p. 205]." The one area where "m" values, the degree of departure from natural fertility, were consistently above .2 was the urban region of Durham and Easington. Furthermore, there was no consistent trend in "m." The level of fertility at ages 20–24, as measured by M, was close to the model natural fertility standard (of 1.000) for Durham and Easington and reasonably close for England and Wales.[28] But Merthyr Tydfil showed a somewhat lower level in these early years of child bearing. Nevertheless, the general impression is one of either a modest degree of control of fertility within marriage or of none at all. Furthermore, there appeared to be little change over time in the application of contraceptive practices of whatever type.

In concluding this section, the central feature of overall fertility in this period was a modest tendency to rise. This was true both for Durham and Easington and for Merthyr Tydfil, as well as for the country as a whole. These small increases were really the product of small changes in marriage age among younger women and some very small adjustments in marital fertility among older women. The latter might well have been caused by changes in natural fertility in the sense that there seemed to be little or no

[28] An exact match to the natural fertility standard occurs when $M = 1.0$.

TABLE V-18 Deviation of Age-Specific Marital Fertility from Natural Fertility as Measured by Coale-Trussell "m" Values. Durham and Easington R.D.'s, England and Merthyr Tydfil, Wales; England and Wales, 1846/1851 - 1866/1871

	M	"m"	Mean square error
A. *Total*			
1. Durham and Easington			
1846/1851	1.001	.239	.0043
1856/1861	.936	.101	.0003
1866/1871	1.026	.293	.0036
2. Merthyr Tydfil			
1846/1851	.780	-.089	.0146
1856/1861	.892	.268	.0007
1866/1871	.861	.097	.0028
3. England and Wales			
1861	.927	.175	.0054
1871	.927	.144	.0047
B. *Rural*			
1. Durham and Easington			
1846/1851	.979	.152	.0054
1856/1861	.938	.020	.0028
1866/1871	1.038	.298	.0039
2. Merthyr Tydfil			
1846/1851	.701	-.216	.0160
1856/1861	.950	.389	.0052
1866/1871	.961	.028	.0143
C. *Urban*			
1. Durham and Easington			
1846/1851	1.158	.755	.0050
1856/1861	.916	.325	.0108
1866/1871	1.000	.288	.0045
2. Merthyr Tydfil			
1846/1851	.823	-.028	.0150
1856/1861	.877	.232	.0010
1866/1871	.850	.102	.0033

Source: Calculated from data in Table V-13, using the method developed by Coale and Trussell (1974, 1978).

deliberate attempt to control fertility on the part of a large part of the population of married women. In terms of differences in overall fertility between Durham and Easington, Merthyr Tydfil, and England and Wales and also between the rural and urban areas within Durham and Easington and Merthyr Tydfil, most were caused by differences in marriage patterns, although marital fertility played some role. It is in this connection that the importance of migration comes again to the fore. Mining and heavy-industrial areas like Durham and Easington and Merthyr Tydfil attracted young adult males, raising sex ratios in these age groups and generally lowering female age at marriage and decreasing permanent female celibacy. This situation was amplified by the lack of employment among married females, stemming from the same economic structures that created the migration imbalances. Male age at marriage was not as much affected.

Thus, again, appears the intimate and complex interaction between fertility, marriage, migration, employment, and economic structures which combined to create the peculiar and distinctive demographic patterns of mining areas. The setting itself was not without importance, since the level of marital fertility in the Welsh area was generally lower than that of the case study from northern England. One might speculate on a particular regional natural fertility pattern, since neither case seemed to deviate a great deal from a model natural pattern. On the other hand, marriage patterns were similar, especially for females, and this was probably dominated more by economic structure that by any regional peculiarity.

Patterns of Mortality

In this final section, some use will be made of the extensive mortality statistics by age, sex, and cause published by the Registrar General for the decades of the 1850s and the 1860s for individual registration districts in England and Wales (England and Wales, 1864, 1875). Age-specific death rates for males and females for the periods 1851–1860 and 1861–1870 are presented in Table V-19 for Durham and Easington, Merthyr Tydfil, and England and Wales. The total death rate is equivalent to the crude death rate. An age-standardized death rate was also calculated, using the actual age-specific death rates for each location at each date standardized to the overall age structure of either males or females in England and Wales at the same date.

As may be seen from Table V-19, the level of mortality in Durham and Easington was quite similar to that for England and Wales as a whole. Only for children and teenagers and, for females, for the peak childbearing years 25–34 were death rates much above the national average. For older ages of males and other ages of females, age-specific mortality in Durham and Easington was below the national average. Further, mortality in these two registration districts in northern England declined relative to the national level, especially for males. In the case of males, the age-standardized death rate was always higher than the crude death rate. The reverse was true for females. The age structure in Durham and Easington was heavily weighted toward adult males in the prime working ages because of migrant selectivity. These were also the ages with mortality which was low relative to the national average. It thus seems reasonable that standardizing to the age structure of all males in England and Wales, with much more weight assigned to children and teenagers (partly because of differential net outmigration of males for the country), should thus raise the death rate for males in Durham and Easington. This was not the case for females, since the female age structure in Durham and Easington was not as weighted toward adults and also because death rates for the ages 25–34 were higher

TABLE V-19 Age-Specific Mortality in Durham and Easington R.D.'s, Merthyr Tydfil R.D., and England and Wales, 1851/1860 and 1861/1870 (per 1000 Population)

Ages of males and females	1851/1860 Durham and Easington	1851/1860 Ratio to England and Wales	1851/1860 Merthyr Tydfil	1851/1860 Ratio to England and Wales	1851/1860 England and Wales	1861/1870 Durham and Easington	1861/1870 Ratio to England and Wales	1861/1870 Merthyr Tydfil	1861/1870 Ratio to England and Wales	1861/1870 England and Wales
Males										
0-4	77.48	107	107.50	148	72.43	72.49	99	84.96	116	73.16
5-9	8.40	99	13.12	154	8.51	9.46	116	12.03	148	8.15
10-14	6.12	125	10.89	223	4.88	6.20	139	8.69	195	4.46
15-19	7.37	110	11.37	170	6.69	7.00	114	9.56	155	6.16
20-24	8.17	93	14.63	166	8.83	7.01	83	11.51	136	8.45
25-34	8.37	87	13.19	138	9.57	7.13	72	11.28	114	9.90
35-44	10.75	86	14.13	113	12.48	9.45	70	14.43	107	13.46
45-54	14.94	83	21.68	121	17.96	15.64	82	20.16	105	19.16
55-64	26.60	86	36.28	118	30.85	28.97	88	38.74	117	33.00
65-74	63.42	97	75.92	116	65.33	64.02	96	83.09	125	66.69
75+	156.30	94	193.00	117	165.40	156.19	95	186.76	113	164.64
Total	22.14	96	29.69	129	23.05	21.39	91	25.96	110	23.61
Age standardized	22.82	99	32.03	139	23.05	22.24	94	28.69	120	23.61
Females										
0-4	68.78	110	92.20	147	62.74	66.03	104	76.57	121	63.43
5-9	9.78	116	13.14	156	8.42	9.62	124	9.82	127	7.76
10-14	4.22	83	6.51	129	5.06	4.77	106	4.59	102	4.48
15-19	5.56	75	8.47	115	7.38	6.42	97	6.52	98	6.62
20-24	8.28	97	10.75	126	8.53	7.42	93	10.18	128	7.96
25-34	10.53	106	13.42	135	9.92	9.83	102	11.08	114	9.68
35-44	11.20	92	15.13	124	12.15	10.87	90	14.15	118	12.03
45-54	14.12	93	15.67	103	15.20	13.75	88	17.28	111	15.55
55-64	23.26	86	24.53	91	27.01	24.08	87	29.84	107	27.77
65-74	53.64	91	56.51	96	58.66	54.51	93	56.45	96	58.80
75+	146.23	94	143.20	92	155.45	151.40	98	145.85	95	154.28
Total	21.68	102	27.39	128	21.32	21.35	100	24.18	114	21.28
Age standardized	21.33	100	26.66	125	21.32	21.11	99	23.97	113	21.28

Source: Calculated from England and Wales, Registrar General, *Supplement to the Twenty-Fifth Annual Report* (1864). *Supplement to the Thirty-Fifth Annual Report* (1875). Standardization was to the age structure of England and Wales for the appropriate sex at each date.

than the national average. Therefore, standardized death rates were below the unstandardized crude death rates.

Merthyr Tydfil had somewhat the same pattern of age-specific mortality relative to national levels, but the overall level of mortality in Merthyr Tydfil was much higher than in either Durham and Easington or in England and Wales. It is quite apparent that the higher mortality in Merthyr was not just occupation or work related, since the higher death rates were characteristic of children as well as adults and of females as well as males. Merthyr Tydfil, it must be concluded, was simply a much less healthy area than either Durham and Easington or the country overall. Standardization to the England–Wales age structure had the same effect as in Durham–Easington: Standardized male death rates were higher than unstandardized, and standardized female death rates were lower. The reasons for these effects were also the same.

In order to explore the possibility that mining and industrial districts had peculiar mortality patterns, which, in turn, might have had some influence on fertility and possibly even marriage, death rates by sex, age, and cause of death were examined for these same two decades. Because of the large bulk of tabular data involved, only the general results are described and no tables are presented. Also, given some of the uncertainties involved with medical diagnosis of cause of death in mid-nineteenth-century Britain, the results must be interpreted with some caution, and more emphasis should be placed on general categories of diseases by age.[29]

Given these caveats about the use of cause of death data, there were some distinguishing features about mortality in both Durham–Easington and in Merthyr Tydfil. The first point is that death rates from respiratory tuberculosis and from "Diseases of the Lungs" among adult males in Durham and Easington were well below the national average. Since it might have been expected that adult males in a mining region would suffer inordinately from afflictions like black lung disease and silicosis, this is somewhat surprising. In Durham and Easington, in fact, death rates from tuberculosis among adult females were closer to the national average than was the case for males. The same was less true in Merthyr Tydfil, although death rates there were generally high. One way to compensate for this is to examine the ratio of male to female deaths from the same cause at various ages. The assumption here is that general mortality conditions, as opposed to specific male

[29] For a description of some of the problems involved with using cause of death statistics for Britain in the middle of the nineteenth century, see McKeown and Record (1962, pp. 95–96). For example, diphtheria and scarlet fever were not reported separately until 1855 and typhus and typhoid were not separated until 1869. There were a number of general categories, such as diseases of the brain, of the heart, of the lungs, of the stomach and liver, of the kidneys, of the joints, and of the skin, which were sometimes used as catchalls when diagnosis was not more precise. Diagnosis of tuberculosis must also have been much less certain in an era prior to chest X-rays or even identification of the bacillus.

occupational-mortality conditions, were reflected in the age-specific female death rates. The ratio of male to female rates in the mining and industrial areas, when compared to the national average, should have reflected any irregular patterns in male mortality. Based on this reasoning, mortality from tuberculosis in both Durham–Easington and Merthyr Tydfil was low for adult males relative to adult females. The male–female ratios for death rates from lung disease were quite close to the national average ratios in both areas as well. Thus, if occupational hazards were prevalent, they did not tend to affect deaths from respiratory conditions.

From the death rates from violence, however, it is clear that occupational hazards were of a much more direct and less subtle form. Most of these deaths from violence were from accidental injury, although the proportions were not reported directly.[30] In 1851–1860, male death rates from violence were 74% above the national average in Durham–Easington and 153% above in Merthyr Tydfil. The differences were 42% and 134%, respectively, for 1861–1870. The death rates for violence for females were, on the other hand, relatively close to the national rates at both dates for both areas. Male death rates from violent causes were generally above the female rates. The national ratios of the male to the female rates for the age group 25–34 were 7.9 in 1851–1860 and 8.0 in 1861–1870. But these ratios were much higher for the two periods in Durham and Easington (35.1 and 20.2, respectively) and in Merthyr Tydfil (19.1 and 18.1, respectively), indicating a very high differential net loss due to accident.

Among the specific diseases enumerated, smallpox and typhus/typhoid were above average for both males and females in both districts from 1851 through 1870. In addition, Merthyr Tydfil seems to have suffered well above average mortality from cholera and diarrheal disease at all ages. Sanitary conditions must have been relatively poor in that rapidly growing and highly urbanized area, subject to crowding and probably inadequate sanitation and water supply. The less urban character of the Durham and Easington area may have contributed to its below-average incidence of deaths from gastrointestinal infection.

Some scrutiny of Table V-19 reveals that at some ages female mortality exceeded male mortality, which contradicts the expected pattern of excess male mortality of all ages. This was true for two reasons. First, because fertility was quite high in Durham and Easington and in Merthyr Tydfil, mortality among women of childbearing age from childbirth and puerperal fever was also well above average. For the age group of women 25–34, maternal mortality was 62 and 59% above the national average for Durham–Easington and Merthyr Tydfil, respectively, during 1851–1861.

[30] In the 1861–1870 statistics, suicides were reported separately from other violent deaths. They were only 5.6% of all deaths from violence of males above age 15 in Durham and Easington and 1.7% in Merthyr Tydfil.

The differentials were 40% and 44% in 1861–1870. And it was indeed in the peak childbearing years (25–44) that female mortality exceeded male mortality (except for Merthyr Tydfil, 1861–1870). It is of some note that the differentials in maternal mortality between Durham–Easington and Merthyr Tydfil versus England and Wales were much larger than the differentials in marital fertility. A second contributing factor was the inordinately high female mortality from tuberculosis. At most ages between 5 and 54, female death rates from tuberculosis exceeded male death rates for both Durham–Easington and Merthyr Tydfil over the 1850s and the 1860s. This was not, however, a phenomenon due to any peculiar circumstances in these mining regions. It appeared to have been true for England and Wales generally that tuberculosis mortality among females between about ages 5 and 35 exceeded that for males. It is not easy to explain this pattern, which might have been due to differential nutrition or childrearing between males and females. But it did exacerbate the mortality excess experienced by females from childbearing.

Finally it should be noted that mortality among children before reaching about age 15 was generally higher relative to the national pattern than at older ages. This was especially true for males and was the case for both Durham–Easington and Merthyr Tydfil (see Table V-19). This was caused by a particularly high incidence, especially for Merthyr Tydfil, of such childhood diseases as diptheria, scarlet fever, measles, nonrespiratory tuberculosis,[31] and sometimes whooping cough. Smallpox, typhus/typhoid, cholera, and diarrheal diseases also took an above-average toll among children as well as adults. Thus, the level of infectious disease, combined with the large numbers of children (as a result of high recent fertility), did serve to create an environment more conducive to childhood mortality. This does not seem to have been a predictable characteristic of mining or industrial regions, however.

In sum, mortality in Durham and Easington was not especially high in relation to the national average, while that in Merthyr Tydfil was well above average. The more urban character of Merthyr Tydfil may have contributed to this in creating an environment with poorer housing conditions, worse sanitation, and more contaminated water supplies. There was not too much evidence of occupationally related respiratory disease mortality among males, but there was an exceedingly high male death rate from accidental causes. Female mortality in the childbearing years sometimes exceeded male mortality, and this was attributable to high maternal mortality and death rates for tuberculosis considerably above male death rates from the same disease. Infectious disease was a major contributor to mortality, especially among children and younger teenagers. Typhus/typhoid, smallpox, cholera (in Merthyr Tydfil), and other gastrointestinal infections took a large

[31] This was designated in the causes of death as "scrofula" and "tabes mesenteria."

number of persons at all ages, in addition to the diseases with a heavy incidence just among children. In general, however, there does not appear to be anything peculiar about the mortality pattern in these two mining/industrial regions that would not have been true for any nineteenth-century urbanized area. The exceptions might have been the high mortality from accidents among adult males and from childbirth among adult females, the latter being a product of the high level of fertility characteristic of mining and heavy-industrial regions. The possibility cannot be ignored, however, that there was substantial interaction between the level of fertility and the level of infant and childhood mortality. Fertility might have been high because of the high incidence of death from infectious disease among children. Parents might have sought to replace children who had died, and some biological, natural fertility interaction between infant mortality and fertility might have assisted in this. But it is also true that large families might have led to less care per child and so a higher incidence of death from childhood disease (Schultz, 1976b, pp. 240–283; Wray, 1971, pp. 409–424). Finally, some interaction between mortality and fertility through marriage might have operated. If more marital unions were broken through adult male or female mortality, then overall fertility might have been lower. This could have been true for Merthyr Tydfil, but, as Table V-14 (page 191) shows, proportions of females married at all ages were generally as high or higher among women there as in Durham and Easington. Thus widows did not remain so for long, and fertility (related to females, at least) was not much affected by adult mortality.

SUMMARY AND CONCLUSIONS

In this chapter, the second group of case studies was presented. The Durham and Easington registration districts from the northern part of County Durham were in the center of the great northeastern coalfield and were selected because of their location, economic structure, and demographic characteristics that indicated they were rather typical of mining areas in England in the middle of the nineteenth century. The other case study was of the Merthyr Tydfil registration district in Glamorganshire in South Wales. It was much more urban than the Durham and Easington districts and had a well-developed iron industry as well as substantial coal and iron mining. The case studies themselves were based on 10% samples of the enumerators' schedules for the 1851, 1861, and 1871 censuses.

Overall and age-standardized child–women ratios were calculated for the total population and for married women with husbands present. There was little change over time in these ratios. For rural–urban differentials, urban fertility was below rural fertility in Durham and Easington, but the differential was closing over the 1850s and 1860s. For Merthyr Tydfil, urban fertility was initially above rural fertility but this had reversed by 1871. Examination of occupational fertility differentials for married women with husband present did confirm that families with husbands in mining did have relatively high current fertility. This was also true for families in farming for 1851 and 1861. Laborers generally had wives with low current marital fertility. Otherwise, the rankings by occupational groups were not very stable over time and gave no consistent patterns. Attempts to examine fertility differentials using the Registrar General's social stratification schemes did not reveal the expected patterns either. Since these stratification schemes were based on occupational groupings, this was not surprising. Fertility differentials by place of birth of spouse were not extremely clear. Locally born wives often had higher fertility, and spouses born in Ireland had apparently slowly increasing marital fertility over the 1850s and 1860s. There was no clear differential by nativity in these districts such as came to exist in the Pennsylvania anthracite region. Finally, working spouses had (with one exception) lower fertility than nonworking spouses, although the proportion of wives working was extremely small. This was quite similar to findings from the Pennsylvania mining counties. Regression analysis applied to these families did little to clarify the differentials.

Extension of the analysis to age-specific fertility required the estimation of age-specific birth rates by own-children methods. These birth rates also showed little change over time. There were some small alterations in marital fertility but no indication of decline between 1846–1851 and 1866–1871. The somewhat lower fertility in Merthyr Tydfil was due to lower age-specific marital fertility and not lower age-specific proportions married. Both areas demonstrated little evidence of fertility control within marriage and both may have been largely natural fertility populations. Rural–urban differentials were due both to differences in age-specific fertility and in marriage practices. Fertility in both Durham–Easington and Merthyr Tydfil was higher than in England and Wales as a whole in 1861 and 1871, and this was due to higher age-specific marital fertility in Durham and Easington in addition to earlier and more extensive marriage in both of the mining and industrial areas.

Durham and Easington and Merthyr Tydfil exhibited many of the expected characteristics of mining and industrial districts with heavy differential adult-male net in-migration, high wages for males, lack of employment for females (especially married females), early and extensive marriage for females, and high marital fertility. Durham and Easington, being more concentrated in coal mining, were much less urban than was Merthyr Tydfil which also specialized in iron manufacture. Mortality was also very high in Merthyr Tydfil relative to Durham and Easington and to the country as a whole. No distinctive occupation-related mortality patterns appeared, other than a very high accident mortality among adult males. Female mortality was very high in the childbearing years because of high maternal mortality (attributable to high fertility) and a heavy incidence of tuberculosis. Infectious disease was the major cause of the higher mortality in Merthyr Tydfil, which was probably partly due to its more urban character and greater population density.

Many expectations about the particular characteristics of mining areas have been confirmed by this study of two areas in Britain. Unfortunately, general patterns of occupational fertility differentials did not appear well established in these areas at mid-century. Also, the period prior to 1871 showed no evidence of secular fertility decline and so permitted no analysis of that phenomenon.

VI

The United States Commissioner of Labor Survey, 1889–1890

THE SURVEY

This chapter will present, as a case study, the results of a survey of industrial families conducted in 1889 and 1890 by the United States Commissioner of Labor and published, virtually in entirety, in the Sixth and Seventh Annual Reports of the Commissioner. The data were collected by one of America's great empirical statisticians, Carroll D. Wright, when he was U.S. Commissioner of Labor (U.S. Commissioner of Labor, 1890, 1891).[1] They were the results of a study of costs of production in nine protected industries (bar iron, pig iron, steel, bituminous coal, coke, iron ore, cotton textiles, woolens, and glass) made in preparation for debate over the highly protective McKinley Tariff of 1890. As a virtual by-product of this effort, information was gathered on the demographic characteristics, occupations, incomes, and expenditure patterns of 8544 families and their family members in these nine industries for 24 states of the United States and five European countries (Belgium, France, Germany, Great Britain, and Switzerland).[2] As may be seen from Table VI-1, all industries were not represented for all areas of residence. A few states (e.g., Kentucky, Louisiana, Missouri, Delaware, South Carolina) were only sampled for single indus-

[1] For a biography of Carroll Wright, see Leiby (1960) and also Williamson (1967).

[2] Part of the data set used here was kindly furnished by Peter Lindert and Allen Kelley, to whom many thanks go out.

TABLE VI-1 Families Classified by Industry and Place of Residence, 1889/1890. Commissioner of Labor Survey (All Families)

	Residence	Industry									
		Pig iron	Bar iron	Steel	Coal	Coke	Iron ore	Cottons	Woolens	Glass	Tota
1.	Alabama	143	39	2	60	30	-	43	-	-	31
	(Column %)	(17.0)	(4.5)	(0.5)	(8.5)	(10.8)	-	(1.6)	-	-	(3.
2.	Georgia	25	-	-	-	-	-	199	-	-	22
		(11.2)	-	-	-	-	-	(7.3)	-	-	(2.
3.	Illinois	40	68	38	-	-	-	-	-	106	25
		(4.8)	(7.8)	(9.9)	-	-	-	-	-	(8.0)	(2.
4.	Indiana	-	-	-	36	-	-	-	-	178	21
		-	-	-	(5.1)	-	-	-	-	(13.4)	(2.
5.	New York	56	41	62	-	-	38	187	214	152	75
		(6.7)	(4.7)	(16.1)	-	-	(20.7)	(6.9)	(17.2)	(11.5)	(8.
6.	Ohio	98	140	8	103	-	29	-	-	245	62
		(11.7)	(16.0)	(2.1)	(14.7)	-	(15.8)	-	-	(18.5)	(7.
7.	Pennsyl-vania	313	277	48	301	187	73	213	213	252	187
		(37.3)	(31.7)	(12.5)	(42.9)	(67.5)	(39.7)	(7.9)	(17.1)	(19.0)	(22.
8.	Tennessee	51	17	-	-	15	9	69	-	-	161
		(6.1)	(1.9)	-	-	(5.4)	(4.9)	(2.5)	-	-	(1.
9.	Virginia	27	35	-	-	-	16	124	-	-	20
		(3.2)	(4.0)	-	-	-	(8.7)	(4.6)	-	-	(2.4
10.	West Virginia	9	6	25	8	17	-	-	-	-	6
		(1.1)	(0.7)	(6.5)	(1.1)	(6.1)	-	-	-	-	(0.
11.	Connecticut	-	-	-	-	-	-	150	146	-	296
		-	-	-	-	-	-	(5.5)	(11.7)	-	(3.5
12.	Kentucky	-	-	-	-	-	-	20	-	-	20
		-	-	-	-	-	-	(0.7)	-	-	(0.2
13.	Louisiana	-	-	-	-	-	-	10	-	-	10
		-	-	-	-	-	-	(0.4)	-	-	(0.1
14.	Maine	-	-	-	-	-	-	164	111	-	275
		-	-	-	-	-	-	(6.0)	(8.9)	-	(3.2
15.	Maryland	-	-	-	-	-	-	164	-	47	211
		-	-	-	-	-	-	(6.0)	-	(3.5)	(2.5
16.	Massachu-setts	-	-	-	-	-	-	400	18	-	418
		-	-	-	-	-	-	(14.7)	(1.4)	-	(4.9
17.	Mississippi	-	-	-	-	-	-	34	-	-	34
		-	-	-	-	-	-	(1.3)	-	-	(0.4
18.	New Hampshire	-	-	-	-	-	-	119	36	-	155
		-	-	-	-	-	-	(4.4)	(2.9)	-	(1.8
19.	North Carolina	-	-	-	-	-	-	148	-	-	148
		-	-	-	-	-	-	(5.5)	-	-	(1.7

tries, as was one of the foreign nations (Switzerland). Some areas, such as Pennsylvania (1877 families) and Great Britain (1024 families) were, on the other hand, well sampled over the range of industries. Another aspect of the study was that the industries themselves were rather unevenly covered with cotton textiles taking 31.8% of the sample (2713 families), while steel, coke, and iron ore combined constituted only 9.9% of the whole data set (845 families).

Of the families in the sample, 8363 (or 97.9%) were male headed and only 180 were female headed. There was one family with no parents. Among the male-headed households, 105 (1.3%) had no spouse. Of the female-headed households, all but three were found in either cottons or woolens. The

TABLE VI-1 (Continued)

Residence	Industry									
	Pig iron	Bar iron	Steel	Coal	Coke	Iron ore	Cottons	Woolens	Glass	Total
20. Rhode Island	-	-	-	-	-	-	55	40	-	95
	-	-	-	-	-	-	(2.0)	(3.2)	-	(1.1)
21. South Carolina	-	-	-	-	-	-	33	-	-	33
	-	-	-	-	-	-	(1.2)	-	-	(0.4)
22. Missouri	-	-	-	-	-	-	-	-	18	18
	-	-	-	-	-	-	-	-	(1.4)	(0.2)
23. New Jersey	-	-	-	-	-	-	-	85	279	363
	-	-	-	-	-	-	-	(6.8)	(21.0)	(4.2)
24. Delaware	-	-	-	-	-	-	-	48	-	48
(Column %)	-	-	-	-	-	-	-	(3.9)	-	(0.6)
United States total	762	623	183	508	249	165	2132	911	1276	6809
(Column %)	(90.8)	(71.3)	(47.7)	(72.4)	(89.9)	(89.7)	(78.6)	(73.2)	(96.2)	(79.7)
(Row %)	(11.2)	(9.1)	(2.7)	(7.5)	(3.6)	(2.4)	(31.3)	(13.4)	(18.7)	(100.00)
25. Belgium	11	75	-	10	4	-	-	-	24	124
	(1.3)	(8.6)	-	(1.4)	(1.4)	-	-	-	(1.8)	(1.5)
26. France	-	40	-	-	-	-	116	179	-	335
	-	(4.6)	-	-	-	-	(4.3)	(14.4)	-	(3.9)
27. Germany	-	22	35	18	10	19	72	24	-	200
	-	(2.5)	(9.1)	(2.6)	(3.6)	(10.3)	(2.7)	(1.9)	-	(2.3)
28. Britain	66	114	166	166	14	-	341	131	26	1024
	(7.9)	(13.0)	(43.2)	(23.6)	(5.1)	-	(12.6)	(10.5)	(2.0)	(12.0)
29. Switzerland	-	-	-	-	-	-	52	-	-	52
	-	-	-	-	-	-	(1.9)	-	-	(0.6)
Europe total	77	251	201	194	28	19	581	334	50	1735
(Column %)	(9.2)	(28.7)	(52.3)	(27.6)	(10.1)	(10.3)	(21.4)	(26.8)	(3.8)	(20.3)
(Row %)	(4.4)	(14.5)	(11.6)	(11.2)	(1.6)	(1.1)	(33.5)	(19.2)	(2.9)	(100.00)
Overall total	839	874	384	702	277	184	2713	1245	1326	8544
(Row %)	(9.8)	(10.2)	(4.5)	(8.2)	(3.2)	(2.2)	(31.0)	(14.6)	(15.5)	(100.0)

Source: Data compiled from U.S. Commissioner of Labor, *Sixth Annual Report* (1890) and *Seventh Annual Report* (1891).

male-headed households without spouses were distributed over all the industries, with the largest number (61) being in cotton textiles.

The study itself was undertaken immediately following legislation creating the Department of Labor. Only protected industries were considered and, of those, several were excluded on the basis of small size or of insufficient concentration to allow reasonably low-cost sampling. (These were sugar, confection, and silk manufacture.) Cooperation was solicited from the firms in the remaining industries and representatives of the Department of Labor were sent to each firm in person to collect information about costs of production and costs of living (U.S. Commissioner of Labor, 1890, pp. 3–8). The sampling of the individual families themselves was not, however, fully clarified. The report stated that:

> *The Department has aimed to secure accounts from a representative number of employees of the establishments covered . . . and also from those families whose surroundings and conditions made them representative of the whole body of employees in any particular establishment. This representative character, however, has been impaired in some measure by two features: first, some families have not been willing to give the information desired, while second, other families, perfectly willing, have not been able to give reasonably exact accounts of their living expenses* [U.S. Commissioner of Labor, 1890, pp. 610–611].

The result was 8544 families containing 44,518 persons. It appears that the sample was stratified by the proportions employed in each industry, but it is not clear whether the sample was, or was intended to be, random. It *is* clear that the plan was to obtain a representative sample, but that certain biases appeared because of nonresponse and ignorance of certain respondents. Exactly how the sample was taken is not explained. John Modell, who has used these data, has speculated that workers may have been approached as they left work (Modell, 1978). At any rate, it seems that the survey is not really random nor representative, since it selected, first, only workers within cooperating firms and, second, only workers within those firms who would or could provide information. Finally, it must be remembered that only industrial workers in families were included.

As a test of the representativeness of the sample, the age distributions of currently married and ever-married males were compared between the sample and census data for the United States. This was done for four industrial groups: mining and quarrying (coal and iron mining in the sample), metals (bar iron, pig iron, steel, and coke in the sample), cotton textiles, and woolen textiles. These categories were determined by data available in the 1890 census of the U.S. (U.S. Bureau of the Census, 1897, pp. 759, 774, 778, 785) and do not, unfortunately, fully correspond to the same groups in the Commissioner of Labor sample. So, for example, metal workers in the census of 1890 included those in nonferrous as well as ferrous metals and in fabricating as well as refining. Textile workers in the census tabulation were only those classified as "operatives." Thus, some differences might be expected.

The percentage distributions by age for currently married and ever-married males from the 1890 census and from the United States portion of the 1889–1890 survey are presented in Table VI-2. As may be seen, the distributions were roughly similar, giving some support to the representativeness of the Commissioner of Labor Survey. Only in the case of the mining population, however, was the survey distribution sufficiently close to the census distribution to give a statistically insignificant chi-square test. For the other categories, the differences were significant. In general, the survey contained too few married males below age 25 and above age 65. In the case of metals and textiles, there were also too few aged 25–34. On the other hand, males aged 35–44 were consistently overrepresented in the survey.

TABLE VI-2 Comparison of Age Distributions of Currently Married and Ever-Married Males in the United States Industrial Workers, by Industry, U.S. Census, 1890, and Commissioner of Labor Survey, 1889/1890

	Age								
	15-24	25-34	35-44	45-54	55-64	65+			
	(Percent distribution)							*N*	$[\chi^2]^a$
A. *Mining*									
1. Currently married									
U.S. Census	6.4	36.1	29.9	18.1	7.4	2.1	100.0	190,718	> 7.90
Sample	5.2	37.4	31.7	16.9	7.9	0.9	100.0	669	
2. Ever married									
U.S. Census	6.1	34.8	29.6	18.6	8.1	2.7	99.9	202,247	> 10.86
Sample	5.2	37.4	31.6	16.8	8.0	1.0	100.0	672	
B. *Metals*									
1. Currently married									
U.S. Census	6.6	37.6	28.5	17.3	7.5	2.5	100.0	196,064	> 41.61*
Sample	5.1	34.8	33.6	18.0	7.8	0.8	100.1	1557	
2. Ever married									
U.S. Census	6.3	36.6	28.3	17.8	8.1	3.0	100.1	206,100	> 46.17*
Sample	5.0	34.5	33.6	18.2	7.8	0.8	99.9	1567	
C. *Cotton Textiles*									
1. Currently married									
U.S. Census	11.9	35.5	25.7	17.6	7.2	2.1	100.0	32,023	> 191.95*
Sample	4.8	29.8	27.6	24.8	10.6	2.4	100.0	1926	
2. Ever married									
U.S. Census	11.5	34.6	25.7	18.0	7.7	2.5	100.0	33,678	> 184.32*
Sample	4.6	29.2	27.3	25.4	10.9	2.6	100.0	1980	
D. *Woolen Textiles*									
1. Currently married									
U.S. Census	7.5	33.9	26.4	19.8	9.0	3.3	99.9	21,692	> 56.54*
Sample	2.0	32.2	33.4	22.3	7.7	2.4	100.0	857	
2. Ever married									
U.S. Census	7.2	33.0	26.0	20.0	9.6	4.1	99.9	22,901	> 58.76*
Sample	2.1	31.8	33.3	22.2	8.0	2.5	99.9	868	

Source: Sample data from U.S. Commissioner of Labor, *Sixth Annual Report* (1890) and *Seventh Annual Report* (1891). Census data from U.S. Bureau of the Census, *Eleventh Census of the United States: 1890*, Vol. 1, Part II (1897), pp. 759, 774, 778, 785.

* $p < .01$.

a The χ^2 test was based on the integer values of the sample and the U.S. census age distribution normalized to equal the size of the 1889/1890 sample. The critical χ^2 value for a 1% confidence limit is 15.09.

Overall, however, the broad similarities were more striking than the differences, and the case for the representativeness of the survey is strengthened.

As far as accuracy in the survey is concerned, some margin for error in the data themselves must be allowed, particularly for detailed financial information, but the general magnitudes seem, with a few exceptions, plausible. There was, for example, apparently a good deal of rounding in the reporting of income and expenditure by detailed category, but this is only to be expected from families who probably kept, at best, rudimentary records. A listing of the information taken from the survey is given in Table VI-3. All other measures were calculated from these basic data.

In many ways the Commissioner of Labor Survey is also valuable for insight into the differences which existed within the industrial labor force of

TABLE VI-3 Information Coded from the 1889/1890 Survey of Worker Families in Nine Industries in the United States and Five European Countries

1. State or country of residence
2. Industry
3. Nationality of family head
4. Number of children at school
5. Number of children at home
6. Number of children at work
7. Presence of boarders
8. Number of boarders and others in the household
9. Occupation of husband
10. Age of husband
11. Age of wife
12. Number of children
13. Ages of children
14. Sex of each child above 10
15. Does the family own their home
16. Husband's income
17. Wife's income
18. Children's income
19. Income from boarders
20. Other income
21. Total income
22. Food expenditures
23. Rent expenditures
24. Other expenditures of which:
    a. Tax expenditures
    b. Labor contributions
    c. Expenditures for sickness and dental
    d. Other
25. Number of rooms in the house or apartment

the United States and Western Europe in the late nineteenth century. There were large differences in income, expenditure, and life style detectable in the survey between unskilled laborers and such skilled groups as iron puddlers and rollers and glass blowers, the "aristocracy of the proletariat."

A few examples should suffice. At the one extreme, some skilled workers were paid amazingly high salaries. The highest salary in the sample was earned by a native-born roller in a bar iron firm in Ohio. He was paid the incredible sum of $4500 per year. This was 8.4 times the average income of male heads of household in the United States portion of the sample ($535) and 6.6 times the average income in the United States bar iron industry sample ($686). One might be tempted to suspect that this was an error in the survey, but other information was consistent with this figure. Comments made by the interviewers were appended to the survey, and for this household the interviewer remarked: "Surplus invested in real estate; own house; live in style." The man was aged 47 and his wife, 46. They had one daughter, at home, aged 21. Their house was one of the few lighted with gas; the family paid $220 in life insurance premiums, quite a rational activity in light of his high income. They made approximately $100 in religious and charitable contributions, spent about $380 on clothing, and saved over $1700 for the year. Surely this was a family living better than most of the middle class.

Other examples were also common:

1. Welsh-born bar iron roller. Ohio. Annual income $3000. Age 48. Wife aged 44. Five children (aged 14, 12, 10, 8, and 5). Four of the five children were in school. The family rented a 13-room house for $400 per year and took in one boarder, which brought in an additional $192. They spent $575 on clothing, $108 on property and life insurance, and $52 on books and newspapers. The family made $171 in charitable and religious contributions and was able to save almost $1200 on the year. The comments were: "Surplus on hand; enterprising man; live in style."
2. English-born glassblower. Illinois. Annual income $2263. Age 31. Wife aged 27. Four children (aged 7, 5, 4 and 2), of whom one was in school. The family owned its own house, spent $165 on clothing, and managed to save almost $1600 on the year. The interviewer remarked: "Have a sewing machine and a small garden."

Overall in the sample, there were 20 cases with income for the head of household over $2000. Of these, 5 were glassblowers, 14 were bar iron workers (rollers, heaters, puddlers), and one was in steel. All were in the United States and a number of nationalities were represented, including native-born Americans, English, Welsh, Irish, Scots, and Germans.

At the other extreme, there were also some interesting stories:

1. Native-born American laborer in the pig iron industry in Georgia. Annual income: $150. (The industry average was $762 in the United States

and $405 in Georgia.) Age 50. Wife aged 21. No children. The family rented a one-room home for $12 per year and heated with wood, despite local coal availability. The family spent $19 on liquor and tobacco and the interviewer commented: "In debt; ignorant and dirty 'Georgia Crackers.' "

2. French-Canadian filling carrier in the cotton textile industry in Maine. Annual income $125. (The industry average was $400 for the United States and $427 for Maine.) Age 62. Wife aged 41. Eight children (aged 19, 18, 16, 15, 13, 11, 8, and 3) of whom four were at work (and contributed $841 to family income), three at school, and one at home. They rented a six-room company house for $90 per year. Expenditures exceeded income by $5. The interviewer commented: "Company tenement; big and cheerless; rooms in basement."

This last case illustrates a common occurrence in the industrial labor force in this era. The husband received quite a low income from a poor, menial job. The family, however, used its children to supply additional labor and earn the extra income to bring the family up to a reasonable level of consumption expenditure. This is an example of a strategy followed by many families at this time in reaction to low or declining earnings of the head of household. This issue, as well as others related to income and family labor supply, will be treated later in this chapter. First, however, differential fertility will be discussed.

DIFFERENTIAL FERTILITY

One of the great advantages of the U.S. Commissioner of Labor Survey is that it provides information on several of the specific industries which have been the focus of discussion in previous chapters, namely coal mining and ferrous metallurgy. In addition, there are also a substantial number of families from two light industries (cotton and woolen textiles) and from a craft industry (glass). As may be seen in Table VI-3, there is not only information on the demographic composition of the family, but also of its economic activity, especially income from various sources. The survey thus furnishes a large quantity of information valuable in assessing differentials in fertility. Because the data are for families only, and because the overall population of women at risk of childbearing is not known, only marital child–woman ratios will be discussed. No attempt will be made to convert them to age-specific marital fertility rates (as was done in Chapters IV and V).

Overall and age-standardized marital child–woman ratios are presented in Table VI-4. The two standardizations are to the age structure of all married women in the survey (Standardization A) and to the age structure of married women in the Pennsylvania anthracite region in 1880 (Standardization B).

The latter was calculated in order to facilitate comparisons with the samples in Chapters IV and V. The ratios are presented for the total subset of families with wives aged 15–49 and for the various dimensions within the United States and Europe.[3] Finally, within Europe, Great Britain was considered separately. The dimensions along which the child–woman ratios are viewed include the industry of the family head, nativity of the family head (for the United States and Britain), country of residence (for Europe), whether the family owned its own home, and whether the wife had worked in the year prior to the survey (i.e., whether she had earned any income).

As Table VI-4 indicates, for the United States, marital child–woman ratios were higher for mining than for metallurgy and higher for the heavy industries than for textiles or for glass. When standardized, mining still maintained its leading position, but iron and steel manufacture dropped behind textiles. As a result, heavy industry as a group (iron, steel, and mining) had standardized ratios below those for textiles. The reason is that the age composition of wives (and also of heads of household) was generally younger in ferrous metallurgy (and also in mining) relative to textiles. This led to higher overall ratios and supports the hypothesis that mining and heavy-industrial employment attracted younger men and favored earlier marriage and childbearing. The glass industry, despite its high average incomes (see Table II-1, pages 43–44), high skill levels, and younger population was consistently the lowest in terms of marital fertility.

For Europe, on the other hand, coal mining lagged behind the iron and steel industries in terms of overall fertility.[4] This was not true, however, when age-standardized ratios were calculated, indicating, somewhat surprisingly, an older population of wives in coal mining than in ferrous metallurgy. For Europe, textiles were below the heavy industries for both overall and age-standardized ratios, which was more the expected pattern. Glass remained the industry with the lowest fertility levels, as in the United States. Within Europe, the highest fertility was found in Germany, followed by France, Belgium, Britain, and Switzerland. (The Swiss case must be considered with caution, in view of the very small number of cases—36.) These results do not have a great deal of significance, however, in view of the differing industry mix within each country. (See Table VI-1.) One alternative would be to standardize for industry composition, which was not done. Instead, multiple regression was applied. These results are discussed later in

[3] The term "family" will be used in this chapter to apply to the primary family of the household sampled in the survey. Since there is no information on the existence or composition of any possible secondary families, this is the only course possible.

[4] The extremely high ratios in iron mining may be attributed to the small sample (only 15 cases for Europe). Given the large sampling error which accompanies such results, they may be unreliable. A test of the significant of the difference between the iron-mining overall average ratio and the population mean revealed, however, that the difference between the ratio for iron mining in Europe and for the whole European sample was statistically significant at a 1% level.

TABLE VI-4 Overall and Standardized Marital Child-Woman Ratios (Children 0-4 per 1000 Married Women 15-49) U.S. Commissioner of Labor Survey 1889/1890. (Married Couples with Husband and Wife Present) (per 1000)

	Overall ratio	N	Standardization[a] A	Standardization[b] B
I. *Total sample*	834.3	7322	834.3	833.8
II. *United States*				
A. Total	843.1	5883	840.5	840.1
B. Industry				
1. Pig iron	870.5	695	838.3	831.3
2. Bar iron	859.0	539	858.2	853.8
3. Steel	942.3	156	850.6	852.5
4. Coke	729.7	222	732.3	712.8
1-4. Iron and steel	854.2	1612	828.2	822.0
5. Coal	997.8	449	969.7	964.4
6. Iron ore	1013.0	154	893.6	924.7
5-6. Mining	1001.7	603	956.1	957.6
1-6. Heavy industry	894.4	2215	863.9	860.4
7. Cottons	820.0	1739	881.0	876.0
8. Woolens	820.3	757	835.2	842.7
7-8. Textiles	820.1	2496	867.1	865.4
9. Glass	795.2	1177	761.1	769.3
C. Nativity of family head				
1. Native-born	803.4	3336	764.1	767.3
2. Foreign-born	895.0	2552	936.4	933.7
a. British	837.7	770	891.9	898.8
b. Irish	849.0	715	955.6	953.8
c. Canadian	1125.0	304	1146.5	1121.5
d. German	885.2	566	879.8	875.3
e. Slavic, Italian, and other	959.4	197	915.7	923.5
D. Home ownership				
1. Home owner	823.2	967	897.8	911.2
2. Not home owner	847.0	4921	832.3	830.9
E. Wife's labor force status				
1. Not working	858.2	5445	860.8	860.4
2. Working	656.9	443	610.0	606.2
III. *Europe*				
A. Total	798.5	1434	804.6	800.8
B. Industry				
1. Bar iron	806.0	67	774.6	775.6
2. Pig iron	829.0	193	854.2	856.0
3. Steel	925.7	175	895.2	874.1
4. Coke	782.6	23	941.4	852.8
1-4. Iron and steel	860.3	458	867.6	857.8
5. Coal	779.1	163	866.2	888.5
6. Iron ore	1600.0	15	1644.9	1637.6
5-6. Mining	848.3	178	931.9	953.9
1-6. Heavy industry	856.9	636	871.9	866.3
7. Cottons	743.9	488	747.4	745.2
8. Woolens	768.1	263	777.8	780.7
7-8. Textiles	752.3	751	761.9	762.7
9. Glass	744.7	47	720.8	708.5

this chapter. For the subset of the European sample from Great Britain, heavy industry ranked ahead of textiles and also, when standardized, ahead of glass. Mining again showed a dramatic rise in the age-standardized child–woman ratios. In the case of standardization to the age structure of married women in the Pennsylvania anthracite region in 1880, coal mining emerged as having the highest ratios, indicating a somewhat older age composition in the population of miners' wives than in the standard population. Overall, then, the high fertility of mining and metallurgical popula-

TABLE VI-4 (Continued)

	Overall ratio	*N*	Standardization[a] A	Standardization[b] B
C. Country				
1. Belgium	795.5	88	801.1	815.4
2. France	829.6	270	802.3	801.8
3. Germany	1171.7	163	1169.2	1153.2
4. Great Britain	730.9	877	748.0	743.0
5. Switzerland	527.8	36	486.3	441.3
D. Home ownership				
1. Home owner	888.9	81	968.1	951.4
2. Not home owner	793.1	1353	793.7	790.5
E. Wife's labor force status				
1. Not working	829.5	1255	858.3	853.6
2. Working	581.0	179	474.9	479.9
IV. *Great Britain*				
A. Total	730.9	877	748.0	743.0
B. Industry				
1-4. Iron and steel	812.5	304	815.2	800.6
5-6. Mining	715.2	144	809.4	834.3
1-6. Heavy industry	781.2	448	790.7	782.4
7-8. Textiles	670.0	403	713.9	716.2
9. Glass	807.7	26	586.5	569.0
C. Nativity of family head				
1. English	729.6	673	746.8	743.6
2. Irish	875.0	32	849.6	824.0
3. Scots	776.8	112	789.5	783.6
4. Welsh	593.2	59	591.4	547.1
D. Home ownership				
1. Home owner	600.0	15	582.9	541.3
2. Not home owner	733.2	862	748.5	743.5
E. Wife's labor force status				
1. Not working	740.9	822	769.5	764.8
2. Working	581.8	55	437.6	416.3

Source: Data compiled from U.S. Commissioner of Labor, *Sixth Annual Report* (1890) and *Seventh Annual Report* (1891).

[a]Standardization A = Standardized to the age structure of all married women with husbands present in the Commissioner of Labor Survey.

[b]Standardization B = Standardized to the age structure of married women in the Pennsylvania anthracite region in 1880.

tions relative to textiles (and glass, a craft industry) was confirmed for Europe but not for the United States.

As far as the other dimensions were concerned, working wives had consistently lower fertility than nonworking wives, which bears out prior expectations. The relationship between home ownership, which is a proxy for wealth, and current fertility was ambiguous. Homeowners had lower overall ratios but higher standardized ratios in the United States, but had uniformly higher ratios (overall and standardized) in Europe. For the British subsample, on the other hand, homeowners had lower child–woman ratios, although the very small proportion of homeowners in the sample (1.7% among the 877 British families in Table VI-4) makes this a somewhat unreliable comparison. Actually, homeownership had an ambiguous relationship to fertility because a family might have owned a home precisely because there were many children (i.e., high current and past fertility) and a need for space. Thus, homeownership might have been a dependent rather than an independent variable. But the relationship should, in general, have been a positive one, both because of this effect and of a pure wealth effect (i.e., higher nonwage income to the family).

Within the United States, ethnic fertility differentials within the survey sample conformed to anticipated patterns. Families with native-born heads had lower current fertility than families with foreign-born heads. This differential was considerably widened by standardization. Within the foreign-born group (about 43% of the whole United States sample) the highest fertility was among Canadians, of whom a substantial proportion were French Canadians.[5] Among the age-standardized ratios, the French Canadians were followed by the Irish, the Slavic–Italian–other group, the British (English, Scottish, Welsh), and finally the Germans. This is somewhat similar to the results found for the anthracite region, although there British ethnicity usually accompanied fertility below all the foreign-born groups. Within Great Britain, the highest child–woman ratios were found among the small number of Irish-headed families, followed by the Scots, English, and finally the Welsh. Again the results are not unexpected.

As in prior chapters, problems arise in considering each dimension in isolation. Since the simultaneous effect of various dimensions can be partially controlled through regression analysis,[6] this was done, and the results are presented in Table VI-5. Equations were estimated for the whole sample, and for the United States, Europe, and Great Britain separately. The units of observation were individual families, using only married couples with husband and wife present and with the wife aged 15–49 at the time of the survey. The dependent variable was the number of young own children aged 0–4 present in the family. The method of estimation was ordinary least-squares regression which, as was shown in Chapter IV, is fairly robust when used with this particular limited value dependent variable.

Among the independent variables in the equation are the age of the wife and the age of the wife squared which, in view of previous results, should have positive and negative signs, respectively. This reflects the curvilinear relationship of fertility to age of woman.[7] Sets of dummy variables were included for the industry, occupation (classed as unskilled; semiskilled;

[5] French Canadians made up 71% of the 304 Canadian families used to calculate the ratios in Table VI-4. The ratios were actually quite similar between the families labeled as having French Canadian heads and those simply having Canadian heads, although there might well have been some heads denoted as simply Canadian who were, in reality, French Canadians.

[6] The term "partially controlled" is used because interaction effects for dummy variables, unless explicitly specified, are not taken into account.

[7] The relationship is, in fact, a parabola which is concave downward (which is implied by a negative sign on the age-of-wife-squared coefficient). The coefficient of age must be positive if age is positive and the age-squared coefficient is negative.

skilled; craftsman; white collar and supervisory; helper and apprentice; other), region within the United States, country within Europe, and ethnicity of head of household for the United States and for Great Britain. As usual with sets of dummy variables in regression equations, one in each set had to be deleted in order to estimate the equation. These dummy variables allow some test of the relationship of fertility to residence, industry, occupation, and ethnicity, while holding other things constant. Homeownership[8] was also entered as an independent variable in order to test the effect of wealth on fertility. The relative income of the husband, defined as the actual money income of the husband divided by the average for his state within the United States or his country within Europe, was included in an attempt to assess not only the absolute income effect but also a relative one. That is, more income from the husband (who presumably has a lower opportunity cost in terms of allocation of time from having additional children) should increase fertility, all other things being held constant (see Mincer, 1963; McCabe and Rosenzweig, 1976). There also might be, however, some relative income effect (Duesenberry, 1949) with respect to fertility, such as has been found for the contemporary United States (Freedman, 1963). This implies that it is income relative to one's environmental norm that is important. Above average relative income should lead to above average fertility and vice versa.

The wife's income was included as an independent variable as some measure of the extent of labor-force participation and opportunity cost, although, for the latter, a "full" income measure would have been desirable. "Full" income is income that would have been earned if the wife worked full time. Since the survey did not provide information on the number of hours worked, it was not possible to calculate this for the wives in the sample. As with a simple labor-force participation measure, there is a problem of simultaneous equation bias. High fertility may be a cause as well as an effect of low labor-force participation outside the home by married women. For data with limited value dependent variables, the theoretical and computational problems have not yet been solved and so, in the absence of techniques analogous to two-stage least squares for limited dependent variables, ordinary least squares was applied. It must be borne in mind, however, that the coefficients for the wife's income variable (and also those coefficients for other independent variables which were highly correlated with wife's income) will be biased. Hopefully the bias is small and will not much alter the results of the significance tests.

One final variable, income from boarders, was added to test the hypothesis that there were forms of economic activity within the home which were partial substitutes (in terms of income) for market work outside the home and which were much more compatible with child rearing. The

[8] Homeownership = 0 if home is not owned and 1 if home is owned.

TABLE VI-5 Regression Equations with Number of Own Children Aged 0-4 Present as the Dependent Variable. Worker Families in Nine Industries. United States, Britain, France, Germany, Belgium, and Switzerland, 1889/1890. (Families with Both Husband and Wife Present. Wife Aged 15-49)

Variables	Total			United States		
	Coefficient	Significance	β-Coefficient	Coefficient	Significance	β-Coefficient
I. *Dependent variable*						
Own children aged 0-4 present						
II. *Independent variables*						
1. Constant	-.8563	NC[a]	NC	-.9856	NC	NI
2. Age of wife	.1487	***	1.3647	.1501	***	1.3784
3. Age of wife squared	-.0027	***	-1.7072	-.0028	***	-1.7287
4. Homeownership	.0846	***	.0344	.0773	***	.0330
5. Industry						
a. Pig iron	-.1300	*	-.0464	-.0588	n.s.	-.0219
b. Bar iron	-.0953	n.s.[c]	-.0334	-.0594	n.s.	-.0198
c. Steel	-.0379	n.s.	-.0092	-.0700	n.s.	-.0130
d. Coal	-.0363	n.s.	-.0117	.0360	n.s.	.0111
e. Coke	-.2299	***	-.0483	-.2134	**	-.0470
f. Cottons	-.0070	n.s.	-.0037	.0207	n.s.	.0711
g. Woolens	-.0815	n.s.	-.0327	-.1051	n.s.	-.0403
h. Glass	-.2145	***	-.0934	-.1590	**	-.0734
6. Relative income of husband	.0168	n.s.	.0092	.0183	n.s.	.0102
7. Occupation						
a. Unskilled	.0222	n.s.	.0117	.0554	n.s.	.0292
b. Semiskilled	.0439	n.s.	.0236	.0558	n.s.	.0295
c. Skilled	.0829	n.s.	.0389	.0967	n.s.	.0447
d. Craftsman	-.0202	n.s.	-.0074	.0311	n.s.	.0110
e. White collar/supervisor	-.0644	n.s.	-.0122	-.0064	n.s.	-.0012
f. Helper/apprentice	.0212	n.s.	.0042	.0728	n.s.	.0149
8. Income from boarders	-.0000	n.s.	-.0036	-.0001	n.s.	-.0126
9. Wife's income	-.0019	***	-.1191	-.0020	***	-.1248
10. United States or Europe	-.0476	*	-.0220	NI	NI	NI
11. Region in United States						
a. New England	NI[b]	NI	NI	.2250	***	.0986
b. Mid-Atlantic	NI	NI	NI	.1459	***	.0836
c. Midwest	NI	NI	NI	-.0987	**	-.0438
12. Ethnicity of husband						
a. American born	NI	NI	NI	-.0913	*	-.0520
b. English/British	NI	NI	NI	-.0392	n.s.	-.0153
c. Irish	NI	NI	NI	.0350	n.s.	.0131
d. Canadian	NI	NI	NI	.1853	*	.0254
e. French Canadian	NI	NI	NI	.1592	*	.0346
f. German	NI	NI	NI	.0037	n.s.	.0013
g. Slavic	NI	NI	NI	.0549	n.s.	.0061
h. Italian	NI	NI	NI	.2758	n.s.	.0144
i. Welsh	NI[b]	NI	NI	NI	NI	NI
j. Scottish	NI	NI	NI	NI	NI	NI
Number of cases		7218			5785	
R^2 adjusted		0.157			0.171	
F-Ratio		65.047			[illegible]	

Variables	Coefficient	Significance	β-Coefficient	Coefficient	Significance	β-Coefficient
I. *Dependent variable*						
Own children aged 0-4 present						
II. *Independent variables*						
1. Constant	.6433	NC[a]	NC	.6791	NC	NC
2. Age of wife	.0871	***	.7855	.0721	**	.6896
3. Age of wife squared	-.0018	***	-1.1627	-.0016	***	-1.0940
4. Homeownership	-.0200	n.s.[c]	-.0056	-.0750	n.s.	-.0125
5. Industry						
a. Pig iron	-.4473	*	-.1152	NI	NI	NI
b. Bar iron	-.4609	**	-.1920	-.0216	n.s.	-.0083
c. Steel	-.4182	*	-.1671	-.0050	n.s.	-.0024
d. Coal	-.4354	**	-.1687	-.0722	n.s.	-.0344
e. Coke	-.4933	*	-.0757	-.2647	n.s.	-.0402
f. Cottons	-.5070	**	-.2932	-.1676	n.s.	-.1019
g. Woolens	-.5021	**	-.2369	-.1456	n.s.	-.0604
h. Glass	-.6581	***	-.1430	-.2617	n.s.	-.0570
6. Relative income of husband	.0035	n.s.	.0018	.0717	n.s.	.0343
7. Occupation						
a. Unskilled	-.1891	n.s.	-.0957	-.3531	*	-.1895
b. Semiskilled	-.0481	n.s.	-.0279	-.3181	n.s.	-.1996
c. Skilled	-.1719	n.s.	-.0867	-.3941	*	-.1920
d. Craftsman	-.1612	n.s.	-.0696	-.3717	*	-.1634
e. White collar/supervisor	-.1672	n.s.	-.0267	-.3983	n.s.	-.0725
f. Helper/apprentice	-.2832	n.s.	-.0495	-.5417	***	-.1223
8. Income from boarders	.0004	n.s.	.0175	-.0003	n.s.	-.0142
9. Wife's income	-.0021	***	-.1325	-.0011	**	-.0702
10. Ethnicity of husband						
a. English/British	NI	NI	NI	.0112	n.s.	.0060
b. Welsh	NI[b]	NI	NI	-.1666	n.s.	-.0536
c. Scottish	NI	NI	NI	-.0681	n.s.	-.0292
11. Country						
a. Belgium	.0874	n.s.[c]	.0256	NI	NI	NI
b. France	.1275	n.s.	.0608	NI	NI	NI
c. Germany	.3975	***	.1540	NI	NI	NI
d. Great Britain	-.0024	n.s.	-.0015	NI	NI	NI
Number of cases		1433			876	
R^2 adjusted		0.186			0.174	
F-Ratio		14.657 ***			9.380 ***	

Source: Data compiled from U.S. Commissioner of Labor, *Sixth Annual Report* (1890) and *Seventh Annual Report* (1891).

[a]NC = Not calculated.

[b]NI = Not included.

[c]n.s. = Not significant at least at a 10% level.

$^{*}p < .1$

$^{**}p < .05$

$^{***}p < .01$

domestic handicraft industry was another such activity (Jaffe and Azum 1960). It is hypothesized that income from boarders should be positively, weakly, related to current fertility.

In looking at the equations in Table VI-5, it is clear that they explaine between 15–20% of total variation in marital child–woman ratios. Much c this variation was, in fact, explained simply by the age of the wife (as may b seen from the very large β-coefficients for age of wife and age of wif squared). Each equation was jointly significant at a 1% level (as may be see from the F-ratios).

In terms of prior expectations, the coefficients for age of wife and age c wife squared had the correct signs and were the most important variables i the sense of having the highest β-coefficients (and hence the greatest impac on the dependent variables). As far as industry of husband was concerned coal mining had a positive effect on fertility in the United States sample an a less negative effect in the overall sample.[9] The same was also true, some what surprisingly, for cotton textiles, although this had been suggeste by the standardized child–woman ratios in Table VI-4. Apparently, control ling for the effects of other variables, such as location, ethnicity, income and homeownership, did not eliminate the peculiarly high fertility amon cotton textile workers in the United States.

The higher fertility among miners' families was also confirmed for Grea Britain but not strongly for the European sample as a whole. For the European and British samples, however, families in cotton textiles did not have high predicted child–woman ratios (relative to the other industries in the sample). In general, having the family head in mining and heavy industry had a positive effect on fertility, while having the family head in textiles or glass had a negative effect. The exceptions to this were the coke industry, which had quite a negative impact on fertility, and the cotton textile industry in the United States, which had a positive effect on current fertility. Overall, prior hypotheses were borne out, although many of the estimated dummy variable coefficients were not significantly different from zero.

For the United States sample and the overall equation (which was dominated by the United States sample), occupation of husband had a very regular relationship to the categories as defined here. That is, skilled workers had the highest fertility, followed by semiskilled, unskilled, craftsmen, and white-collar–supervisory personnel. This contradicts all or part of the view that occupation and skill were good proxies for social class, that social class

[9] The effect of dummy variables is to create an adjustment to the constant term that is equal to the size of the coefficient. In the case of industry here, all the dummy variables in the overall equation can logically be negative, because the adjustments are all to reduce the size of the constant term (holding all other things constant). Therefore, in this case, a small negative coefficient is equivalent to having a positive effect on fertility.

as positively related to skill levels, and that fertility was negatively related to ocial class. These views were encountered in Chapter V in connection with ocial stratification schemes used by the Registrar General for England and Vales. The relationships for the British and European samples were even ss clear. It must be remembered, however, that all such schemes are ensitive to the classification typology used.

Relative income of husband turned out to have the expected positive sign n all cases, but was statistically insignificant (and had relatively small -coefficients) in all four equations. Wife's income, on the other hand, was onsistently negative and significant and had relatively large β-coefficients or all the equations. The estimated coefficient here is actually thus the sum f a negative substitution or price effect (because a wife must give up ncome to have more children) and a positive income effect (because a igher income means that more children can be afforded) (Mincer, 1963). Thus the negative sign implies that the substitution effect dominates. The oefficient on income from boarders was always insignificant and the sign vas negative in the United States, British, and overall equations, but not for he European equation. The expected relationship was positive, so that this ariable did not reveal a consistent or plausible connection between fertility nd this particular measure of nonmarket work opportunity for wives.

The residence variables showed some interesting patterns. In the overall equation, European residence clearly had a negative effect on fertility.[10] This probably reflected, as much as anything else, the composition of the survey, since available evidence indicates that fertility rates in the United States were, by about 1890, not greatly different from Britain, although they were well above those for France.[11] As the standardized ratios in Table VI-4 show, marital child–woman ratios for the United States were above those for France, Belgium, Britain, and Switzerland and only below those for Germany. Within the United States, quite surprisingly, residence in New England (Maine, New Hampshire, Massachusetts, Connecticut, Rhode Island) had a more positive effect on fertility than residence in the Middle Atlantic states (New York, New Jersey, Delaware, Pennsylvania). The Middle Atlantic states in turn showed a higher fertility than the Midwestern states in the sample (Illinois, Indiana, Michigan, Ohio). The omitted dummy variable was for the Southern states. The high fertility of the New England states might have been due to the heavy representation of cotton textiles in those states (see Table VI-1), although the existence of a separate dummy variable for cotton textiles should have controlled for this effect.

[10] This is implied by a negative coefficient for the "U.S. or Europe" variable, which was 0 if residence was in the U.S. and 1 if residence was in Europe.

[11] Compare a total fertility rate of 3.93 for the white population of the United States in 1889–1891 (Coale and Zelnik, 1963, p. 36) with one of 4.080 for England and Wales in 1891 and of 2.988 for France in 1889–1893 (calculated from Keyfitz and Flieger, 1968, pp. 322–524).

For the European sample, German residence strongly and positively affected marital fertility, while, at the other extreme, residence in Great Britain had a weakly negative effect.

Ethnicity or nativity of the husband was also a factor considered in the regressions for the United States and for Great Britain. In the United States a significant negative effect on fertility was created by having a native-born family head, and a smaller negative effect was created by having a British-born (English, Scottish, or Welsh) family head. All other ethnic origins had a positive effect on fertility, those for Canadians, French Canadians, and Italians being the largest. These results conform to expectations about the effects of nativity on fertility in the United States in the late nineteenth century, with the immigrant groups from Eastern and Southern Europe having the highest fertility and native-born Americans having the lowest. (The Canadians were exceptional in this respect.) Within the subsample for Great Britain, English nativity had a positive effect on current fertility whereas Scottish and Welsh nativity had a negative effect. (The omitted dummy variable was for Irish, for whom there were only a few observations.)

The application of regression analysis in this case has largely confirmed the results suggested in the tabulations in Table VI-4. Heavy industry and mining were generally associated with higher current marital fertility, except for the notable exception of cotton textiles in the United States. Working women definitely had smaller families, although causality was likely in both directions. Homeownership was positively associated with fertility in the United States, but was not significantly related to it in the European sample. Region seemed to make a difference, with marital child–woman ratios being significantly higher in the United States and, within the United States, in New England. For the United States, nativity of the family head also seemed to play a role, with native Americans having the lowest predicted fertility and Canadians and French Canadians the highest. Additional variables related to income and occupation were tested, with relatively inconclusive results.

One final test was conducted in connection with fertility. All nonhomeowners were selected from the whole sample and from the United States, European, and British subsamples, and the regressions were rerun. Instead of the variable on homeownership, a variable on number of rooms in the home was substituted.[12] Most of the results were broadly similar to the sample including both homeowners and nonhomeowners (which is not surprising since 77% of both the United States and European samples were nonhomeowners). The variable on number of rooms was positively and significantly related to fertility in the overall sample and also for the European and British subsamples. This implies that space constraints may have

[12] Information on number of rooms was included in the original survey only for nonhomeowners.

affected fertility decisions, but the causality might have as easily been reversed. A larger number of children might have induced a family to move to more spacious quarters. The latter, in fact, appears most plausible. For the United States, however, an insignificant negative relation between the number of rooms and fertility appeared.

LABOR-FORCE ACTIVITY

The Commissioner of Labor Survey is especially useful for examining patterns of labor-force activity and how they might relate to other demographic behavior. There are two major and interrelated issues which are relevant here. The first is that relating to age–earnings profiles for male heads of families and the second is the pattern of labor-force participation of secondary wage earners (i.e., wives and children). Patterns in the latter can, as it turns out, usefully be viewed as a response to the former.

As was pointed out in Chapter II, manual workers usually experience a relatively early peak in earnings with respect to age. This was amply illustrated by data from the Commissioner of Labor Survey presented in Table II-1 (pages 43–44). This phenomenon existed in all the industries—metallurgy, mining, textiles, and glass—and was true for the American as well as the European portions of the survey. This feature of age–earnings profiles remains true for blue-collar workers in the contemporary United States (Oppenheimer, 1974), although the profiles now tend to peak early and remain at a rough plateau, rather than decline, as they did in the nineteenth century. The situation is illustrated in Figure VI-1 for the United States and Europe separately, where it is clear in both cases that the average husband's income peaked out between ages 30–39. This may also be seen in Table VI-6, where it is also shown that husbands' incomes declined from approximately 90% of total family income for husbands aged 20–29 to approximately 50% for husbands aged 60 and over.[13] And it must be kept in mind that this was for families with husbands still employed in these industries. It does not include families for which the male head was forced to find still less reliable and less remunerative employment elsewhere.

The reasons for declining earnings as industrial workers became older, such as an obsolescence of skills among older workers because of increased education among younger worker cohorts or because older workers are simply less strong and less productive, cannot be discerned with these data.[14]

[13] The averages and the number of cases differ slightly from those in Table II-1 because only families with some incomes for the husband were included in Table II-1.

[14] It must be remembered that these are cross-sectional data. The relationship observed in the cross-section may not actually hold for cohorts over time. But the existence of these wage differentials by age in the cross-section may have influenced families to behave as *if* they existed over time, because younger males would see older males as their future reference group.

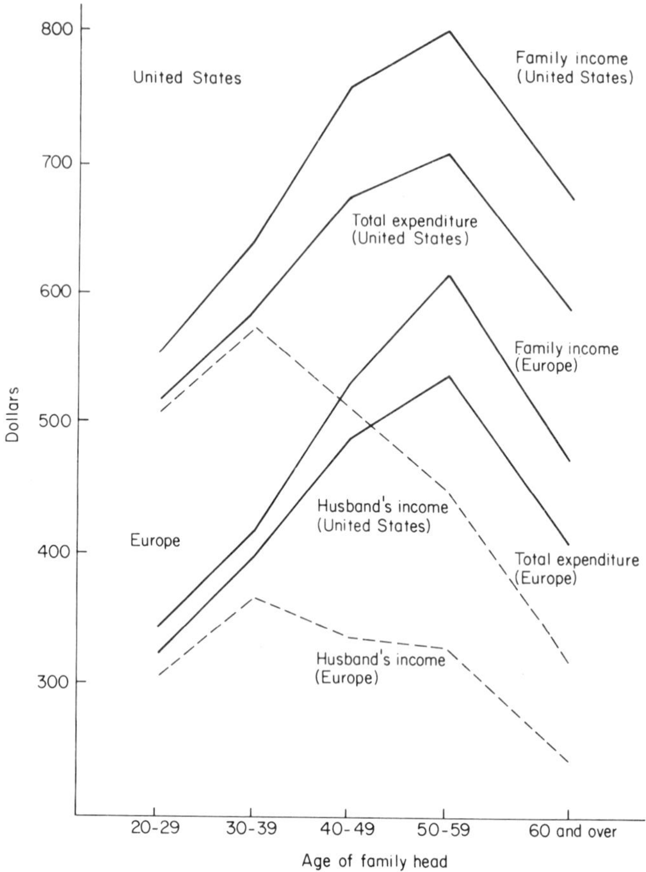

FIGURE VI-1 Income and expenditure profiles by age of male family head in nine industries, United States and five European countries (Britain, France, Germany, Belgium, and Switzerland), 1889–1890.

In order to test a few other hypotheses, however, one regression was run with the United States data alone (Table VI-7). For one thing it was found that the relationship of income to age was indeed strongly quadratic.[15] The age of head and age of head squared coefficients were highly significant, had the correct signs, and had the largest β-coefficients. In addition, as might be expected from the results in Table II-1 (pages 43–44), the highest incomes were found in glass manufacture and ferrous metallurgy. Coal mining was the

[15] The equation was specified in natural logarithms of income in order to reduce the impact of extreme income observations. This specification implies Income $= \exp(B_0 + \Sigma_{i=1}^{n} B_iX_i)$, where B_0 is the constant term, the X_is are the various independent variables, and the B_is are their estimated coefficients. The results, in terms of significance, signs, and β-coefficients were not greatly different from a simple linear specification.

owest. Craftsmen, semiskilled, and skilled workers did better than unskilled workers and apprentices–helpers. Rather surprisingly, white-collar workers did not do as well as skilled workers or craftsmen. Living in New England and the Midwest was beneficial to income, whereas living in the Middle Atlantic states or in the South was detrimental. Being native born, British, or Irish was better from the point of view of expected income than being Canadian (largely French Canadian), German, or especially Slavic. Language difficulties could have been a barrier to higher incomes.

Whenever other sources of income were larger, the husband's income was lower. But which was cause and which effect? One might argue that the husband needed to work harder if there were fewer sources of other income (i.e., from the wife, from children, from boarders, or from wealth), or when need was greater, such as when more children were present. This is substantiated by the positive coefficient for the total number of children, which implies that a heavier burden of family responsibility might indeed have induced a husband to work harder.[16] Another argument is that the alternative sources of income were sought because the husband's income was so low. In effect, this induced women and especially children to go out into the labor force.

This latter point is what is suggested by Table VI-6 and Figure VI-1. As the family head became older and as his income began to decline, children were sent out into the labor force and, increasingly, boarders were taken in. As Table VI-6 shows, the percentage of families taking in boarders and with children working increased steadily with the age of the family head. In the United States, the percentage of families with income from children rose from virtually nothing for families with the head aged 20–29 to 58% for families with the head aged 50–59. For Europe, the increase was from 7 to 78%. For the United States, where boarder income was more important, the percentage of families with boarder income rose from 12% for families with the head aged 20–29 to 34% for families with the head aged 60 and over.

All this points to a possible family-formation strategy in which a family, perceiving unfavorable or uncertain income prospects for the male head of family, would decide to have more children. The expectation would be that these children would go out into the labor force, usually when they became teenagers, and contribute to the support of the family. As has been recently noted for the United States:

> *Today, parents look at middle age as a time when their teenage children will place an extraordinary drain on family resources. In 19th-century families the opposite was true; teenage children were economic assets and were expected to compensate by their earnings for the fact that they had been economic liabilities when young* [Kett, 1977, p. 169].

[16] The causality might also have been reversed here. A husband's higher income might have encouraged higher fertility through an income effect, which was suggested in the last section.

TABLE VI-6 Composition of Mean Family Income by Age of Family Head. Nine Industries. United States, Britain, France, Germany, Belgium, and Switzerland, 1889/1890

Family income	Age of family head: Below 20	20-29	30-39	40-49	50-59	60 and over	Total
	Mean income						
Total sample							
Total income	$326	$519	$600	$714	$766	$631	$641
a. Husband	197	475	532	479	427	304	481
b. Wife	10	19	16	15	7	3	14
c. Children	33	2	27	180	253	221	106
d. Boarder	78	17	15	28	60	76	29
e. Other	8	6	11	15	17	27	11
N	6	1578	2955	2329	1199	424	8491
	Percent shares						
Total income	100.00	100.00	100.00	100.00	100.00	100.00	100.00
a. Husband	60.43	91.52	88.67	67.09	55.74	48.18	75.04
b. Wife	3.07	3.66	2.67	2.10	0.91	0.48	2.18
c. Children	10.12	0.38	4.50	25.21	33.03	35.02	16.54
d. Boarder	23.93	3.28	2.50	3.92	7.83	12.04	4.52
e. Other	2.45	1.16	1.83	2.10	2.22	4.28	1.72
	Number with some income						
Total income	6	1578	2955	2329	1199	424	8491
a. Husband	5	1576	2929	2239	1130	358	8237
b. Wife	1	187	250	141	53	11	643
c. Children	1	15	385	1276	753	251	2681
d. Boarder	2	168	273	350	320	122	1235
e. Other	2	174	405	379	190	86	1236
	Percent of total with some income						
Total income	100.00	100.00	100.00	100.00	100.00	100.00	100.00
a. Husband	83.33	99.87	99.12	96.14	94.24	84.43	97.01
b. Wife	16.67	11.85	8.46	6.05	4.42	2.59	7.57
c. Children	16.67	0.95	13.03	54.79	62.80	59.20	31.57
d. Boarder	33.33	10.65	9.24	15.03	26.69	28.77	14.54
e. Other	33.33	11.02	13.70	16.27	15.85	20.28	14.56
	Mean income of those who have income						
Total income	$326	$519	$600	$714	$766	$631	$641
a. Husband	237	475	537	499	453	360	495
b. Wife	60	163	191	243	168	132	191
c. Children	200	179	208	329	403	373	336
d. Boarder	234	157	167	189	227	266	197
e. Other	21	56	80	93	108	133	88
Income per working child	$200	$ 93	$121	$160	$174	$186	$162
Number of children working	1	29	664	2625	1749	505	5573

TABLE VI-6 (Continued)

Family income	Age of family head						Total
	Below 20	20-29	30-39	40-49	50-59	60 and over	
	Mean income						
United States							
Total income	$346	$557	$646	$765	$806	$674	$684
a. Husband	192	511	575	515	454	320	517
b. Wife	12	18	16	16	8	4	15
c. Children	40	2	26	183	253	226	106
d. Boarder	94	20	19	34	72	91	34
e. Other	8	6	10	17	19	33	12
N	5	1298	2345	1859	939	338	6784
	Percent shares						
Total income	100.00	100.00	100.00	100.00	100.00	100.00	100.00
a. Husband	55.49	91.74	89.01	67.32	56.33	47.48	75.58
b. Wife	3.47	3.23	2.48	2.09	0.99	0.59	2.19
c. Children	11.56	0.36	4.02	23.92	31.39	33.53	15.50
d. Boarder	27.17	3.59	2.94	4.44	8.93	13.50	4.97
e. Other	2.31	1.08	1.54	2.22	2.36	4.90	1.75
	Number with some income						
Total income	5	1298	2345	1859	939	338	6784
a. Husband	4	1296	2319	1771	873	278	6541
b. Wife	1	132	184	107	40	11	475
c. Children	1	13	275	943	550	195	1977
d. Boarder	2	156	252	322	290	114	1136
e. Other	2	146	330	314	162	74	1028
	Percent of total with some income						
Total income	100.00	100.00	100.00	100.00	100.00	100.00	100.00
a. Husband	80.00	99.85	98.89	95.27	92.97	82.25	96.42
b. Wife	20.00	10.17	7.85	5.76	4.26	3.25	7.02
c. Children	20.00	1.00	11.73	50.73	58.57	57.70	29.14
d. Boarder	40.00	12.02	10.75	17.32	30.88	33.73	16.74
e. Other	40.00	11.25	14.07	16.89	17.25	21.89	15.15
	Mean income of those who have income						
Total income	$346	$557	$646	$765	$806	$674	$684
a. Husband	240	512	582	541	488	389	536
b. Wife	60	177	207	279	186	132	211
c. Children	200	167	225	361	432	392	364
d. Boarder	234	163	173	193	233	268	203
e. Other	21	58	85	101	115	145	95
Income per working child	$200	$ 80	$128	$171	$186	$198	$172
Number of children working	1	27	483	1991	1280	386	4168

TABLE VI-6 (Continued)

Family income	Below 20	20-29	30-39	40-49	50-59	60 and over	Total
	Age of family head						
	Mean income						
Europe							
Total income	$224	$344	$420	$535	$618	$475	$471
a. Husband	224	308	367	338	330	244	337
b. Wife	0	26	16	9	6	0	13
c. Children	0	2	30	169	254	201	106
d. Boarder	0	4	3	9	19	21	8
e. Other	0	4	4	6	9	9	7
N	1	280	610	470	260	86	1707
	Percent shares						
Total income	100.00	100.00	100.00	100.00	100.00	100.00	100.00
a. Husband	100.00	89.53	87.38	63.18	53.40	51.37	7.15
b. Wife	0.00	7.56	3.81	1.68	0.97	0.00	2.76
c. Children	0.00	0.58	7.14	31.59	41.10	42.32	22.51
d. Boarder	0.00	1.16	0.71	1.68	3.07	4.42	1.70
e. Other	0.00	1.16	0.95	1.12	1.46	1.89	1.49
	Number with some income						
Total income	1	280	610	470	260	86	1707
a. Husband	1	280	610	468	257	80	1696
b. Wife	0	55	66	34	13	0	168
c. Children	0	2	110	333	203	56	704
d. Boarder	0	12	21	28	30	8	99
e. Other	0	28	75	65	28	12	208
	Percent of total with some income						
Total income	100.00	100.00	100.00	100.00	100.00	100.00	100.00
a. Husband	100.00	100.00	100.00	99.57	98.85	93.02	99.36
b. Wife	0.00	19.64	10.82	7.23	5.00	0.00	9.84
c. Children	0.00	7.14	18.03	70.85	78.09	65.12	41.24
d. Boarder	0.00	4.29	3.44	5.96	11.54	9.30	5.80
e. Other	0.00	10.00	12.30	13.83	10.77	13.95	12.19
	Mean income of those who have income						
Total income	$224	$344	$420	$535	$618	$475	$471
a. Husband	224	308	367	340	334	263	340
b. Wife	0	130	146	129	114	0	135
c. Children	0	258	164	239	326	308	258
d. Boarder	0	84	92	144	162	231	138
e. Other	0	44	56	56	64	62	56
Income per working child	0	$258	$100	$126	$141	$145	$129
Number of children working	0	2	181	634	469	119	1405

Source: Data compiled from U.S. Commissioner of Labor, *Sixth Annual Report* (1890) and *Seventh Annual Report* (1891).

TABLE VI-7 Regression with the Income per Working Male Family Head as the Dependent Variable. Worker Families in Nine Industries. United States 1889/1890

Variables	United States only[a]		
	Coefficient	Significance	β-Coefficient
I. *Dependent variable*			
Natural logarithm of income of male family head			
II. *Dependent variables*			
1. Constant	5.6823	NC[b]	NC
2. Age of head	.0254	***	.4984
3. Age of head squared	-.0004	***	-.5948
4. Homeownership	.1189	***	.0863
5. Wife's income	-.0009	***	-.0875
6. Children's income	-.0004	***	-.1756
7. Boarder income	-.0002	***	-.0327
8. Other income	-.0000	n.s.[c]	-.0007
9. Number of children	.0078	***	.0315
10. Industry			
a. Pig iron	.6029	***	.3667
b. Bar iron	.7783	***	.4312
c. Steel	.5783	***	.1805
d. Coal	.2542	***	.1288
e. Coke	.5002	***	.1812
f. Cottons	.3692	***	.3181
g. Woolens	.4377	***	.2804
h. Glass	.8473	***	.6345
11. Occupation			
a. Unskilled	-.2950	***	-.2588
b. Skilled and semi-skilled	-.0308	n.s.	-.0292
c. Craftsman	.1603	*	.0940
d. White collar and supervisory	-.1308	n.s.	-.0443
e. Apprentice and helper	-.3139	***	-.1042
12. Region in United States			
a. New England	.0347	n.s.	.0253
b. Middle Atlantic	-.0106	n.s.	-.0100
c. Midwest	.0081	n.s.	.0057
d. South	-.2132	***	-.1452
13. Ethnicity			
a. Born in United States	-.0884	***	-.0833
b. British	-.0276	n.s.	-.0154
c. Irish	-.0816	***	-.0528
d. Canadian	-.1174	***	-.0491
e. German	-.1110	***	-.0629
f. Slavic	-.1867	***	-.0340

Source: Data compiled from U.S. Commissioner of Labor, *Sixth Annual Report* (1890) and *Seventh Annual Report* (1891).

[a] Number of cases, 6538; R^2 adjusted, 0.410; *F*-ratio, 147.323; ***.

[b] NC = Not calculated.

[c] n.s. = Not significant at least at a 10% level.

*p < .1.

***p < .01.

One implication was that families with lower and/or more uncertain future income would have more children and that fewer of their children would attend school as teenagers. Another implication is that married women would leave the labor force outside the home (if they had not already done so at marriage) and shift their allocation of time first to child rearing and later to economic activity within the home, such as taking in boarders or domestic handicrafts. It is apparent in Table VI-6 that married women did leave the labor force as the family became older. For the United States families in the survey, about 10% of families with the head aged 20–29 had the wife working. This had dropped to about 3% by the time the head was aged 60 and over. For the European sample, the decline in labor-force participation of married females was from almost 20% for families with the head aged 20–29 to about 5% for families with the head aged 50–59. No European wives were working in the sample of families with the head aged 60 and over. (See "Percentage of Total with Some Income" in Table VI-6.) This situation was very much unlike that which prevailed in the United States in 1960 when, faced with a relatively flat age–earnings profile, blue-collar families sent wives out into the labor market to help bring the earnings profile in line with the expenditure profile. This has been called the "life cycle squeeze [Oppenheimer, 1974]." The situation which was common to late nineteenth-century working-class families was different in one crucial respect. As Figure VI-1 shows, expenditures did peak late in the family cycle while the head's earnings peaked early as was the case 70 years later. The difference was made up by the earnings from children, from boarders, and from other sources, some of which was almost certainly from domestic handicraft manufacture.[17] It was not, however, made up from wife's market earnings, as in the mid-twentieth century.

The contention that children's contribution to family income arose from necessity can be supported from the Commissioner of Labor Survey. Regressions run for families with both husband and wife present and at least one child over age 10 show for both the United States and Europe that the number of children working per family was strongly negatively associated with the relative income of the husband (see Table VI-8).[18] Also, the number of children working per family (holding family composition constant) was negatively associated with the presence of boarders and a working wife. The negative coefficient for the number of children in school indicated that there was some tradeoff between keeping children in school and sending them to work. Economic necessity frequently intervened. As the coefficients for children of various ages and sexes make clear, it was the older children who were more likely to work and males were more likely to

[17] Wife's income was, in the Commissioner of Labor Survey, from market wage income only.

[18] The results are presented and discussed in much greater detail in Haines (1979).

be working outside the home than females.[19] Child labor-force participation was higher in families in the textile industries, which provided both lower adult-male wages than glass, ferrous metallurgy, or coal mining (see Table II-1, pages 43–44) and also more opportunities for child labor.

This is not to say that families were totally free to exploit their children indefinitely. In Preston in mid-nineteenth-century England, for example, children did, it seems, leave home if not given a reasonable share of their income (Anderson, 1971, Chaps. 4 and 5). For the Commissioner of Labor Survey, an older family was associated, as might be expected, with older children and greater income per working child. (See Tables VI-6 and VI-8, and Haines, 1979.) The number of working children *per family*, however, peaked out for families with the head aged 50–59. It is quite apparent that children were beginning to leave the family after that point, although some of the attrition can be attributed to mortality.[20] Thus children did indeed leave the family, but did not object to spending some considerable period of their adolescence contributing their earnings to the family. They also undoubtedly shared some of the benefits of the high expenditure peak. This pattern of child labor-force activity was not independent of institutions and customs. Work by children was less frequent in the United States for states with child labor and/or compulsory schooling laws (e.g., in the South) (Haines, 1979). It was also less, controlling for income, industry, residence, and family composition, within native American, British or German households in the United States and higher in Irish and Canadian families (see Table VI-7).

A final further exploration of the wife's labor-force participation outside the home is made in Table VI-9, which presents ordinary least squares and maximum likelihood logit regressions for the total sample and the United States subsample, with the dependent variable as a zero–one dummy vari-

[19] The use of variables for the age and sex composition of the children in families was necessary because the survey only gave information on the total number of children working per family, but did not identify which children were actually working.

[20] The number of working children per family (with both husband and wife present) was:

Age of head	Total sample	U.S.	Europe
40–49	1.13	1.07	1.35
50–59	1.46	1.36	1.80
60 and over	1.19	1.14	1.38

If one assumes a West model life table Level 11 ($\mathring{e}_0 = 42.5$ years for females and 41.116 years for males), which is similar to the 1890 Massachusetts table (Glover, 1921) and slightly below the 1891 table for England and Wales (Keyfitz and Flieger, 1968, p. 524), then among males who reach age 15, only about 6.4% die before reaching age 25. The percentage for females is very similar (6.3%). Since the number of working children per family declined 18.5% for the total sample, 16.2 for the United States sample and 23.4% for the European sample, only about 25 to 40% of the decline in number of working children per family can have been due to mortality.

TABLE VI-8 Regression Equations with Number of Children Working as the Dependent Variable for Worker Families in Nine Industries. United States, Britain, France, Germany, Belgium, and Switzerland, 1889/1890. (Families with Both Husband and Wife Present and with at Least One Child Aged 10 or Over)

	Total[a]			United States[b]			Europe[c]		
	Coefficient	Significance	β-Coefficient	Coefficient	Significance	β-Coefficient	Coefficient	Significance	β-Coefficient
I. *Dependent variable*									
Number of children working									
II. *Independent variables*									
1. Constant	1.3333	NC[d]	NC	1.7456	NC	NC	1.5090	NC	NC
2. Number of children in school	-.0999	***	-.1084	-.0078	***	-.0838	-.0403	n.s.	-.0451
3. Are boarders present?	-.1782	***	-.0567	-.1799	***	-.0599	-.4411	***	-.1048
4. Wife aged below 25	-.4165	*	-.0208	-.4277	*	-.0236	.1070	n.s.	-.0027
5. Wife aged 25-34	-.4956	***	-.1447	-.3649	***	-.1079	-1.0296	***	-.2873
6. Wife aged 35-44	.0096	n.s.[f]	.0036	.1227	*	.0463	-.3598	***	-.1441
7. Wife aged 45-54	.3235	***	.1100	.3116	***	.1043	.2363	**	.0853
8. Mining	-.2987	***	-.0726	-.3918	***	-.0905	-.4615	*	-.1303
9. Metal	-.3640	***	-.1221	-.5286	***	-.1709	-.4316	*	-.1612
10. Cotton	.7646	***	.2774	.5388	***	.1940	.3640	n.s.	.1364
11. Woolen	.2652	***	.0709	.0413	n.s.	.0103	.3899	n.s.	.1247
12. Does the wife work?	-.7208	***	-.1247	-.5844	***	-.0962	-.8636	***	-.1732
13. Home ownership	-.1230	***	-.0366	-.0753	*	-.0237	.1740	n.s.	.0378
14. Number of children 0-4	.0847	***	.0486	.0878	***	.0506	-.0794	n.s.	.0449
15. Relative income of husband	-.5443	***	-.2017	-.6838	***	-.2514	-.2076	***	-.0789
16. Number of boys 10-13	.1522	***	.0590	.0988	***	.0380	.1661	**	.0672
17. Number of boys 14-15	.3270	***	.1007	.2659	***	.0809	.3634	***	.1172
18. Number of boys 16-17	.4008	***	.1132	.3356	***	.0932	.4838	***	.1460
19. Number of boys 18 and over	.3369	***	.1360	.3508	***	.1266	.2271	***	.1184
20. Number of girls 10-13	.0684	**	.0264	.0560	n.s.	.0214	-.0115	n.s.	-.0046
21. Number of girls 14-15	.0764	*	.0238	.0727	n.s.	.0228	-.0114	n.s.	-.0035
22. Number of girls 16-17	.1935	***	.0563	.1571	***	.0462	.2241	**	.0631
23. Number of girls 18 and over	.1635	***	.0765	.1290	***	.0592	.1447	***	.0727

24.	United States or Europe	.2038	***	.0671	NI	NI	NI	NI	NI	NI
25.	Alabama	NI[e]	NI	NI	.1005	n.s.	.0140	NI	NI	NI
26.	Georgia	NI	NI	NI	.6130	***	.0794	NI	NI	NI
27.	Illinois	NI	NI	NI	-.5247	***	-.0707	NI	NI	NI
28.	Indiana	NI	NI	NI	-.0961	n.s.	-.0119	NI	NI	NI
29.	New York	NI	NI	NI	.0218	n.s.	.0055	NI	NI	NI
30.	Ohio	NI	NI	NI	-.2886	*	-.0612	NI	NI	NI
31.	Pennsylvania	NI	NI	NI	-.2277	n.s.	-.0772	NI	NI	NI
32.	Tennessee	NI	NI	NI	.2201	n.s.	.0248	NI	NI	NI
33.	Virginia	NI	NI	NI	.4329	***	.0580	NI	NI	NI
34.	West Virginia	NI	NI	NI	-.1470	n.s.	-.0111	NI	NI	NI
35.	Connecticut	NI	NI	NI	-.1618	n.s.	-.0271	NI	NI	NI
36.	Maine	NI	NI	NI	-.1423	n.s.	-.0206	NI	NI	NI
37.	Maryland	NI	NI	NI	.1211	n.s.	.0169	NI	NI	NI
38.	Massachusetts	NI	NI	NI	-.1742	n.s.	-.0302	NI	NI	NI
39.	New Hampshire	NI	NI	NI	-.3128	*	-.0393	NI	NI	NI
40.	North Carolina	NI	NI	NI	.6538	***	.0780	NI	NI	NI
41.	Rhode Island	NI	NI	NI	-.4227	*	-.0314	NI	NI	NI
42.	New Jersey	NI	NI	NI	-.3957	**	-.0668	NI	NI	NI
43.	Delaware	NI	NI	NI	-.4730	n.s.	-.0220	NI	NI	NI
44.	Husband American-born	NI	NI	NI	-.1973	***	-.0746	NI	NI	NI
45.	Husband British-born	NI	NI	NI	-.0974	n.s.	-.0226	NI	NI	NI
46.	Husband Irish-born	NI	NI	NI	.0374	n.s.	.0105	NI	NI	NI
47.	Husband Canadian-born	NI	NI	NI	.3623	***	.0642	NI	NI	NI
48.	Husband German-born	NI	NI	NI	-.1226	n.s.	-.0283	NI	NI	NI
49.	Husband Slavic-born	NI	NI	NI	-.3268	n.s.	-.0205	NI	NI	NI
50.	Belgium	NI	NI	NI	NI	NI	NI	.5037	**	.1118
51.	France	NI	NI	NI	NI	NI	NI	.0473	n.s.	.0150
52.	Germany	NI	NI	NI	NI	NI	NI	-.0067	n.s.	-.0017
53.	Britain	NI	NI	NI	NI	NI	NI	.1846	n.s.	.0731

Source: Data compiled from U.S. Commissioner of Labor, *Sixth Annual Report* (1890) and *Seventh Annual Report* (1891).

*$p < .1$.
**$p < .05$.
***$p < .01$.

[a] Number of cases, 4203; R^2 adjusted, 0.382; *F*-ratio, 113.742 ***.
[b] Number of cases, 3171; R^2 adjusted, 0.455; *F*-ratio, 57.337 *** .
[c] Number of cases, 1032; R^2 adjusted, 0.327; *F*-ratio, 20.291 *** .
[d] NC = Not calculated.
[e] NI = Not included.
[f] n.s. = Not significant at least at a 10% level.

TABLE VI-9 Regression[a] Equation with Female Labor Force Participation[b] as the Dependent Variable. Worker Families in Nine Industries. United States, Britain, France, Germany, Belgium, and Switzerland, 1889/1890

	Total sample				United States only			
	OLS		LOGIT		OLS		LOGIT	
	Coefficient	Significance	Coefficient	Significance	Coefficient	Significance	Coefficient	Significance
I. *Dependent variables*								
Is spouse working?								
II. *Independent variables*								
1. Constant	.1186	***	-1.941	***	.0679	***	-2.823	***
2. Age of wife	.0063	***	.1529	***	.0069	***	.1846	***
3. Age of wife squared	-.0001	***	- .0025	***	-.0001	***	- .0029	***
4. Home ownership	.0055	n.s.[c]	- .0566	n.s.	-.0146	***	- .2614	n.s.
5. Industry								
a. Iron and steel	-.0723	***	-2.085	***	-.0470	***	-1.594	***
b. Mining	-.0900	***	-2.464	***	-.0624	***	-1.931	***
c. Textiles	.0961	***	1.141	***	.0601	***	.5929	***
6. Relative income of husband	-.0009	***	- .0252	***	-.0009	***	- .0296	***
7. Boarder income	-.0002	***	- .0043	***	-.0002	***	- .0052	***
8. Other income	-.0001	n.s.	- .0023	*	-.0001	**	- .0039	***
9. Childrens' income	-.0002	***	- .0043	***	-.0002	***	- .0047	***
10. Children 0-4 present	-.0178	***	- .0341	***	-.0202	***	- .3935	***
11. United States or Europe	.0362	***	.3678	***	NI	NI	NI	NI
12. Region in United States								
a. New England	NI[d]	NI	NI	NI	.1546	***	2.150	***
b. South	NI	NI	NI	NI	.0653	***	1.221	***
c. Border	NI	NI	NI	NI	-.0051	n.s.	.0857	n.s.
13. Nativity of husband								
a. Born in United States	NI	NI	NI	NI	-.0076	n.s.	- .1512	n.s.
b. Irish	NI	NI	NI	NI	.0165	*	.2564	n.s.
c. Slavic	NI	NI	NI	NI	.0098	n.s.	.7687	n.s.
Number of cases	8144		8144		6431		6431	
R^2 adjusted	0.113				0.139			
F-ratio	65.823 ***				26.140 ***			

[a]Both ordinary least squares (OLS) and dichotomous logit (LOGIT) were used.

[b]Female labor force participation was coded as 0=not in labor force, 1=in labor force.

[c]n.s. = Not significant at least at a 10% level.

[d]NI = Not included

*$p < .1$.

**$p < .05$.

***$p < .01$.

able. The reason for the use of the logit transformation is that the dependent variable is in this case not only bounded by zero and one, but also badly skewed.[21] Only about 7.5% of all married women were working in the total sample, and only about 7% in the United States subsample. The logit transformation can compensate for this (although not for the simultaneity problems discussed earlier). From the standpoint of estimation, it is encouraging to note that the results using ordinary least squares are quite similar in terms of hypothesis testing, signs, and relative magnitudes of the coefficients to the maximum likelihood logit estimates. The equations "explained" only about 10 to 15% of total variation in wives' labor-force participation, but they were jointly significant at a 1% level.

The equations in Table VI-9 show that labor-force participation of wives declined with age and that the relationship was somewhat curvilinear (i.e., quadratic with respect to age). Women were more likely to work when the husband was employed in textiles or if the family was located in Europe and were less likely to work if the husband was employed in heavy industry. This supports earlier contentions about the limited opportunities for female employment in heavy-industrial and mining areas. Wives were also less likely to work when the husband's income was higher, when boarders were taken in, when children were working, or when young children were present in the house. This reaffirms the view that wives worked only when necessity dictated and that other sources of income (i.e., children and boarders) were often resorted to in place of the wife's entering the labor force. The low labor-force participation of wives in the late nineteenth century was also a symptom of this. As has been noted for the United States: "Most of the married women who worked outside the home had little choice; they were the victims of one misfortune or another which had deprived them of adequate support by a husband. . . . Around the turn of the century, in short, when a married woman worked it was usually a sign that something had gone wrong [Smuts, 1959, pp. 51, 55]." Also of note for the United States subsample was that native American families were less likely to have wives working than some of the foreign born, particularly the Irish. With respect to fertility, the result was again confirmed that the presence of young children (i.e., higher recent fertility) had a depressing effect on the labor-force activity of married women.

Overall, then, the Commissioner of Labor Survey furnishes valuable information not only on differential fertility among mining and industrial populations in the late nineteenth century, but also on possible strategies of labor-force participation by wives and children to compensate for stagnant, reduced, and/or uncertain future income for the head of household. It appears that unfavorable future income prospects for some industrial work-

[21] For a discussion of these problems, see Nerlove and Press (1973) and Maddala (1977, Chap. 9).

ers might have induced them to opt for higher fertility because children were a most definite economic asset later in the life cycle. This strategy would mean that the wife would have been even less likely to help the family by entering the labor force outside the home, because of the extreme demands of childbearing and child rearing. Early in the life cycle, the family would have numerous young children and would have been extremely dependent on the earnings of the family head. This vulnerable and difficult stage may have prompted even greater exertions by the head to gain more income, thus accentuating the peak in earnings in the 30s. This kind of activity might even be viewed as a form of increased real savings and capital formation, aimed at increasing income later in the life cycle. The capital would have been in the form of children.

SUMMARY AND CONCLUSIONS

This 1889–1890 survey of families employed in nine industries in Europe and America is a valuable and important social document from many points of view. Carroll D. Wright, first U.S. Commissioner of Labor, was mandated by the United States Congress to conduct a study of cost of production in protected industries in the United States and in industrial Europe. Fortunately for posterity, Wright interpreted his charge broadly and collected detailed information concerning 8544 families employed in the industries selected for analysis. Even more remarkable was the fact that he deemed it appropriate to publish the original data virtually complete. While the criteria for sampling the families were not clearly delineated, it does appear that the sample was roughly representative of families in these industries in the United States at least. Hence, conclusions drawn from analysis of this sample are reasonably general.

An analysis of overall and age-standardized marital child–woman ratios of families in ferrous metallurgy, coal and iron mining, cotton and woolen textiles, and the glass industry revealed that heavy industry did indeed have higher marital fertility than textiles or glass (a craft industry). One exception was the cotton-textile industry in the United States which had relatively high levels of marital fertility. Application of multivariate analysis to the individual families as units of analysis confirmed this finding, while controlling for a number of other features of the family (such as occupation, ethnicity, and relative income of family head; homeownership; residence of family; income from the wife or from boarders). Further exploration of labor-force activity suggested a further aspect to the problem of occupational fertility differentials. A characteristic of industrial employment in the late nineteenth century was an age–earnings profile for adult-male wage earners which peaked relatively early (i.e., on average when males were 30–39) and then declined.

A response to this was to send secondary wage earners into the labor market. In the late nineteenth century, this almost always meant older children. Married women were more likely to take in boarders or engage in domestic handicraft work than to enter the labor market outside the home. Their task was to raise the children who were later to become an economic asset and, when the children had grown, to contribute through taking in boarders or making things at home. Such a situation thus would create fertility differentials across industries depending on the steepness of the decline of husband's income and the availability of employment for children versus that for women. Some calculations with the data in Table II-1 (pages 43–44) show that the industries with steeper declines at the oldest age group were metallurgical and especially mining.[22] Also, for the United States, the cotton industry had a steep decline relative to woolens and glass. Furthermore, the textile industries could provide more employment of women as well as children. Mining and metallurgy provided very little for women. These factors make it appear that the uncertainties of life, as reflected in male incomes, could have prompted families in some industries to have had more children. Thus, again, fertility was dependent on economic structures.

[22] The income of family head relative to peak earnings (at whatever age) is as follows:

Age of head	Pig iron	Bar iron	Steel	Coal	Coke	Iron ore	Cottons	Woolens	Glass
				United States					
20–29	.885	.864	1.000	.982	.905	.882	.906	.912	.892
30–39	1.000	.992	.973	.958	.889	1.000	1.000	1.000	1.000
40–49	.930	1.000	.841	1.000	.970	.919	.872	.996	.963
50–59	.946	.892	.700	.884	1.000	.988	.804	.877	.929
60 and over	.687	.736	.714	.678	.641	.483	.701	.777	.743
				England					
20–29	.901	.797	.754	.952	.934	1.000	.840	.789	
30–39	1.000	1.000	.998	1.000	1.000	.961	1.000	.842	
40–49	.832	.986	1.000	.928	.821	.868	.897	.932	
50–59	.811	.966	.919	.974	.950	.825	.954	.882	
60 and over	.788	.669	.454	.696	.806	—	.817	1.000	

VII

Patterns of Similarity: Demographic Patterns among Mining and Industrial Populations across Space and Time

This chapter concludes the exploration into historical patterns of population change during the process of industrialization. The purpose here is to draw together some of the findings and to interpret them in light of the model presented in Chapter II. The major focus has been occupational fertility, particularly the high fertility of populations engaged in mining and heavy industry. In the course of investigating and explaining this phenomenon, however, it was necessary to explore the structure of fertility (i.e., age-specific fertility), marriage practices, mortality levels and differentials, migration patterns, population composition, and labor-force activity. The related issue of fertility decline was also addressed when appropriate. The inquiry is largely confined to the nineteenth century, although some census data from the twentieth century confirm the continued existence of the occupational fertility differentials observed in the previous century.

The types of evidence considered included published census tabulations (Chapter I), multivariate analysis of cross-sectional published census and vital data for small geographic areas (Chapter III), and use of samples from nineteenth-century census manuscripts (Chapters IV and V). Chapter VI made use of a rather unusual data set, a survey of family composition, budgets, and expenditures for industrial families in 1889–1890 in which the original data were actually published. The basic findings confirmed many of the original expectations and predictions of the model (Chapter II). Although the results were not always exactly as expected, the general tendencies were clear.

One of the most consistent findings was that regions specializing in mining and/or heavy-industrial activity (especially metallurgy) had higher overall fertility than other regions or national units. This was confirmed for England and Wales in 1851, 1861, and 1871 and for Prussia in periods around the occupational censuses of 1882, 1895, and 1907 (Chapter III). This was also true in comparing fertility estimates for the Pennsylvania anthracite region between about 1850 and 1900 with independent estimates for the whole United States (Chapter IV). Some confirmation of this may be seen by comparing the Total Fertility Rates (TFRs) of the anthracite region with the Coale and Zelnik (1963) estimates for the whole United States in Table VII-1. The same was also true for England and Wales for the periods around the censuses of 1851, 1861, and 1871. The mining districts of Durham and Easington in northern England and the mining and metallurgical district of Merthyr Tydfil in South Wales both had TFRs and GRRs (Gross Reproduction Rates) consistently higher than those for England and Wales as a whole (Table VII-1). The net reproduction rate (NRR) in Merthyr Tydfil was below that for England and Wales, however, because of the particularly high mortality in that district.

There was some variation between the regions. This is to be expected, since many factors varied across regions, such as ethnic composition, extent of urbanization, exact labor-force structure, etc. So, for example, the TFRs and GRRs for the Pennsylvania anthracite region were well above those for Durham–Easington and for Merthyr Tydfil for the 1850–1851 and 1860–1861 censuses. Durham and Easington had TFRs which rose somewhat between 1851 and 1871, while that for the Pennsylvania anthracite region declined. Thus, by 1870–1871, the Durham–Easington districts had overall fertility higher than that for the main Pennsylvania anthracite mining counties. The variation among mining districts was, however, less than among other districts, as indicated by the coefficients of variation for I_f for the samples in Chapter III for England and Wales (1851, 1861, 1871). The coefficients of variation were uniformly lower for the sample of mining districts than for the random sample of all districts. The shapes of the age-specific fertility schedules were also reasonably similar, peaking (with one exception) at ages 25–29. There were, however, noticeable variations in the age-specific rates from census to census as well as between areas.

There were fewer differences in marital fertility between the different regions. In Chapter III, it was observed for England and Wales for 1851, 1861, and 1871 that the coefficient of variation for the index of marital fertility (I_g) was always less than that for the index of overall fertility (I_f). This was true for both the mining samples and the random samples of registration districts. Similar results may be observed in the age-specific marital fertility rates in Table VII-1 and in the age-standardized marital child–woman ratios in Table VII-2. Whereas the TFRs for England and

TABLE VII-1 Comparison of Age-Specific Overall and Marital Fertility Rates. Pennsylvania Anthracite Region; Durham and Easington, England; Merthyr Tydfil, Wales; England and Wales; 1846/1850 - 1896/1900

	Age									
	15-19	20-24	25-29	30-34	35-39	40-44	45-49	TFR	GRR	NRR
I. *Total fertility*										
A. Pennsylvania Anthracite Region										
1846/1850	74.5	256.8	308.3	268.0	222.8	129.4	39.7	6420.	3132.	2026.
1856/1860	80.0	260.4	309.7	258.1	206.5	132.2	30.3	6310.	3078.	2050.
1866/1870	66.6	226.9	291.1	268.2	192.0	89.4	16.6	5696.	2778.	1849.
1876/1880	69.8	226.3	276.6	233.6	179.2	97.1	8.7	5411.	2639.	1670.
1896/1900	59.4	180.9	225.8	215.3	138.5	44.4	8.1	4328.	2111.	1451.
B. Durham and Easington										
1846/1851	36.9	181.8	280.9	301.3	222.3	92.9	45.0	5733.	2755.	1518.
1856/1861	53.3	214.6	291.7	272.6	229.7	117.5	18.3	5935.	2876.	1707.
1866/1871	59.6	237.2	308.3	288.6	234.3	91.9	10.4	6101.	2957.	1782.
C. Merthyr Tydfil										
1846/1851	39.2	176.0	254.1	223.4	220.1	146.9	7.6	5296.	2551.	1170.
1856/1861	47.8	198.7	290.7	265.9	184.4	90.2	19.2	5432.	2655.	1320.
1866/1871	43.3	199.6	277.4	245.8	213.5	112.2	17.0	5497.	2684.	1450.
D. England and Wales										
1861	27.3	154.5	224.3	217.0	181.5	100.2	NA[a]	4614.	2256.	1393.
1871	26.8	159.0	231.2	224.9	188.1	103.9	NA	4698.	2308.	1419.
1881	22.5	156.0	227.2	223.6	183.2	97.9	NA	4552.	2233.	1536.
1891	17.5	136.9	212.1	203.3	162.3	84.0	NA	4080.	2002.	1360.
1901	8.3	120.1	190.5	175.0	131.9	63.8	NA	3448.	1690.	1208.
E. United States										
1850	NA	NA	NA	NA	NA	NA	NA	5420.	NA	NA
1856/1860	NA	NA	NA	NA	NA	NA	NA	5256.	NA	NA
1866/1870	NA	NA	NA	NA	NA	NA	NA	4538.	NA	NA
1876/1880	NA	NA	NA	NA	NA	NA	NA	4312.	NA	NA
1886/1890	NA	NA	NA	NA	NA	NA	NA	4018.	NA	NA
1896/1900	NA	NA	NA	NA	NA	NA	NA	3628.	NA	NA
	Age									
	15-19	20-24	25-29	30-34	35-39	40-44	45-49	TMFR[b]	M	"m"
II. *Marital fertility*										
A. Pennsylvania Anthracite Region										
1846/1850	661.3	469.5	370.5	306.9	243.1	148.1	46.9	7925.	.921	.110
1856/1860	866.7	450.4	359.6	280.7	237.6	150.6	34.7	7568.	.870	.075
1866/1870	781.7	407.6	336.4	301.6	214.7	103.4	20.5	6921.	.870	.243
1876/1880	879.5	421.4	360.0	260.5	200.0	115.4	10.2	6842.	.867	.237
1896/1900	663.7	382.6	317.5	256.2	166.4	52.5	9.5	5924.	.898	.645
B. Durham and Easington										
1846/1851	1028.4	455.1	377.0	375.1	259.0	112.2	54.6	8165.	1.001	.239
1856/1861	1000.6	437.4	390.7	338.4	267.1	138.4	24.9	7984.	.936	.101
1866/1871	843.3	467.7	389.9	344.8	267.3	104.8	12.9	7937.	1.026	.293
C. Merthyr Tydfil										
1846/1851	1113.3	391.5	359.3	267.1	258.5	169.3	10.2	7280.	.780	-.089
1856/1861	982.1	397.4	364.2	304.7	213.0	101.3	24.9	7028.	.892	.268
1866/1871	980.1	412.0	366.7	287.6	251.6	131.1	20.7	7348.	.861	.097
D. England and Wales										
1861	895.4	466.2	366.1	297.6	237.3	131.8	NA	7495.	.927	.175
1871	849.4	463.3	370.6	305.8	245.6	137.0	NA	7612.	.927	.144

Source: Tables IV-18, 19, 21, 23, 28. V-12, 13, 18.

[a] NA = Not available.

[b] Excludes ages 15-19.

TABLE VII-2 Comparison of Standardized Marital Child-Woman Ratios.[a] Pennsylvania Anthracite Region; Durham and Easington R.D.'s, Endland; Merthyr Tydfil R.D., Wales, Commissioner of Labor Survey, 1850-1900. (Married Women with Husband Present) (per 1000 Women)

	Pennsylvania anthracite region					Durham and Easington			Merthyr Tydfil			Commissioner of Labor Survey (1889/1890)		
	1850	1860	1870	1880	1900	1851	1861	1871	1851	1861	1871	United States	Europe	Britain
Total	1093	1093	1070	984	901	1006	1059	1037	895	898	953	834	801	743
Occupation of husband														
1. Farmer, farm laborer	1225	1056	1042	901	879	981	1222	1027	(857)[e]	828	(468)	NA	NA	NA
2. Laborer	1067	1159	1124	976	873	933	1084	969	775	784	763	NA	NA	NA
3. Miner, mine worker	1163	1109	992	1180	1038	1062	1076	1057	930	923	967	NA	NA	NA
4. Manufacturing, crafts, construction	1057	1153	1043	816	825	935	1004	1029	945	858	942	NA	NA	NA
5. Mercantile, food, lodging, transport, servants	1037	938	965	890	797	917	1044	975	700	930	1065	NA	NA	NA
6. Professional, clerical[f]	868	749	856	622	514	1056	929	1001	(958)	883	1044	NA	NA	NA
7. Other						(928)	1176	932	(530)	(614)	(388)	NA	NA	NA
Industry of husband														
1. Metallurgy	NA[b]	NA	NA	NA	NA	NA	NA	NA	859	868	970	822	858	801
2. Mining	1163	1109	992	1180	1038	1062	1076	1057	930	923	967	958	954	834
3. Textiles	NA	NA	NA	NA	NA	NA	NA	NA	NA[b]	NA	NA	865	763	716
4. Glass	NA	NA	NA	NA	NA	NA	NA	NA	NA	NA	NA	769	708	569
Nativity of parents[c]														
1. Native	1092	1037	956	831	796	NA	NA	NA	NA	NA	NA	767	NA	NA
2. Foreign born	1060	1144	1064	1167	1004	NA	NA	NA	NA	NA	NA	934	NA	NA
Wife working[d]														
1. Not working	NA	1139	1076	981	910	1004	1070	1040	900	908	951	860	854	765
2. Working	NA	(909)[e]	(500)	(0)	(153)	(768)	866	795	(693)	721	(1014)	606	479	416
Residence														
1. Rural	1115	1126	1036	1003	902	1036	1102	1043	858	922	1112	NA	NA	NA
2. Urban	1013	941	1012	940	871	871	940	1019	914	897	937	NA	NA	NA

Source: Tables IV-8, V-8, V-9, and VI-4.

[a]Standardized to the age structure of married women in the Pennsylvania anthracite region in 1880.

[b]NA = Not available.

[c]For the Pennsylvania anthracite region, both parents native versus both parents foreign. For the Commissioner of Labor Survey, place of birth of husband.

[d]Unstandardized ratios for the Pennsylvania anthracite region.

[e]Numbers in parentheses are based on fewer than 30 cases.

[f]For professional, clerical and other, together, for the Pennsylvania anthracite region.

Wales were well below those for the two mining and industrial districts, marital fertility was higher in 1861 and 1871 in the country as a whole than in Merthyr Tydfil. Marital fertility in Durham and Easington, however, remained above the national average. Marital fertility was also higher in Durham and Easington than in the Pennsylvania anthracite counties for 1850–1851 and 1860–1861, even though total fertility had been higher in the anthracite region. This may be readily seen in the Total Marital Fertility Rate (TMFR) in Table VII-1. By 1870–1871, marital fertility was even higher in Merthyr Tydfil and in England and Wales as a whole than in the Pennsylvania mining region.

The differences in the results for total and marital fertility are attributable to differences in marriage patterns for females among the various areas. For example, the proportion of total females who were married at ages 20–24 was 58% in the Pennsylvania anthracite region in 1860, whereas it was only 47% in Durham and Easington and in Merthyr Tydfil and 33% in England and Wales in 1861. Thus some differences in nuptiality could and did exist among the different mining regions. By 1871, the equations explaining variation in the index of proportions married (I_m) were much more successful than those explaining marital fertility (I_g) for the two samples of English and Welsh registration districts (Chapter III). Female nuptiality in mining and heavy-industrial areas was also quite early and extensive in comparison with other areas. This has been pointed out in Chapters IV and V. In Chapter III, it was found that the average index of proportions married (I_m) was significantly higher in the sample of mining districts than a random sample of all districts for 1861 and 1871.

From the evidence of marital fertility, it also appears that the degree of control of fertility within marriage in the Pennsylvania anthracite region, Durham–Easington, and Merthyr Tydfil was relatively small from the late 1840s through the late 1860s. This may be seen from the Coale and Trussell (1974, 1978) "m" values in Table VII-1. According to Coale and Trussell (1978, p. 205), values of "m" below about .2 denote little intramarital fertility control. Also, values between .2 and .3 indicate only a very modest degree of control. Thus none of the regions exhibited a tendency to extensive deliberate modification of fertility within marriage within the periods considered. One exception was the Pennsylvania anthracite region which, by 1896–1900, had given strong indications of fertility decline. During the mid-nineteenth century the level of natural fertility[1] itself also appeared to vary. The M values in Table VII-1 suggest this. This measure assumes that women aged 20–24 were in a natural fertility condition.[2] If this were true,

[1] Natural fertility is defined as fertility subject to no *deliberate*, *voluntary* limitation. A more technical definition is that birth rates are independent of parity.

[2] An M value of 1.000 means that the population in question has a level of "natural" fertility of ages 20–24 equal to the average of the schedules used by Coale and Trussell (1974) to construct their model natural fertility schedule.

there was then considerable variation between regions and also across time within the same region. The overall conclusion must be, however, that marital fertility was subject to only modest deliberate limitation in all three of these mining and industrial areas in the mid-nineteenth century. Modifications in overall fertility were accomplished much more through variations in marriage. Substantial control of fertility within marriage only began to appear later, after 1880. This is indicated for the Pennsylvania counties, but not directly for the Durham–Easington, Merthyr Tydfil, or England and Wales. There is evidence that I_g did begin to decline in the English case, however, after 1881 (see Table V-5, page 161). The somewhat belated decline in marital fertility in mining and industrial regions may be characteristic, but there is not enough evidence on the subject here to draw firm conclusions.

In terms of mining and industrial populations, as opposed to regions, Table VII-2 shows that wives of miners and mine workers did have relatively high standardized marital child–woman ratios within mining and industrial areas, despite the existence of only moderate fertility limitation within marriage. In some cases, wives of miners and mine workers were not the most fertile, but the rankings were usually high. Comparing marital fertility among the mining/industrial areas, spouses of miners had higher fertility in the eastern Pennsylvania coalfield than in either Durham–Easington or in Merthyr Tydfil. One exception was 1871 when the Durham–Easington miners' families had higher standardized ratios. In 1889–1890, United States miners also were more fertile than in Britain, but, in both areas, wives of miners and mine workers had relatively more young children present than other groups. Among other occupational groups, farmers and farm laborers generally had wives with higher child–woman ratios than most other groups, but the ratios were often absolutely higher in Pennsylvania than in Durham–Easington or in Merthyr Tydfil. Laborers often had above average fertility in the United States case, but below average fertility in the British case studies. As mentioned in Chapter V, however, this may have been due to the more precise occupational descriptions in the British censuses. Many laborers in the United States might well have been workers in other, economically better off, fields. The Professional–Clerical categories showed rather high fertility in British cases relative to the Pennsylvania anthracite region. This is puzzling, since the higher-status groups might have been expected to have had smaller families, a pattern found later in Britain. Such was not the case in the mid-nineteenth century in these British mining–industrial areas. Finally, wives of metallurgical workers generally had marital child–woman ratios below, but not too far from, the miners' wives. This was confirmed for Merthyr Tydfil and for the U.S. Commissioner of Labor Survey of 1889–1890. One surprising result of the Commissioner of Labor Survey was the relatively high marital fertility among families of textile workers in the United States. This was not true for Britain, which conformed more closely to the expected pattern. Glass workers, members of a craft industry, had wives with the lowest fertility.

Several other dimensions besides occupation and industry were examined in Chapters IV–VI. Some of these are presented in Table VII-2. Among these, marital fertility among rural wives was, with one exception (Merthyr Tydfil in 1851), higher than urban fertility. Working wives, with the exception of Merthyr Tydfil in 1871, had lower fertility than nonworking wives. Also notable was the very small number of working wives in these samples of mining and industrial populations and regions. For the United States after 1850, migration status was important. Families with both parents foreign born had higher fertility than those with native-born parents in both the Pennsylvania anthracite region and the United States portion of the Commissioner of Labor Survey. Migration status in Durham–Easington and Merthyr Tydfil did not produce any such striking results.

It should be noted that the existence of substantial differentials in marital fertility is consistent with a relatively modest degree of fertility control within marriage. For one thing, at levels of fertility closer to natural fertility, intramarital fertility control does not have to be too extensively and efficiently applied to achieve differentials. Furthermore, some groups might have been using deliberate birth spacing and family limitation more assiduously than others, although the overall average use of family limitation might have been very modest. An example of this is the Pennsylvania anthracite region in about 1870 or 1880, when the overall degree of family limitation was rather low while that of the native-born population was considerably higher.

Despite the fact that various geographic areas were studied at varying points in time, it does emerge that the demographic behavior of mining and industrial populations was distinctive and was influenced by characteristic economic structures. As shown earlier, mining and heavy-industrial populations and areas were characterized by high total fertility. This was, in turn, due partly to high marital fertility but also due to very early and extensive marriage in mining areas. This early marriage was most characteristic of females, although there is some evidence that it did extend to particular occupational groups among males, notably miners. The reason that males did not experience such early marriage was that the selective heavy net in-migration of young adult males into mining and heavy-industrial areas created a marriage market much more favorable to females than to males. Sex ratios well above 100 (males per 100 females) in the young adult years were characteristic of such labor markets and were consistently found for the regions studied. They were an obvious manifestation of the interaction of economic opportunity, migration marriage, and fertility. These results support the contention of Wrigley (1961) that it was low female age of marriage that was important with respect to high overall fertility in mining and heavy-industrial areas. He chose, however, to minimize the importance of specific male occupational nuptiality differentials. Some of the evidence presented in the preceding chapters indicates that this too was a significant phenomenon.

The same industrial structures that favored male employment also created earnings profiles that peaked early for males in manual work. The U.S. Commissioner of Labor Survey, with its unusual income and expenditure data, provided insights into this area. Incomes in industrial work did peak early, usually when a male was in his 30s, and then declined. This encouraged the selective net in-migration of young adult males and also earlier marriage. In contrast to males, married females had very limited labor-force participation outside the home in these male-dominated labor markets. This reduced opportunity costs of childbearing and led to higher fertility. (As shown in Table VII-2, working wives generally did have lower fertility than nonworking wives.) Multivariate analysis with areal data for Britain and Prussia (Chapter III) and with microdata from the Commissioner of Labor Survey (Chapter VI) tended to confirm this. On the other hand, children in industrial working-class families were, in the late nineteenth century, an important source of income for the family, as was demonstrated by the Commissioner of Labor Survey. This factor raised the value of children in this context and created still greater motives for the wife to remain at home and rear children. As a consequence, the economic contribution of wives was often to take in boarders or engage in handicraft manufacture. There was ample demand for boarding and lodging in these areas of rapid economic growth with many recently arrived single male workers. These patterns were common to the Pennsylvania anthracite region and also to Durham–Easington and Merthyr Tydfil. Again, the economic structure promoted greater childbearing.

One factor that seemed to affect the fertility patterns of mining and industrial regions was the extent of urbanization. Urban fertility was usually below rural fertility. Mining areas were usually less urban than most industrial regions, at least in the early stages of development. This was due to the resource location constraints imposed on the mining industry, but it helped to encourage the higher fertility of mining areas, which enjoyed some of the benefits of rural life, including cheaper housing and the availability of garden plots. Lack of urbanization, or the isolated urbanization such as occurred in many mining areas, may have slowed changes in general social norms and favored differentially high fertility of mining areas when fertility in general was declining.[3]

One area that produced less certain results was that of differential mortality. Analysis of the 1900 census for the Pennsylvania anthracite region

[3] The geographic and social isolation of many of the small mining towns in the Pennsylvania anthracite field has been noted in Chapter IV. The isolation of mining populations in modern day Britain has been documented for Yorkshire in a book by Dennis, Henriques, and Slaughter (1956, Chap. V).

revealed that miners and mine workers had especially heavy mortality among infants and young children. Mortality among children 0–4 appeared to have been above the national average in Durham–Easington and in Merthyr Tydfil for the 1850s and the 1860s. This particular mortality pattern may thus have been more common among mining populations and in mining areas in the past and itself stimulated higher fertility to replace children who had died. The possibility cannot be ignored, however, that high infant and child mortality may have been an effect as well as a cause of high fertility. An examination of adult mortality by age and cause for Durham–Easington and for Merthyr Tydfil for the decades 1851–1860 and 1861–1870 showed excessive mortality among adult males from accidents but not from tuberculosis or other lung diseases, as might have been expected. Adult females experienced high mortality from childbearing, as might have been anticipated in a very fertile population. These were the only distinctive patterns of mortality which seemed to be common to these particular mining and industrial areas. The very high general level of mortality in Merthyr Tydfil was probably as much due to its high level of urbanization, with concomitant poor sanitary conditions and crowding, as to its industrial character. The high male mortality from accident does suggest, however, that many injuries occurred which were not fatal, only debilitating. This fact might have encouraged earlier marriage and closer spacing of children among the most accident-prone groups, especially those in mining and metallurgy, if children were indeed a form of social and accident insurance. The evidence from Chapter VI suggests that this probably was true. The negative effect of high adult male mortality on fertility, through interruption of marital unions, did not seem too important since widowed females apparently remarried quickly in the favorable marriage market of these mining and industrial areas.[4]

CONCLUDING COMMENTS

It is notable that occupational fertility differentials, in this case with reference to coal mining and heavy industry, should persist with such

[4] The incidence of widows in the childbearing years was not excessive, despite the higher mortality in Merthyr Tydfil. As an indication, the ratio of widowed to married women in 1861 indicates the following:

Age	Durham–Easington	Merthyr Tydfil	England and Wales
25–34	.0356	.0405	.0423
35–44	.0795	.0988	.1032

Given the much higher level of male mortality in Merthyr Tydfil, considerable remarriage of widows is implied.

regularity across time and, more particularly, across national boundaries. This is encouraging from the point of view of causal factors because it indicates a rather general or similar response to the socioeconomic and demographic conditions within individual occupations and industries, at least in Western society. The fact that regularities were also found within the mining and industrial regions themselves is also a strong indication that the differentials in fertility and marriage observed in these areas were partly (or even largely) a function of particular economic structures common to these regions.

It should be further noted that the study of the interaction of fertility, marriage, migration, and mortality with occupation and economic structure can be usefully viewed at two levels of analysis. First, the specific setting of each occupation had a series of general or expected characteristics which influenced fertility and nuptiality behavior. In the case of coal mining and metallurgy these included a relatively lower level of extrahousehold female labor-force participation than in many other nonagricultural populations, relatively high sex ratios in the young adult years because of differential male net in-migration, very favorable male income-earning opportunities, and higher mortality and debility levels, both for children and adults. The level of urbanization was also related to the type of economic activity, often being considerably lower in areas concentrating on mining alone than in regions that also had heavy industry. Second, however, there were characteristics which varied with the specific context of each given region at each date which affected the relationship of fertility, marriage, migration, and occupation. These included ethnic composition, religion, levels of literacy, and similar personal characteristics. The specific cultural setting also played a role. While it has not always been possible to analyze all suggested variables at all the dates considered, both levels of analysis have been pursued, though not always distinctly.

It was pointed out in Chapter I that the study of occupation can be useful beyond the conventional areas of labor-force, social-stratification, and mobility studies. An analysis of fertility, nuptiality, and mortality is one such case. Although occupation itself may have little residual effect on fertility, for example, once education, income, age, and residence are taken into account (Bogue, 1969, p. 705), it is still useful to study occupation historically. Information on such variables as income and education are frequently lacking for historical populations, while occupational data are more abundant. Individual occupations or occupational groupings, each with its own set of attributes and accompanying socioeconomic structures, thus provide interesting dimensions for historical analysis of population, economy, and society.

Finally, the importance of fertility and marriage decisions to an historical study of the family needs no emphasis. The fact that these decisions have been cast here in a social and economic framework whose basis is utility naximization in no way detracts from the human and personal aspects of he dynamics of the family. Children, for example, are desired for many easons, and these chapters have tried to approach the issue of why some amilies, influenced by social, economic, and other environmental circumtances, might want a greater or a smaller number than other families. But, is the evidence indicates, great personal individual variations in preference iave influenced, and will continue to influence, these crucial decisions.

Bibliography

Agarwala, S. N.
1962 *Age at marriage in India*. Allahabad: Kitab Mehal.

Anderson, M.
1971 *Family structure in nineteenth century Lancashire*. Cambridge, England. Cambridge Univ. Press.

Anderson, M.
1972 Household structure and the Industrial Revolution: Mid-nineteenth century Preston in comparative perspective. In P. Laslett (Ed.), *Household and Family in Past Time*. Cambridge, England: Cambridge Univ. Press. Pp. 215–235.

Anderson, M.
1976 Marriage patterns in Victorian Britain: An analysis based on registration district data for England and Wales 1861. *The Journal of Family History*, *1*(1), pp. 55–78.

Andrews, F. M., J. N. Morgan, J. A. Sonquist, and L. Klem
1973 *Multiple classification analysis* (2nd ed.). Ann Arbor, Michigan: Institute for Social Research, Univ. of Michigan.

Ariès, P.
1948 *Histoire des populations françaises et de leurs attitudes devant la vie depuis le XVIIIe siècle*. Paris: Editions Self.

Aris, N.
1976 "Status of own children fertility estimates for Malaysia." Paper presented at Second Own Children Method Workshop, East–West Population Institute, Honolulu, October 18–22.

Armstrong, W. A.
1972 The use of information about occupation. In E. A. Wrigley (Ed.), *Nineteenth century society: Essays in the use of quantitative methods for the study of social data*. Cambridge, England: Cambridge Univ. Press. Pp. 191–310.

Arnold, F., M. Phananiramai, R. Retherford and L.-J. Cho
1976 "Estimates of fertility in Thailand: An application of own-children estimates." Paper presented at Second Own Children Method Workshop, East–West Population Institute, Honolulu, October 18–22.

Arretx, C.
1976 "The application of the own children methods to measure fertility in Latin America." Paper presented at the Second Own Children Method Workshop, East–West Population Institute, Honolulu, October 18–22.

Ashenfelter, O.
1969 Some statistical difficulties in using dummy dependent variables. In W. G. Bowen and T. A. Finegan (Eds.), *The economics of labor force participation*. Princeton, New Jersey: Princeton Univ. Press. Pp. 644–648.

Avery, R.
1976 "Estimation of individual fertility histories using own children present, children ever born and children surviving, with examples from Costa Rica." Paper presented at Second Own Children Method Workshop, East–West Population Institute, Hawaii, October 18–22.

Becker, G. S.
1960 An economic analysis of fertility. In *Demographic and economic change in developed countries*. Princeton, New Jersey: Princeton Univ. Press. Pp. 209–231.

Becker, G.
1965 A theory of the allocation of time. *Economic Journal*, 75(September), pp. 493–517.

Benjamin, B.
1965 *Social and economic factors affecting mortality*. Paris: Mouton.

Ben-Porath, Y.
1973 Economic analysis of fertility in Israel: Point and counterpoint. *Journal of Political Economy*, *81* (2, Part II), pp. 202–233.

Berger, L.
1912 Untersuchungen über den Zusammenhang zwischen Beruf und Fruchtbarkeit unter besonderer Bürucksichtigung des Königreichs Preussen. *Zeitschrift des preussischen statistischen Büreaus*, Bd. 52, pp. 225–250.

Berthoff, R.
1965 The social order of the anthracite region, 1825–1902. *Pennsylvania Magazine of History and Biography*, 89(3), pp. 261–291.

Blake, J.
1965 Demograhpic science and the redirection of population policy. In M. C. Sheps and J. C. Ridley (Eds.), *Public health and population change*. Pittsburgh: Univ. of Pittsburgh Press. Pp. 41–69.

Blake, J.
1968 Are babies consumer durables? *Population Studies*, 22(1), pp. 5–25.

Bogue, D.
1969 *Principles of demography*. New York: Wiley.

Bowley, A. L.
1900 *Wages in the United Kingdom in the nineteenth century*. Cambridge, England: Cambridge Univ. Press.

Brass, W.
1975 *Methods for estimating fertility and mortality from limited and defective data*. Chapel Hill, North Carolina: Laboratories for Populations Statistics, Carolina Population Center.

Brass, W. and A. J. Coale
1968 Methods of analysis and estimation. In W. Brass *et al.* (Eds), *The demography of Tropical Africa*. Princeton, New Jersey: Princeton Univ. Press. Pp. 88–142.

Brepohl, W.
1948 *Der Aufbau des Ruhrvolkes im Züge der ost-west Wanderung*. Recklinghausen: Bitter & Co.

Brepohl, W.
1957 *Industrievolk im Wandel von der agraren zur industriellen Daseinsform dargestellt am Ruhrgebiet*. Tübingen: J. C. B. Mohr.

Broehl, W. G., Jr.
1964 *The Molly Maguires*. Cambridge, Massachusetts: Vintage–Chelsea House.

Bry, G.
1960 *Wages in Germany, 1871–1945*. National Bureau of Economic Research, No. 68, General Series. Princeton, New Jersey: Princeton Univ. Press.

Burstein, A.
1975 "Residential distribution and mobility of Irish and German immigrants in Philadelphia, 1850–1880." Unpublished Ph.D. dissertation, Univ. of Pennsylvania.

Cain, G.
1966 *Married women in the labor force: An economic analysis*. Chicago: Univ. of Chicago Press.

Cain, G. G. and M. D. Dooley
1976 Estimation of a model of labor supply, fertility, and wages of married women. *The Journal of Political Economy*, 84(4, Part 2), pp. S179–199.

Cain, G. G. and A. Weininger
1973 Economic determinants of fertility: Results from cross-sectional aggregate data. *Demography*, 10(2), pp. 205–224.

Cameron, R.
1958 Economic growth and stagnation in France, 1815–1914. *The Journal of Modern History*, 30(1), pp. 1–13.

Carrier, N. and J. Hobcraft
1971 *Demographic estimation for developing societies: A manual of techniques for the detection and reduction of errors in demographic data*. London: London School of Economics, Population Investigation Committee.

Chambers, J. D.
1968 *The workshop of the world: British economic history from 1820 to 1880* (2nd ed.). London: Oxford Univ. Press.

Charles, E. and P. Moshinsky
1938 Differential fertility in England and Wales during the past two decades. In L. Hogben (Ed.), *Political arithmetic*. New York: Macmillan.

Cho, L.-J.
1971 On estimating annual birth rates from census data on children. *Proceedings of the American Statistical Association, Social Statistics Section*. Pp. 86–96.

Cho, L.-J.
1973 The own-children approach to fertility estimation: An elaboration. IUSSP. *International Population Conference: Liège, 1973* (Vol. 2). Liège. Pp. 263–279.

Cho, L.-J., W. H. Grabill, and D. J. Bogue
1970 *Differential current fertility in the United States*. Chicago: Community and Family Study Center, Univ. of Chicago.

Chow, G.
1960 Tests of equality between sets of coefficients in two linear regressions. *Econometrica*, 28(3), pp. 591–605.

Cipolla, C. M.
1965 *The economic history of world population* (3rd ed.). Baltimore: Penguin Books.

Cipolla, C. M.
1969 *Literacy and development in the West*. Baltimore: Penguin Books.

Clapham, J. H.
1936 *The economic development of France and Germany, 1815–1914* (4th ed.). Cambridge, England: Cambridge Univ. Press.
Coale, A. J.
1967 Factors associated with the development of low fertility: An historic summary. In United Nations, *World Population Conference: 1965* (Vol. II). New York: United Nations. Pp. 205–209.
Coale, A. J.
1974 The demographic transition reconsidered. IUSSP. *International Population Conference: Liège, 1973* (Vol. 1). Liège: International Union for the Scientific Study of Population. Pp. 53–72.
Coale, A. J. and P. Demeny
1966 *Regional model life tables and stable populations*. Princeton, New Jersey: Princeton Univ. Press.
Coale, A. J. and T. J. Trussell
1974 Model fertility schedules: Variations in the age structure of childbearing in human populations. *Population Index*, 40(2), pp. 185–258.
Coale, A. J. and T. J. Trussell
1978 Technical note: Finding the two parameters that specify a model schedule of marital fertility. *Population Index*, 44(2), pp. 203–213.
Coale, A. J. and M. Zelnik
1963 *New estimates of fertility and population in the United States: A study of annual white births from 1855 to 1960 and of completeness of enumeration in the censuses from 1880 to 1960*. Princeton, New Jersey: Princeton Univ. Press.
Cole, G. D. H. and R. Postgate
1961 *The British common people: 1746–1946*. London: Methuen.
Cottrell, F.
1955 *Energy and society: The relation between energy, social change, and economic development*. New York: McGraw-Hill.
Courthéoux, J. P.
1959 Privilèges et misères d'un métier sidé-rurgique au XIXe siècle: Le puddleur. *Révue d'histoire économique et sociale*, 37, pp. 161–184.
Crafts, N. F. R.
1978 Average age at first marriage for women in mid-nineteenth century England and Wales: A cross-section study. *Population Studies*, 32(1), pp. 21–25.
Crafts, N. F. R. and J. Ireland
1976 A simulation of the impact of changes in age at marriage before and during the advent of industrialization in England. *Population Studies*, 30(3), pp. 495–510.
Davis, K.
1967 Population policy: Will current programs succeed? *Science*, 158(November 10), pp. 730–739.
Davis, K. and J. Blake
1956 Social structure and fertility. *Economic Development and Cultural Change*, 4(3), pp. 211–235.
Davis, L. *et al*.
1972 *American economic growth: An economist's history of the United States*. New York: Harper and Row.
Deane, P. and W. A. Cole
1969 *British economic growth 1688–1959: Trends and structure* (2nd ed.). Cambridge, England: Cambridge Univ. Press.
Dennis, N., F. Henriques, and C. Slaughter
1956 *Coal is our life: An analysis of a Yorkshire mining community*. London: Eyre and Spottiswoode.

Desai, A. V.
1968 *Real wages in Germany, 1871–1913*. Oxford: Oxford Univ. Press.
Disraeli, B.
1845 *Sybil, or the two nations*. London.
Dixon, R. B.
1976 The roles of rural women: Female seclusion, economic production, and reproductive choice. In R. G. Ridker (Ed.), *Population and development: The search for selective interventions*. Baltimore: The Johns Hopkins Univ. Press. Pp. 290–321.
Dubester, H. J.
1948 *State censuses: An annotated bibliography of censuses of population taken after the year 1790 by states and territories of the United States*. Washington, D.C.: Government Printing Office.
Dublin, L. I., A. J. Lotka, and M. Spiegelman
1949 *Length of life: A study of the life table* (Rev. ed.). New York: The Ronald Press.
Duesenberry, J. S.
1949 *Income, saving, and the theory of consumer behavior*. Cambridge, Massachusetts: Harvard Univ. Press.
Easterlin, R. A.
1968 *Population, labor force, and long swings in economic growth*. New York: National Bureau of Economic Research.
Easterlin, R. A.
1970 Towards a socioeconomic theory of fertility: A survey of recent research on economic factors in American fertility. In S. J. Behrman, L. Corsa, Jr., and R. Freedman (Eds.), *Fertility and family planning: A world view*. Ann Arbor: The Univ. of Michigan Press. Pp. 127–156.
Easterlin, R. A.
1971 Does human fertility adjust to the environment? *American Economic Review*, *61*(2), pp. 399–407.
Easterlin, R. A.
1976 Population change and farm settlement in the northern United States. *The Journal of Economic History*, *XXXVI*(1), pp. 45–75.
Easterlin, R. A.
1977 Population issues in American economic history: A survey and critique. In R. E. Gallman (Ed.), *Recent developments in the study of business and economic history: Essays in honor of Herman E. Krooss*. Greenwich, Connecticut: JAI Press. Pp. 131–158.
Easterlin, R. A.
1978 The economics and sociology of fertility: A synthesis. In C. Tilly (Ed.), *Historical studies of changing fertility*. Princeton, New Jersey: Princeton Univ. Press.
Easterlin, R. A., G. Alter, and G. A. Condran
1978 Farms and farm families in old and new areas: The Northern states in 1860. In T. K. Hareven and M. A. Vinovskis (Eds.), *Family and population in nineteenth-century America*. Princeton: Princeton Univ. Press. Pp. 22–84.
Engels, F.
1958 *The condition of the working class in England*. Translated by W. O. Henderson and W. H. Chaloner. London: Basil Blackwell. (Originally published in 1845).
England and Wales. Registrar General
1864 *Supplement to the Twenty-Fifth Annual Report*. "Mortality 1851–60." London: Eyre and Spottiswoode.
England and Wales. Registrar General
1875 *Supplement to the Thirty-Fifth Annual Report*. "Mortality 1861–70." London: Eyre and Spottiswoode.

England and Wales. Registrar General
1885 *Supplement to the Thirty-Fifth Annual Report*. "Mortality 1861–70." London: Eyre and Spottiswoode.

England and Wales. Registrar General
1887 *Forth-Ninth Annual Report*. (1886). London: Eyre and Spottiswoode.

England and Wales. Registrar General
1923 *Census of England and Wales: 1911* (Vol. 13. "Fertility of Marriage." Part II). London His Majesty's Stationery Office.

Engracia, L.
1976 "Own children fertility estimates based on Philippines 1970 census." Paper presented at Second Own Children Method Workshop, East–West Population Institute, Honolulu, October 18–22.

Espenshade, T. T.
1972 The price of children and socioeconomic theories of fertility: A survey of alternative methods of estimating the parental cost of raising children. *Population Studies*, *26*(2), pp. 207–221.

Evans, E. W.
1961 *The miners of South Wales*. Cardiff: Univ. of Wales Press.

Farr, W.
1865 On infant mortality, and on alleged inaccuracies of the census. *Journal of the Statistical Society of London*, *XXVIII*, pp. 125–149.

Feeney, G.
1976 "Estimating infant mortality rates from child survivorship data by age of mother. Honolulu: East–West Population Institute, (September). Mimeo.

Forster, C. and G. S. L. Tucker
1972 *Economic opportunity and white American fertility ratios, 1800–1860*. New Haven: Yale Univ. Press.

France
1918 Ministère du Travail et de la Prévoyance Sociale. Statistique des familles et des habitations en 1911. In *Statistique générale de la France*. Paris: Imprimerie Nationale.

Freedman, D.
1963 The relation of economic status to fertility. *American Economic Review*, *53*(3), pp. 414–427.

von Fircks, A.
1889 Die Berufs-und Erwerbsthätigkeit der eheschliessenden Personen in ihrem Einflüsse auf deren Verheiratbarkeit, die Wahl des Gatten bezs. der Gattin, das durchschnittliche Heiratsalter, die ehelich und uneheliche Fruchtbarkeit sowie das Geschlecht und die Lebensfähigkeit der Kinder, *Zeitschrift des preussischen statistischen Büreaus*. Bd. 29. Pp. 165–203.

Friedlander, D.
1973 Demographic patterns and socioeconomic characteristics of the coal-mining population in England and Wales in the nineteenth century. *Economic Development and Cultural Change*, *22*(1), pp. 39–51.

Gillet, M.
1969 The coal age and the rise of coalfields in the north and Pas-de-Calais. (Translated by C. H. Kent.) In F. Crouzet, W. H. Chaloner, and W. M. Stern, *Essays in European economic history, 1789–1914*. New York: St. Martin's. Pp. 179–202.

Girard, A.
1955 Aspects statistiques du probleme familial. In *Sociologie comparée de la famille contemporaine*. Colloques Internationaux du Centre National de la Recherche Scientifique: Paris.

Glasco, L.
1973 "Ethnicity and social structure: Irish, Germans, and native born of Buffalo, New York, 1850–1860." Unpublished Ph.D. dissertation: SUNY, Buffalo.
Glass, D. V.
1938 Changes in fertility in England and Wales, 1851–1931. In L. Hogben (Ed.), *Political arithmetic*. London: George Allen and Unwin. Pp. 173–191.
Glass, D. V.
1951 A note on the underregistration of births in Britain in the nineteenth century. *Population Studies*, 5(1), pp. 70–80.
Glass, D. V. and E. Grebinik
1954 *The trend and pattern of fertility in Great Britain: A report on the Family Census of 1946*. London: Her Majesty's Stationery Office.
Glover, J. W.
1921 *United States life tables, 1890, 1901, 1910 and 1901–10*. Washington, D.C.: U.S. Government Printing Office.
Goldberger, A.
1964 *Econometric theory*. New York: Wiley.
Goldstein, S.
1972 The influence of labor force participation and education on fertility in Thailand. *Population Studies*, 26(3), pp. 419–436.
Grabill, W. H. and L.-J. Cho
1965 Methodology for the measurement of current fertility from population data on young children. *Demography*, 2, pp. 50–73.
Grabill, W. H., C. Kiser, and P. K. Whelpton
1958 *The fertility of American women*. New York: Wiley.
Great Britain
1949 *Report of the Royal Commission on Population* (Vol. 1). London: His Majesty's Stationery Office.
Great Britain. General Register Office
1959 *Census: 1951, England and Wales*. "Fertility Report." London: Her Majesty's Stationery Office.
Great Britain. General Register Office
1966 *Census: 1961, England and Wales*. "Fertility Tables." London: Her Majesty's Stationery Office.
Great Britain. Parliament
1842– Report of the Commission of Inquiry of Children and Young Persons in Mines and
1843 Collieries . . . (Ashley Commission). First Report (1842), Second Report (1843). *Parliamentary Papers* (1842–1843), Vols. XV–XVII.
Greenberg, S.
1977 "Industrialization in Philadelphia: The relationship between industrial location and residential patterns, 1880–1970." Unpublished Ph.D. dissertation, Temple Univ.
Gregory, P. R., J. M. Campbell, and B. S. Cheng
1972 A simultaneous equations model of birth rates in the United States. *Review of Economics and Statistics*, 54(4), pp. 374–380.
Griffin, C.
1972 Occupational mobility in nineteenth-century America: Problems and possibilities. *Journal of Social History*, 5, pp. 310–330.
Gronau, R.
1973 The effect of children on the housewife's value of time. *Journal of Political Economy*, 81(2, Part II), pp. S168–199.
Gronau, R.
1976 The allocation of time of Israeli women. *Journal of Political Economy*, 84(4, Part 2), pp. S201–220.

Habakkuk, H. J.
1972 *Population growth and economic development since 1750*. Leicester, England: Leicester Univ. Press.
Haines, M. R.
1975 Fertility and occupation: Coal mining populations in the nineteenth and early twentieth centuries in Europe and America. *Cornell University Western Societies Program. Occasional Paper No. 3*. Ithaca, New York: Center for International Studies, Cornell Univ.
Haines, M. R.
1976 Population and economic change in nineteenth century Eastern Europe: Prussian Upper Silesia, 1840–1913. *The Journal of Economic History*, 36(2), pp. 334–358.
Haines, M. R.
1977 Fertility, marriage, and occupation in the Pennsylvania anthracite region, 1850–1880. *Journal of Family History*, 2(1), pp. 28–55. (a)
Haines, M. R.
1977 Fertility, nuptiality, and occupation: A study of coal mining populations and regions in England and Wales in the mid-nineteenth century. *The Journal of Interdisciplinary History*, 8(2), pp. 245–280. (b)
Haines, M. R.
1977 Mortality in nineteenth century America: Estimates from New York and Pennsylvania census data, 1865 and 1900. *Demography*, 14(3), pp. 311–331. (c)
Haines, M. R.
1977 A model life table system for the United States, 1850–1910. *Cornell University Department of Economics Working Paper No. 151* (September). Mimeo. (d)
Haines, M. R.
1978 *Economic demographic interrelations in developing agricultural regions: A case study of Prussian Upper Silesia, 1840–1914*. New York: Arno.
Haines, M. R.
1979 Industrial work and the family life cycle, 1889/90. *Research in Economic History*, 4 (in press).
Hajnal, J.
1953 Age at marriage and proportions marrying. *Population Studies*, 7(3), pp. 111–136.
Hajnal, J.
1965 European marriage patterns in perspective. In D. V. Glass and D. E. C. Eversley (Eds.), *Population in history*. London: Arnold. Pp. 101–143.
Hareven, T. and M. A. Vinovskis
1975 Marital fertility, ethnicity and occupation in urban families: An analysis of South Boston and the South End in 1850. *Journal of Social History* (Spring), pp. 69–93.
Harvey, K. A.
1969 *The best dressed miners: Life and labor in the Maryland coal region, 1835–1910*. Ithaca, New York: Cornell Univ. Press.
Hawthorn, G.
1970 *The sociology of fertility*. London: Collier–Macmillan.
Heckman, J. J.
1974 Effects of child-care programs on women's work effort. *Journal of Political Economy*, 82(2, Part II), pp. S136–163.
Hendry, J. B.
1961 The bituminous coal industry. In W. Adams (Ed.), *The structure of American industry* (3rd ed.). New York: Macmillan. Pp. 74–112.
Hershberg, T., M. Katz, S. Blumin, L. Glasco, and C. Griffin
1974 Occupation and ethnicity in five nineteenth century cities: A collaborative inquiry. *Historical Methods Newsletter*, 7(3), pp. 174–216.

Hewitt, M.
1958 *Wives and mothers in Victorian industry*. London: Rockliff.

Higgs, R.
1973 Mortality in rural America, 1870–1920: Estimates and conjectures. *Explorations in Economic History*, *10*(2), pp. 177–195.

Hill, K. and J. Trussell
1977 Further developments in indirect mortality estimation. *Population Studies*, *31*(2), pp. 313–334.

Himes, N. E.
1936 *Medical history of contraception*. Baltimore: Williams & Wilkins.

Holsinger, D. B. and J. D. Kasarda
1976 Education and Human Fertility: Sociological Perspectives. In R. G. Ridker (Ed.), *Population and development: The search for selective interventions*. Baltimore: The Johns Hopkins Univ. Press. Pp. 154–181.

Hopkin, W. A. B. and J. Hajnal
1947 Analysis of births in England and Wales, 1939, by father's occupation. *Population Studies*, *1*(Parts 2 and 3), pp. 187–203; 275–300.

House, J. W.
1954 *Northeastern England: Population and the landscape since the early nineteenth century*. Research Series No. 1. Newcastle upon Tyne: Department of Geography, King's College in the Univ. of Durham.

Hunter, L. C.
1951 The heavy industries before 1860. In H. F. Williamson (Ed.), *The growth of the American economy*. Englewood Cliffs, New Jersey: Prentice-Hall. Pp. 172–189. (a)

Hunter, L. C.
1951 Products of the earth, 1866–1918. In H. F. Williamson (Ed.), *The growth of the American economy*. Englewood Cliffs, New Jersey: Prentice-Hall. Pp. 454–473. (b)

Innes, J. W.
1938 *Class fertility differentials in England and Wales, 1876–1934*. Princeton, New Jersey: Princeton Univ. Press.

Innes, J. W.
1941 Class birth rates in England and Wales, 1921–1931. *The Milbank Memorial Fund Quarterly*, *19*(1), pp. 72–96.

Jacobson, P. H.
1957 An estimate of the expectation of life in the United States in 1850. *The Milbank Memorial Fund Quarterly*, 35(2), pp. 197–201.

Jaffe, A. J. and K. Azumi
1960 The birth rate and cottage industries in underdeveloped countries. *Economic Development and Cultural Change*, 9, pp. 52–63.

John, A. H.
1950 *The industrial development of South Wales, 1750–1850*. Cardiff: Univ. of Wales Press.

Johnston, J.
1972 *Econometric methods* (2nd ed.). New York: McGraw-Hill.

Jones, E.
1914 *The anthracite coal combination in the United States*. Cambridge, Massachusetts: Harvard Univ. Press.

Kasarda, J. D.
1971 Economic structure and fertility: A comparative analysis. *Demography*, 8(3), pp. 307–317.

Katz, M. B.
1972 Occupational classification in history. *The Journal of Interdisciplinary History*, (Summer) 3(1), pp. 63–88.

Katz, M. B.
1975 *The People of Hamilton, Canada West: Family and class in a mid-nineteenth century city*. Cambridge, Massachusetts: Harvard Univ. Press.

Kett, J. F.
1977 *Rites of passage: Adolescence in America, 1790 to the present*. New York: Basic Books.

Keyfitz, N. and W. Flieger
1968 *World population: An analysis of vital data*. Chicago: Univ. of Chicago Press.

Kindleberger, C. P.
1964 *Economic growth in France and Britain, 1851–1950*. Cambridge, Massachusetts: Harvard Univ. Press.

Kitagawa, E. M. and P. M. Hauser
1973 *Differential mortality in the United States: A study in socioeconomic epidemiology*. Cambridge, Massachusetts: Harvard Univ. Press.

Knodel, J.
1974 *The fertility decline in Germany, 1871–1939*. Princeton, New Jersey: Princeton Univ. Press.

Koellman, W.
1958 Binnenwanderung und Bevölkerungs strukturen der Ruhrgebiets grosstädte im Jahre 1907. *Soziale Welt*, 9.

Koellman, W.
1965 The population of Barmen before and during the period of industrialization. In D. V. Glass and D. E. C. Eversley, *Population in history*. London: Edward Arnold. Pp. 588–607.

Krause, J. T.
1958 Changes in English fertility and mortality 1781–1850. *Economic History Review*, Series 2, *XI*(August), pp. 52–70.

Kucynski, R. R.
1935 *The measurement of population growth: Methods and results*. London: Sidgwick and Jackson.

Landes, D. S.
1969 *The unbound Prometheus: Technological change and industrial development in Western Europe from 1750 to the present*. Cambridge, England: Cambridge Univ. Press.

Lebergott, S.
1964 *Manpower in economic growth: The American record since 1800*. New York: McGraw-Hill.

Leet, D. R.
1976 The determinants of fertility transition in ante-bellum Ohio. *The Journal of Economic History*, 36(2), pp. 359–378.

Leiby, J.
1960 *Carroll Wright and labor reform: The origin of labor statistics*. Cambridge, Massachusetts: Harvard Univ. Press.

Levasseur, E.
1897 *L'enseignement primaire dans les pays civilisés*. Paris–Nancy: Berger–Levrault.

Lewis, B.
1971 *Coal mining in the eighteenth and early nineteenth centuries*. London: Longman Group.

Lewis, E. D.
1959 *The Rhondda Valleys: A study in industrial development, 1800 to the present day*. London: Phoenix House.

Lindert, P.
1973 "The relative cost of American children." Discussion Paper ED73-18. University of Wisconsin, Graduate Program in Economic History.

Lindert, P.
1978 *Fertility and scarcity in America*. Princeton, New Jersey: Princeton Univ. Press.
Llewellyn, R.
1940 *How green was my valley*. New York: Macmillan.
Lorimer, F.
1967 The economics of family formation under different conditions. In *World population conference: Belgrade* (Vol. II). New York: United Nations. Pp. 92–95.
Maddala, G. S.
1977 *Econometrics*. New York: McGraw-Hill.
Manschke, R.
1916 Beruf und Kinderzahl. *Schmollers Jahrbuch*, Bd. 40, pp. 1867–1937.
Massachusetts, Bureau of Statistics of Labor
1888 *Census of Massachusetts: 1885* (Vol. I). Population and social statistics. Boston: Wright and Potter.
Mathias, P.
1969 *The first industrial nation: An economic history of Britain, 1700–1914*. New York: Charles Scribner's Sons.
McCabe, J. L. and M. R. Rosenzweig
1976 Female employment creation and family size. In R. G. Ridker (Ed.), *Population and development: The search for selective interventions*. Baltimore: The Johns Hopkins Univ. Press. Pp. 322–355.
McKeown, T. and R. G. Record
1962 Reasons for the decline of mortality in England and Wales during the nineteenth century. *Population Studies*, *XVI*(Part 2), pp. 94–122.
McLaughlin, V. Yans
1971 Patterns of work and family organization: Buffalo's Italians. *The Journal of Interdisciplinary History*, 2(2), pp. 299–314.
Meeker, E.
1972 The improving health of the United States, 1850–1915. *Explorations in Economic History*, 9(4), pp. 353–373.
Meinert, R.
1956 *Die Entwicklung der Arbeitszeit in der deutschen Industrie, 1820–1956*. Unpublished Ph.D. dissertation, Univ. of Münster.
Meitzen, A. and F. Grossman
1901 *Der Boden und die landwirtschaftliche Verhältnisse des preussischen Staates*. Bd. 6. Berlin: Paul Parey.
Michael, R. T.
1973 Education and the derived demand for children. *Journal of Political Economy*, 81(2, Part II), pp. S128–164.
Mincer, J.
1962 Labor Force Participation of Married Women. In *Aspects of labor economics*. Universities-National Bureau Committee for Economic Research. Princeton, New Jersey: Princeton Univ. Press. Pp. 63–97. ["Comment" by C. D. Long, pp. 98–105.]
Mincer, J.
1963 Market prices, opportunity costs, and income effects. In C. F. Christ (Ed.), *Measurement in economics: Studies in mathematical economics and econometrics in honor of Yehuda Grunfeld*. Stanford, California: Stanford Univ. Press. Pp. 67–82.
Mincer, J.
1974 *Schooling, experience and earnings*. New York: Columbia Univ. Press.
Mincer, J. and S. Polachek
1974 Family investments in human capital: Earnings of women. *Journal of Political Economy*, 82(2, Part II), pp. S76–108.

Minchinton, W. E. (Ed.)
1969 *Industrial South Wales, 1750–1914: Essays in Welsh economic history*. London: Frank Cass.
Mitchell, B. R. and P. Deane
1971 *Abstract of British historical statistics*. Cambridge, England: Cambridge Univ. Press.
Modell, J.
1978 Patterns of consumption, acculturation, and family income strategies in late-nineteenth-century America. In T. K. Hareven and M. A. Vinovskis (Eds.), *Family and population in nineteenth-century America*. Princeton: Princeton Univ. Press. Pp. 206–240.
Modell, J. and T. K. Hareven
1973 Urbanization and the malleable household: An examination of boarding and lodging in American families. *Journal of Marriage and the Family*, 35, pp. 467–479.
Moriyama, I. M. and L. Guralnick
1956 Occupational and social class differences in mortality. In *Trends and differentials in mortality*. New York: Milbank Memorial Fund. Pp. 61–73.
Mott, F. L.
1972 Fertility, life cycle stage and female labor force participation in Rhode Island: A retrospective overview. *Demography*, 9(1), pp. 173–185.
Mueller, E.
1976 The economic value of children in peasant agriculture. In R. G. Ridker (Ed.), *Population and development: The search for selective interventions*. Baltimore: The Johns Hopkins Univ. Press. Pp. 98–153.
Nef, J. U.
1932 *The rise of the British coal industry* (2 vols.). London: Routledge.
Nelder, J. A. and R. W. M. Wedderburn
1972 Generalized linear models. *Journal of the Royal Statistical Society*. Series A, 135, pp. 370–384.
Nerlove, M.
1974 Household and economy: Toward a new theory of population and economic growth. *Journal of Political Economy*, 82(2, Part II), pp. S200–218.
Nerlove, M. and S. J. Press
1973 *Univariate and multivariate loglinear and logistic models*. Santa Monica, California: Rand Corp., R-1306-EDA/NIH.
Notestein, F. W.
1953 The economics of population and food supplies. I. The economic problems of population change. *Proceedings of the Eighth International Conference of Agricultural Economists*. London: Oxford Univ. Press.
Ogburn, W. F.
1912 *Progress and uniformity in child-labor legislation: A study in statistical measurement*. Columbia Univ. Studies in History, Economics, and Public Law. Vol. XLVIII, No. 2. New York: Longmans, Green.
Okun, B.
1958 *Trends in birth rates in the United States since 1870*. Baltimore: The Johns Hopkins Univ. Press.
Oppenheimer, V. K.
1970 *The female labor force in the United States: Demographic and economic factors governing its growth and changing composition*. Population Monograph Series No. 5. Berkeley, California: University of California, Institute of International Studies.
Oppenheimer, V. K.
1973 Demographic influence on female employment and the status of women. *American Journal of Sociology*, 78(4), pp. 946–961.

Oppenheimer, V. K.
1974 The life-cycle squeeze: The interaction of men's occupational and family life cycles. *Demography*, *11*(2), pp. 227–245.

Orwell, G.
1937 *The road to Wigan Pier*. New York: Harcourt, Brace.

Parker, E. W.
1905 Coal. *Twelfth census of the United States, 1900. Special reports: Mines and quarries: 1905*. Washington, D.C.: Government Printing Office.

Poedjastoeti, S.
1976 "On estimating fertility using 1976 intercensal survey data, a case for Indonesia." Paper presented at Second Own Children Method Workshop, East–West Population Institute, Honolulu, October 18–22.

Potter, J.
1965 The growth of population in America, 1700–1860. In D. V. Glass and D. E. C. Eversley (Eds.), *Population in history*. Chicago: Aldine. Pp. 631–688.

Pounds, N. J. G., and W. N. Parker
1957 *Coal and steel in Western Europe*. Bloomington: Univ. of Indiana Press.

Preston, S. H.
1972 Female employment policy and fertility. In R. Parke, Jr. and C. Westoff (Eds.), *Aspects of population growth policy*. Vol. VI of Research Reports. U.S. Commission on Population Growth and the American Future. Washington, D.C.: U.S. Government Printing Office. Pp. 375–393.

Preston, S. H.
1976 Estimating child survival rates from data on women's reproductive histories. *Technical report*, Department of Sociology, Univ. of Washington, Seattle, Washington. Mimeo.

Prussia
1885 Statistisches Landesamt. *Preussische Statistik*. Band 76, Teil II.

Redford, A.
1964 *Labour migration in England, 1800–1850* (2nd ed.). Edited and revised by W. H. Chaloner. Manchester, England: Manchester Univ. Press.

Repetto, R. G.
1976 Direct economic costs and value of children. In R. G. Ridker (Ed.), *Population and development: The search for selective interventions*. Baltimore: The Johns Hopkins Univ. Press. Pp. 77–97.

Retherford, R. D. and L.-J. Cho
1974 Comparative analysis of recent fertility trends in East Asia. IUSSP. *International Population Conference: Liège, 1973* (Vol. 2). Liège: International Union for the Scientific Study of Population. Pp. 163–181.

Roberts, P.
1901 *The anthracite coal industry: A study of the economic conditions and relations of the cooperative forces in the development of the anthracite coal industry of Pennsylvania*. New York: Macmillan.

Roberts, P.
1904 *Anthracite coal communities: A study of the demography, the social, educational and moral life of the anthracite regions*. New York: Macmillan.

Rosenzweig, M. S.
1976 Female work experience, employment status, and birth expectations: Sequential decision-making in the Philippines. *Demography*, *13*(3), pp. 339–356.

Sargant, W. L.
1865 Inconsistencies of the English census of 1861. *Journal of the Statistical Society of London*, *28*, pp. 73–124.

Schaefer, D. F.
1977 *A quantitative description and analysis of the growth of the Pennsylvania anthracite coal industry, 1820 to 1865*. New York: Arno.

Schofer, L.
1975 *The formation of a modern labor force: Upper Silesia, 1865–1914*. Berkeley, California: Univ. of California Press.

Schultz, T. P.
1969 An economic model of family planning and fertility. *Journal of Political Economy*, 77(2), pp. 153–180.

Schultz, T. P.
1976 Determinants of fertility: A microeconomic model of choice. In A. J. Coale (Ed.), *Economic factors in population growth*. New York: Wiley. Pp. 89–124. (a)

Schultz, T. P.
1976 Interrelationships between mortality and fertility. In R. G. Ridker (Ed.), *Population and development: The search for selective interventions*. Baltimore: The Johns Hopkins Univ. Press. Pp. 239–289. (b)

Schultz, T. W. (Ed.)
1975 *Economics of the family: Marriage, children and human capital*. Chicago: Univ. of Chicago Press.

Smuts, R. W.
1959 *Women and work in America*. New York: Columbia Univ. Press.

Spagnoli, P. G.
1977 High fertility in mid-nineteenth century France: A multivariate analysis of fertility patterns in the arrondissement of Lille. *Research in Economic History*, 2. Pp. 281–336.

Spengler, J. J.
1930 The fecundity of native and foreign-born women in New England. *Brookings Institution Pamphlet Series, II*(1).

Stearns, P. N.
1967 *European society in upheaval: Social history since 1800*. New York: Macmillan.

Stearns, P. N.
1970–1971 National character and European labor history. *The Journal of Social History*, 4(2), pp. 95–124.

Stevenson, T. H. C.
1920 The fertility of various social classes in England and Wales from the middle of the nineteenth century to 1911. *Journal of the Royal Statistical Society*, 83(Part III), pp. 401–444.

Stycos, J. M. and R. H. Weller
1967 Female working roles and fertility. *Demography*, *1*, pp. 210–217.

Sullivan, J. M.
1972 Models for the estimation of the probability of dying between birth and exact ages in early childhood. *Population Studies*, 26(1), pp. 79–97.

Sweet, J. A.
1970 Family composition and the labor force activity of American wives. *Demography*, 7(2), pp. 195–209.

Sweet, J. A.
1973 *Women in the labor force*. New York: Seminar Press.

Taeuber, C. and I. B. Taeuber
1958 *The changing population of the United States*. New York: Wiley.

Taylor, A. J.
1951 The taking of the census, 1801–1851. *British Medical Journal*. (April 7).

Taylor, C. E., J. S. Newman, and N. U. Kelly
1976 The child survival hypothesis. *Population Studies*, 30(2), pp. 263–278.

Teitelbaum, M. S.
1974 Birth underregistration in the constituent counties of England and Wales: 1841–1910. *Population Studies*, 28(2), pp. 329–343.

Temin, P.
1964 *Iron and steel in nineteenth century America: An economic inquiry*. Cambridge, Massachusetts: M.I.T. Press.

Terry, G. B.
1975 Rival explanations in the work–fertility relationship. *Population Studies*, 29(2), pp. 191–206.

Theil, H.
1971 *Principles of econometrics*. New York: Wiley.

Thernstrom, S. and P. R. Knights
1971 Men in motion: Some data and speculations about urban population mobility in nineteenth century America. In T. K. Hareven (Ed.), *Anonymous Americans: Explorations in nineteenth century social history*. Englewood Cliffs, New Jersey: Prentice-Hall. Pp. 17–47.

Thomas, B.
1930 The migration of labour into the Glamorganshire coalfield, 1861–1911. *Economica*, *10*, pp. 275–294.

Thompson, W. S. and P. K. Whelpton
1933 *Population trends in the United States*. New York: McGraw-Hill.

Tillott, P. M.
1972 Sources of inaccuracy in the 1851 and 1861 censuses. In E. A. Wrigley (Ed.), *Nineteenth century society: Essays in the use of quantitative methods for the study of social data*. Cambridge, England: Cambridge Univ. Press. Pp. 82–133.

Tilly, L. A.
1977 "Occupational structure, women's work and demographic change in Anzin and Roubaix, 1872–1906." Unpublished manuscript.

Tilly, L. A., J. W. Scott, and M. Cohen
1976 Women's work and European fertility patterns. *The Journal of Interdisciplinary History*, 6(3), pp. 447–476.

Trussell, T. J.
1975 A re-estimation of the multiplying factors for the Brass technique for determining childhood survivorship rates. *Population Studies*, 29(1), pp. 97–107.

Turchi, B. A.
1975 *The demand for children: The economics of fertility in the United States*. Cambridge, Massachusetts: Ballinger. (a)

Turchi, B. A.
1975 Microeconomic theories of fertility: A critique. *Social Forces*, 54(1), pp. 107–125. (b)

United Nations
1953 Department of Economic and Social Affairs. *The determinants and consequences of population trends*. New York: United Nations.

United Nations
1967 Department of Economic and Social Affairs. *Manuals on methods of estimating population. Manual IV*. Methods of estimating basic demographic measures from incomplete data. *Population Studies*, 42. New York: United Nations.

United Nations
1973 *The determinants and consequences of population trends: New summary of findings on interaction of demographic, economic and social factors*. New York: United Nations.

U.S. Bureau of the Census
1893 Population (Vol. 1, Part 2). *Eleventh Census of the United States: 1890*. Washington, D.C.: U.S. Government Printing Office.

U.S. Bureau of the Census
1892 Report on the mineral industries of the United States, 1889 (Vol. 7). *Eleventh census of the United States: 1890*. Washington, D.C.: U.S. Government Printing Office.

U.S. Bureau of the Census
1943 Differential fertility, 1940 and 1910: Fertility for states and large cities. *U.S. census of population: 1940*. Washington, D.C.: U.S. Government Printing Office. (a)

U.S. Bureau of the Census
1943 Differential fertility, 1940 and 1910: Women by number of children ever born. *U.S. census of population: 1940*. Washington, D.C.: U.S. Government Printing Office. (b)

U.S. Bureau of the Census
1960 *Historical statistics of the United States, colonial times to 1957*. Washington, D.C.: U.S. Government Printing Office.

U.S. Bureau of the Census
1964 Women by number of children ever born. *U.S. census of population: 1960*. Subject Reports. Washington, D.C.: U.S. Government Printing Office. PC(2)-3A.

U.S. Bureau of the Census
1971 *The methods and materials of demography* (Vols. 1,2). H. S. Shryock, J. S. Siegal, and Associates. Washington, D.C.: U.S. Government Printing Office.

U.S. Bureau of the Census
1973 Women by number of children ever born. *U.S. census of population: 1970*. Subject Reports. Washington, D.C.: Government Printing Office. (a)

U.S. Bureau of the Census
1973 *Population and Housing Inquiries in U.S. Decenial Censuses, 1790–1970*. Working Paper No. 39. Washington, D.C.: U.S. Government Printing Office. (b)

U.S. Bureau of the Census
1975 *Historical Statistics of the United States, Colonial Times to 1970* (Parts 1 and 2). Washington, D.C.: Government Printing Office.

U.S. Commissioner of Labor
1890 *Sixth annual report of the commissioner of labor, 1890*. Part III: Cost of living. U.S. Congress, House of Representatives, House Executive Document 265, 51st Congress, 2nd Session.

U.S. Commissioner of Labor
1891 *Seventh annual report of the commissioner of labor, 1891*. Part III: Cost of living. U.S. Congress, House of Representatives, House Executive Document 232, 52nd Congress, 1st Session, Vols. I and II.

U.S. Department of Labor
1934 Bureau of Labor Statistics. *Bulletin of the United States Bureau of Labor Statistics*. No. 604: History of wages in the United States from colonial times to 1928. (Revision of Bulletin No. 499 with Supplement, 1929–1933.) Washington, D.C.: U.S. Government Printing Office.

Uselding, P.
1976 In dispraise of the Muckrakers: United States occupational mortality, 1890–1910. *Research in Economic History*, *1*, pp. 334–371.

Van de Walle, E.
1968 Marriage and marital fertility. *Daedalus*, 97(2), pp. 486–501.

Vinovskis, M.
1972 Mortality rates and trends in Massachusetts before 1860. *The Journal of Economic History*, 32(1), pp. 184–213.

Vinovskis, M.
1976 Socioeconomic determinants of interstate fertility differentials in the United States in 1850 and 1860. *The Journal of Interdisciplinary History*, 6(3), pp. 375–396. (a)

Vinovskis, M. A.
1976 "The Jacobson life table of 1850: A critical re-examination from a Massachusetts perspective." Paper presented at the meeting of the Social Science History Association. Philadelphia. (October). (b)

Ware, H.
1976 Fertility and work force participation: The experience of Melbourne wives. *Population Studies*, 30(3), pp. 413–427.

Weber, A. F.
1899 *The growth of cities in the nineteenth century: A study in statistics* (Vol. XI). Studies in History, Economics and Public Law. Columbia Univ. New York: Macmillan.

Williamson, H. F. (Ed.)
1951 *The growth of the American economy*. Englewood Cliffs, New Jersey: Prentice-Hall.

Williamson, J. G.
1967 Consumer behavior in the nineteenth century: Carroll D. Wright's Massachusetts workers in 1875. *Explorations in Entrepreneurial History* (Second Series.), 4(2), pp. 98–135.

Wray, J. D.
1971 Population pressure on families: Family size and child spacing. In National Academy of Sciences, *Rapid Population Growth*. Baltimore: The Johns Hopkins Univ. Press. Pp. 403–361.

Wright, C. D. and William C. Hunt.
1900 *The history and growth of the United States census*. Washington, D.C.: U.S. Government Printing Office.

Wrigley, E. A.
1961 *Industrial growth and population change: A regional study of the coalfield areas of north–west Europe in the later nineteenth century*. Cambridge, England: Cambridge Univ. Press.

Wrigley, E. A.
1969 *Population and history*. New York: McGraw-Hill.

Yasuba, Y.
1962 *Birth rates of the white population of the United States, 1800–1860: An economic analysis*. Baltimore: The Johns Hopkins Univ. Press.

Yearley, C. K., Jr.
1962 *Enterprise and anthracite: Economics and democracy in Schuylkill county 1820–1875*. Baltimore: The Johns Hopkins Univ. Press.

Zola, E.
1885/1970 *Germinal* (1970 ed., translated by S. & E. Hochman). New York: The New American Library. (Originally published, 1885.)

Subject Index

Y

Z

STUDIES IN SOCIAL DISCONTINUITY

Under the Consulting Editorship of:

William A. Christian, Jr. Person and God in a Spanish Valley

Joel Samaha. Law and Order in Historical Perspective: The Case of Elizabethan Essex

John W. Cole and Eric R. Wolf. The Hidden Frontier: Ecology and Ethnicity in an Alpine Valley

Immanuel Wallerstein. The Modern World-System: Capitalist Agriculture and the Origins of the European World-Economy in the Sixteenth Century

John R. Gillis. Youth and History: Tradition and Change in European Age Relations 1770 – Present

D. E. H. Russell. Rebellion, Revolution, and Armed Force: A Comparative Study of Fifteen Countries with Special Emphasis on Cuba and South Africa

Kristian Hvidt. Flight to America: The Social Background of 300,000 Danish Emigrants

James Lang. Conquest and Commerce: Spain and England in the Americas

Stanley H. Brandes. Migration, Kinship, and Community: Tradition and Transition in a Spanish Village

Daniel Chirot. Social Change in a Peripheral Society: The Creation of a Balkan Colony

Jane Schneider and Peter Schneider. Culture and Political Economy in Western Sicily

Michael Schwartz. Radical Protest and Social Structure: The Southern Farmers' Alliance and Cotton Tenancy, 1880-1890

Ronald Demos Lee (Ed.). Population Patterns in the Past

Charles P. Cell. Revolution at Work: Mobilization Campaigns in China

Frederic L. Pryor. The Origins of the Economy: A Comparative Study of Distribution in Primitive and Peasant Economies

Harry W. Pearson. The Livelihood of Man by Karl Polanyi

Richard Maxwell Brown and Don E. Fehrenbacher (Eds.). Tradition, Conflict, and Modernization: Perspectives on the American Revolution

Juan G. Espinosa and Andrew S. Zimbalist. Economic Democracy: Workers' Participation in Chilean Industry 1970-1973

Arthur L. Stinchcombe. Theoretical Methods in Social History

Randolph Trumbach. The Rise of the Egalitarian Family: Aristocratic Kinship and Domestic Relations in Eighteenth-Century England

Tamara K. Hareven (Ed.). Transitions: The Family and the Life Course in Historical Perspective

Henry A. Gemery and Jan S. Hogendorn (Eds.). The Uncommon Market: Essays in the Economic History of the Atlantic Slave Trade

Keith Wrightson and David Levine. Poverty and Piety in an English Village: Terling, 1525-1700

Michael Haines. Fertility and Occupation: Population Patterns in Industrialization

In preparation

Harvey L. Graff. The Literacy Myth: Literacy and Social Structure in the Nineteenth-Century City

Elizabeth Hafkin Pleck. Hunting for a City: Black Migration and Poverty in Boston, 1865-1900

Lucile H. Brockway. Science and Colonial Expansion: The Role of the British Royal Botanic Gardens

James Lang. Portuguese Brazil: The King's Plantation